HUMAN STRESS:
ITS NATURE AND CONTROL

Roger J. Allen
University of Maryland
College Park, Maryland

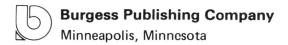
Burgess Publishing Company
Minneapolis, Minnesota

Editorial: Wayne Schotanus, Sharon Harrington, Anne Heller
Copy editor: Kathleen Wolter
Production: Melinda Radtke, Morris Lundin, Pat Barnes, Judy
    Vicars
Cover photograph: Used with permission from the Film Stills
    Archive of the Museum of Modern Art, New York
Cover design: Melinda Radtke

Library of Congress Cataloging in Publication Data

Allen, Roger J.
    Human stress.

    Includes bibliographies and index.
    1. Stress (Psychology)   2. Stress (Physiology)
I. Title.
BF575.S75A44   1983   158'.1   83-2601
ISBN 0-8087-0083-9

Burgess Publishing Company
7108 Ohms Lane
Minneapolis, Minnesota 55435

J   I   H   G   F   E   D   C

My work on this book is dedicated to the spirit of people like Galilaeo Galilaei Lynceo. The book itself, however, seems dedicated to the spirit of people like Popes Paul V and Urban VIII.

Contents

Preface

   This is a book about human stress. My aim in composing this text was to help you to come to an understanding of stress and how to control it effectively in your life. Devouring a lot of factual information is not particularly important. A conceptual understanding of the ideas that this book explores is far more valuable. I tried to fill the book with ideas and not weigh it down with academic trivia. When you read this text, I do not want you to walk away with a skull full of facts with which to impress someone or to make a glittering show on an essay examination. I want you to understand. I wish to give you a conceptual realization of why stress is a part of your life, how it affects you, and what you can do about it. This is not a reference book but a tool to help you rise to a new level of personal well-being.

   I begin this understanding and cognitive growth process by discussing the nature of stress—what it is, what factors predispose us to encounter it, and the payments we must make for having experienced it in life. The first half of the book establishes a sound base of knowledge. The theory is that if you first understand stress, you will be in a more effective position to learn to gain control over it. The second half of the book covers a broad variety of stress management techniques and strategies. Since everyone is different, no single stress control strategy is effective or desirable for all people.

   The book is an organized smorgasbord of ideas about stress and stress control. I tried to cover a lot of ground, so I made brief presentations of some detailed issues. I tried to explore the main issues and relevant ideas of each area discussed. If you find any of the areas particularly relevant, interesting, or provocative, I encourage you to pursue them further. The references at the end of each chapter will help you to do this.

   The book has two fundamental viewpoints. The first viewpoint is conceptual. The book does not completely help you to explore how the concepts discussed operate in *your* life nor does it provide enough personal guidance to create a strong stress management program for your personal use. A book that does perform this task is *Investigations in Stress Control* by Allen and Hyde (Ed. 2, Burgess Publishing Company, 1981), a workbook designed to guide you through the comprehensive creation of a stress control plan tailored to your personality and life-style. The book and workbook are intended to be used in combination, with the book providing the concepts, ideas, and understanding and the workbook making these ideas functional in your life.

The second viewpoint is a physiological perspective of stress and stress control. Stress is a physiological phenomenon. Therefore, I focus discussion of predisposing factors on those that actually change the body and produce somatic disease. I also approach stress management in terms of reducing psychophysiological arousal. I look at stress control from a somewhat medical perspective and what we can do to lower the probability of encountering stress-related disease. There are other valid approaches to the study of stress and its regulation, most notably the psychosocial approach. I, however, use biological integrity as the performance criterion.

Finally, there is more behind the activities used to control stress than simply reducing physical disease incidence. Stress control is just a first step in attaining human health and human potential. First, learn what stress is. Then learn to control it, begin to cleanse your mind and body of maladaptive tension, and realize states of greater mental and physical health and positive integration. Then you will begin to understand.

Acknowledgments

I would like to acknowledge the valuable contributions made to this text by the work of the following individuals:

Beverly Battle, M.A.
Thomas Nelson Community College

Mark Fink
University of Maryland

Barry Gruber, Ph.D.
University of Maryland

David Hyde, M.S.
Howard University

Joann Icangelo
University of Maryland

Kathy Lynch, B.S.
University of Maryland

Nancy O'Hara, M.A.
University of South Carolina

Jackie Spadt, B.A.
University of Maryland

Robert Voight, Ph.D.
McNesse State College

Special thanks go to Jeanie and Chris for their heroic typing.
Enjoy the book.

Introduction

We learn things in life either by personal experience or by accepting the wisdom of others. As the *Chicago Tribune* says, "Only some of us can learn by other people's mistakes . . . the rest of us have to be the other people." Sometimes—most of the time—experience can be a painful lesson. Most of us choose the hard road to attain knowledge, but where stress is concerned, that path can be damaging, often resulting in disease. That is too heavy a price to pay.

Not all stress is damaging. Some stress is essential to life and growth; for example, the stress performers are under to do their best. This stress does not work against them, but rather stimulates them to perform at an optimal level. We are more concerned with the "bad" stress and its detrimental effects. In the long run, learning about the nature of stress by considering the wisdom of others is a lot less painful. Once we have acquired a better understanding of what stress is and how it affects the body, we can learn to manage stress effectively in our lives.

What is the importance in learning about the nature and control of stress? Is it really a problem or an issue? Three widespread, glaring manifestations of stress in our culture indicate an urgent need to understand and deal with it as a problem of vast significance and scope: the incidence of psychosomatic disease, the economic loss to business due to stress, and the alarming prevalence of seriously maladaptive coping measures.

According to Harrison's *Principles of Internal Medicine*, 50 to 80 percent of all physical disease is psychosomatic or stress related in origin. This is rapidly becoming a conservative figure in medical texts. Many now express the opinion that psychogenic stress is a potentially significant factor for *any* physical disease in its etiology, process, or rate of healing.

Cardiovascular disorders are the cause of more deaths in this country each year than all other causes combined. Stress attacks every physiological facet of cardiovascular functioning, so it may be a principal cause in most forms of cardiovascular disease.

Cancer is the second leading cause of death in the United States. Stress can weaken the natural defense mechanisms of the body, thereby giving cancer an open door to develop and spread. Stress does not cause cancer, but it plays a major role in setting up the internal conditions conducive to its appearance.

The experience of human stress can either cause or exacerbate a host of other diseases, including diabetes, epilepsy, asthma, arthritis, infectious diseases, muscular dysfunctions, gastrointestinal ulcers and related problems, skin disorders, allergic responses, sexual dysfunctions, and metabolic alterations. One can argue medically that all of these conditions (and most somatic diseases overall) are merely the long-term, severe symptoms of stress. In fact, owing to the central role that psychogenic stress is capable of playing in the etiology of the most prevalent life-threatening diseases, we may defensibly argue that stress is the true number one killer of people in the United States.

Health is a growing business concern because of the wear and tear to which job stress can subject the body. This wear and tear, or stress, can hinder the performance of the backbone of any industry—the human machine. Stress can lead to both the physical and the mental breakdown of the body. Machine failure, even that of the human machine, means money to a business. Many stress-related disorders can become costly to a business, such as loss of motivation, absenteeism, slower working rates, decrease in productivity and quality performance, diminished creativity, and of course, illness and death.

On-the-job stress is a major cause of heart disease according to reports from the Department of Health, Education, and Welfare. The American Heart Association approximates that recruiting replacements for executives who have died of heart disease costs $700 million a year. Absenteeism due to heart-related diseases amounts to a loss of $8.6 billion in wages per year. Estimates range from $17 to $20 billion in annual losses to American industry directly due to stress-related disease. This is greater than the combined annual profits of *Fortune's* top five corporations. Stress is expensive!

Aside from the serious incidence of life-threatening, stress-related disease and the high economic costs from the effects of stress, one of the most striking indications of our stress problem is the ubiquitous use of maladaptive coping schemes. In 1976, 144 million new prescriptions were written for psychoactive drugs. More than half of these were for Valium and Librium. According to some estimates, one third of the total population of the United States is taking Valium. John Peckanen, of the Drug Abuse Council, has said that enough Valium and Librium was sold in 1973 for every child, woman, and man in this country to have 20 pills. Psychopharmacologist Oakley Ray says that "Americans are spending almost half a billion dollars a year on a drug to relieve their anxiety—a fact that is in itself a considerable cause for anxiety." These huge numbers and statistics are fun to throw around, but the point is that the scope of the use of tranquilizers in this country indicates that stress is playing havoc with a massive segment of the population. First our mind and body get strung out from stress, and then we turn to Valium to finish ourselves.

A fascinating statistic is that only about 25 to 30 percent of Valium prescriptions are for patients diagnosed as having anxiety or related mental disorders. Around 70 percent of Valium prescriptions are for somatic conditions—physical disease problems. Clearly, the most massive use of Valium is for symptomatic treatment of physical disorders resulting from psychogenic stress. From this we can reason that the medical profession recognizes the role of maladaptive mental states in the onset and exacerbation of physical disease. A massive stress problem exists, but the treatment approach is wrong. According to Ray, "The antianxiety agents may in fact decrease anxiety, but they also reduce all kinds of emotional responsiveness. . . . Rats drugged with antianxiety agents fail to increase tolerance for frustration shown by undrugged animals trained in the same way. This implies that any drug which reduces the experience of anxiety is also likely to reduce one's capacity to develop behavioral methods of coping with stress." How ironic! We take a drug to help us reduce anxiety and pain, but in fact, it only serves to make us more susceptible to them.

Evidence suggests that some people take more direct and complete action to rid themselves of stress. At least 25,000 Americans commit suicide each year—almost 70 per day—about one every 20 minutes. Clearly it is not only depressed people who commit suicide. For our population, however, the general suicide rate peaked in the depression of the 1930s. People choose suicide as life's final option for many reasons. Certainly a terminally desperate inability to cope is a significant portion of the dark fabric. Many victims of suicide may actually be victims of stress. The excessively high suicide rate (25,000 too many each year) is another factor pointing to the importance of learning to handle the stress of life.

The above data are only indicators. This is not the real issue. You already know that stress is a problem, or you would not be reading this book now. You have already seen human beings suffer the mental and physical pains that stress creates. No doubt you have already seen at least one person die too young from a heart attack. Most important, you know that stress is a problem in need of solutions, because you can feel it in yourself. You may not yet have encountered a stress-related disease personally, but you have felt the pain in life that stress can inflict.

In this book, we are going to try to understand what stress is, what it does, and how to control it effectively. Many ideas in this book are of worth because they may help you to improve the quality of your life. You probably will read and forget most of them, but some of them are too important to lose. Listed below are the basic concepts that form this text. Read them now. Remember them tomorrow. Someday you will profit from them.

1. Stress may be the most serious, life-threatening disease facing individuals in this culture.
2. We should not try to avoid stress, but to learn to control it so that it stimulates growth and life instead of disease and death.
3. The mind and body are not independent, unrelated entities. They are constantly involved in a dynamic interaction. The character and manifestations of that interaction have now become a threat to human health. Through understanding this exchange and learning to work with it, we can turn the mind-body interplay into a powerful tool to prevent disease and enhance high-level human health.
4. To a large extent, you are personally responsible for your own health. You have the capacity to take control over your mental and physical well-being and the overall quality of your life. You are not a helpless leaf blowing in a hostile wind.
5. If you are going to manage stress in your life, you must make it a personal priority and exert the effort yourself. No one else can do it for you. The tools that work are described in this book. Whether you use them is your choice.
6. Human health can be contagious. It transcends mere diseaselessness. Once you have realized an integrated state of health, you can begin to spread it to others. By recognizing and manifesting more of our vast human potential, we can begin to direct our quality of life. We can decide between disease, death, competition, suffering, and holocaust or health, life, cooperation, growth, and positive evolution.

PART I

The Nature
of Human Stress

What exactly is human stress? How did it evolve to become a part of the human organism and why can it have damaging consequences? How can states of mind influence the body to produce psychogenic stress? The first section of this text addresses these questions through an exploration of the nature of human stress. Besides exploring the developmental basics of the human stress concept, we will look at the theoretical interactions of the mind-body interplay. The aim of these first two chapters is to help you develop an understanding of why human stress exists and how it operates in our sociobiological setting. The rationale behind this initial theoretical presentation is that the more you understand about how the human organism operates, the greater is your ultimate capacity to gain control over your biological destiny, personal health, and quality of life.

CHAPTER 1

What Is This Thing Called Stress?

Modern man has retained many physiological and mental attributes ill-suited to civilized life, just as he has retained useless anatomical vestiges from his evolutionary past. As a result, he must meet the challenges of today with biological equipment largely anachronistic. Many forms of organic and mental disease originate from the responses that man's Paleolithic nature makes to the condition of modern life.

René Dubos

A logical place to begin a presentation on the nature and control of human stress is to define the concept. In this chapter, we shall look at more than just definitions of stress, however. We shall explore the underlying biological conditions that have created this problem in humans, tracing the discovery of the stress concept, evaluating the relationship of contemporary life to our biological design, and discussing the distinctions between damaging and growth-promoting stress, all in an effort to begin to understand this ubiquitous human phenomenon.

Ken Pelletier has expressed the opinion that the more you understand about your body and the factors influencing its level of distress or well-being, the more you can take command of your personal health. We begin, therefore, by building an understanding of the nature of stress. If you first understand the factors that contribute to the existence of this condition, you will be prepared to learn to control it effectively.

DEFINING STRESS

Most authors would agree that Hans Selye was the pioneer who is credited as the first to note the existence of human stress, describe its qualities, define the concept, and give the phenomenon an appropriate name.

2

Several definitions have been offered over the years to describe stress as a biological, human phenomenon. Selye (1976) presented the most direct way of defining stress:

In its medical sense, stress is essentially the rate of wear and tear in the body.

This definition fits well with our common notion of stress. When we think of stress, we associate the idea with damage to the body or such unpleasant mental states as anxiety, frustration, and exhaustion or both. This initial definition implies that stress is merely a condition of damage in the body. This simplistic notion has many critical flaws that we shall explore later in this chapter.

Fortunately, Selye has given us another definition that helps clarify the nature of stress. Beginning with his early work and observations, Selye began to view stress as a physiological response that was associated with the process of adaptation. The efforts or work of the body to adapt to changing internal or external conditions produce the characteristic pattern of somatic responses that we call stress. Therefore, Selye's (1946) most widely accepted definition of stress is:

Stress is the nonspecific response of the body to any demand made upon it to adapt whether that demand produces pleasure or pain.

Several elements in this definition require clarification. First, stress is a "response of the body." This means that stress is a *physical* condition, a physiological response. It is physical, not cognitive. Stress is a physiological state; it is not worry, anxiety, depression, or frustration. These mental conditions may serve as triggers for the physiological response, but they themselves are not stress. Some psychological literature may equate anxiety with stress, but they are not the same. Anxiety may precipitate stress, but stress itself is a physical reaction. Also, since stress is a reaction or "response," it is not to be equated with the agents that trigger it. Being forced to stop for a red light when you are late is not stress. Stress is the response of your body to that event. Environmental agents or stimuli that trigger the stress response are termed "stressors." A stressor is the cause, and stress is the physiological effect or result.

Another important element in Selye's definition is the term nonspecific. This term may be interpreted here to mean that stress is nonspecific both in cause and in effect. Nearly anything can trigger the stress reaction—as Selye said, *"any* demand to adapt." Anything that changes conditions for the body to which it must then adapt produces stress. This is different from other problematic physical conditions that largely have a singular cause, such as *Treponema pallidum* being the only agent capable of causing syphilis.

Stress also produces nonspecific effects; it alters the activity of all organ systems in the body, not just one. Stress does not simply attack your heart, or your liver, or your nose. Rather, it has the potential to affect everything. Stress is a physiological pattern of changes that can be triggered by nearly anything and can affect any or all aspects of human biological functioning.

Selye's definition indicates both pleasure and pain as being capable of evoking a stress response. As we shall discuss further, the human body does not (in a general sense) recognize the distinction between pleasure and pain. Both change the circumstances under which the body must operate. Hence, both elicit an adaptation response. Both pleasure and pain therefore stimulate an undifferentiated stress response in the body.

Selye borrowed the term stress from physics. If he had used an exact parallel, however, we would now call the response strain. This is because, in engineering, stress is the load placed on a structure and strain is the response of the structure. The stressor-stress dichotomy is analogous to the stress-strain terminology of physics and engineering.

When Selye was first experimenting and developing the stress concept, he worked mainly with physical stressors. His early research involved inducing stress in animals by altering the hormone balance of their bodies and injecting cellular toxins. His initial conceptualizations of stress were thus drawn from purely physical perspectives.

Most stress conditions that we experience, however, are not physically derived. The stressors for people in this culture, the events that seem to distort our lives and bodies, are more cognitive in origin. Our principal stress triggers are events that by themselves cannot produce physical change in the body, but affect us because of the way we interpret them. Our aroused state of mind therefore becomes the dominant stimulus for the physiological stress response. Therefore, we must extend Selye's conceptualization of stress to embrace the fact that events that trigger mental or cognitive arousal in many cases are the direct trigger for stress. This kind of stress we label **psychogenic** (psyche: mind; genesis: origin; of mental origin). Psychogenic stress is an adaptive, physical response of the body that was initiated by cognitive arousal. This means that the mind is placed in a position in which it must adapt, and then a physical response follows. This implies a critical mind-body link that is explored in detail in the next chapter.

These definitions raise two questions. First, what are the origins and reasons for the existence of this adaptive response pattern? Second, how is it theoretically possible that states of mental arousal could trigger a physiological response? To answer these questions, let us explore one of the basic biological responses with which most animals meet the challenge of daily survival.

THE FIGHT OR FLIGHT RESPONSE

There can be little argument with the idea that stress is currently a contributor to many life-threatening disease conditions. Interestingly, the physiological response mechanism that initiates this pathogenic stress reaction evolved as a response to facilitate physical survival in primitive settings. The initial phase of the psychogenic stress response gives us a survival advantage in the face of physical threats. It is called the **fight or flight response**.

Walter B. Cannon, this century's premier physiologist, first described the fight or flight response. Through early experimentation with decerebrate cats under sham rage conditions, Cannon uncovered a pattern of physiological mobilization elicited during times of cerebral arousal. This response seemed to prepare the animal's body for vigorous physical activity. Cannon reasoned that this collective pattern of reactions was designed to help the animal survive physical threats or attack.

To understand the biological reasoning behind this response pattern, consider the options available to an organism that encounters a physical threat to survival in a primitive setting. When faced with a physical threat to its survival, an animal must either fight off its attacker or flee the dangerous situation if it is to survive.

Both fighting and fleeing require the same response on the part of the internal organs of the body. The visceral organs must mobilize for skeletal muscle activity. The fight or flight response prepares the body for vigorous muscular activity to meet a physical threat. This is a preparatory response. When an animal perceives any possible survival threat, the response is triggered. The body gets ready for action. It makes absolutely no difference whether the threat is real or imagined. If the animal thinks a threat is present, the response happens. Actual physical contact or damage is not required to initiate the fight or flight response. This triggering by the mind gives the animal an edge by preparing its body for the demand before the threat is physically upon it. As soon as a threat is perceived, the body mobilizes so that if real danger actually arrives, the animal is already well prepared. Clearly, a preparatory response of this type can give animals a survival advantage in primitive settings. This response evolved into our bodies during a time when physical threats and challenges were a part of everyday life.

Precisely what happens during the fight or flight response? How does this response pattern change the activity of the body? To help you conceptualize the physiological character of the response, simply remember its purpose—to prepare the body for vigorous, muscular activity in response to perceived danger. The fight or flight response changes the activity of internal organs to facilitate a high level of activity of the skeletal muscles.

Internal Reactions

Fight or flight produces many visceral changes, most of which involve increasing internal organ activity. In the cardiovascular system, heart rate increases, the force of contraction of the myocardium (heart muscle) increases, and stroke volume of the heart (amount of blood pumped out per beat) subsequently rises, all resulting in increased cardiac output (amount of blood pumped by the heart per unit time). The reason for these cardiac changes is to speed up delivery of blood flow to the muscles. Because they will soon need increased oxygen, nutrients, energy, and waste removal, the heart steps up its pumping activity to meet the demand.

Other cardiovascular changes involve the vasomotor activity of the arteries. Arteries supplying blood to deep muscle tissue expand (vasodilation) and arteries to the skin surface contract (vasoconstriction). The reason for vasodilation in deep muscle tissue is clearly to help increase blood supply where it is needed. The reasons for vasoconstriction of superficial arteries are somewhat less obvious. First, restricted blood flow to non-essential areas makes more blood, oxygen, and other essentials available to the muscles. Also since you may be injured in a fight or flight situation and may even bleed, vaso-constriction helps to minimize blood loss by restricting blood flow to the surface of the skin.

Have you ever noticed your hands getting cold in tense or anxious situations? This is due to vasoconstriction during fight or flight. When blood flow to the skin surface is restricted, the blood is no longer bringing the internal heat of the body interior to the surface. Therefore, your hands feel cold.

Both the cardiac and vascular changes occurring during fight or flight have their own discrete reasons for happening, but together they contribute to another effect—an increase in blood pressure. The combination of elevated cardiac output and peripheral vasoconstriction serves to raise both systolic and diastolic arterial blood pressure. This is an important effect of fight or flight arousal that is discussed in Chapters 5 and 6.

The cardiovascular system is only one of several that display profound changes in this fight or flight mobilization effort. Significant activity occurs in the respiratory system. Some of these changes include increases in respiration rate and depth, oxygen consumption, and carbon dioxide production. Bronchodilation, an expansion of the air passageways (bronchioles) in the lungs to allow greater airflow, also occurs. The respiratory changes facilitate increased delivery of needed oxygen to the muscles and other body tissues during physical demand.

Also, the skeletal muscles display an increase in basal tension and strength capacity during fight or flight.

Surface Reactions

Three alterations are readily observable on the body surface. Pupillary dilation, an increase in the diameter of the pupil of the eyes, allows more light to enter and enhances the ability of the animal to perceive movement. This reaction is a good way to tell if someone is excited. No matter how cool a person appears to be, the eyes will always reveal the inner self.

A second visible reaction is perspiration. We can only speculate as to why we sweat when we sense physical threat. One opinion is that, since sweating makes the body surface more slippery, you could more readily escape the grasp of a predator. It is also true that perspiration helps cool the body. With superficial vasoconstriction, body heat is being kept deep inside. This is why your hand surfaces will feel cold. Body metabolism is increasing and heat is being retained, so there is a good possibility of overheating. If perspiration accompanies vasoconstriction, it will serve to keep the body cool. That is why your hands become cold and sweaty when you are nervous.

A third interesting visible response is piloerection. Piloerection means the hair on the body stands up. All mammals display this response, even humans. You have seen cats respond this way, no doubt. In some animals with sparse hair, it is difficult to observe, but it is happening. Why do you suppose it happens? Remember the purpose of the whole response—protection from threat. Often, physical threat comes from another animal. Piloerection makes an animal appear larger than it really is; it appears to be a more formidable entity and is thus less likely to be attacked.

The skeletal muscles work with piloerection to enhance the effect. Watch someone during a heated argument. Notice the subtle sign of hair on the forearms standing on end. Notice how the muscles tense; a person may clench his fists, raise his shoulders, puff out his chest. Some people even stand on their toes. These are all unconscious components of the fight or flight response. They are subtle, unconscious, bodily behaviors that we have inherited from our early biological design.

Inhibitions

Not all organ systems are aroused during the fight or flight response; some are inhibited. The organ systems that perform bodily functions that do not contribute immediately to muscular action shut down. The reproductive and the digestive, or gastrointestinal, systems fall into this category. The reproductive system is suppressed in a long-term sense in the latter phases of the stress response. This will be discussed in Chapter 5 as the pituitary shift theory.

Shutdown of the gastrointestinal system is a classic example of organ inhibition that is necessary during times of high general arousal. When you are fighting or fleeing, you do not need to be processing and digesting food. The resources of the body such as blood flow, oxygen, and energy must go to the skeletal muscles and for a time may be diverted from the stomach and intestines. Part of the fight or flight response acts to temporarily shut down the activity of the gastrointestinal system. Decreases occur in gastric (stomach) movement, intestinal peristalsis (the wavelike intestinal motion that moves food through the gut), and blood flow to the system.

The one exception to this reduction in gastrointestinal system activity is sphincter contraction. Sphincters are relatively small, doughnut-shaped muscles that serve to close off or open tubes and passageways within the body. They act like drawstrings. During fight or flight, the intestinal sphincters all contract. This prevents movement of products through the intestines and waste excretion. The reasoning is simple. If you are running away from wild animals, you do not want to leave a trail.

Summary of Changes

You should by now have a basic idea as to the qualitative nature of physiological changes that happen during the fight and flight response. Other more specific changes do occur, and, because individuals and circumstances vary, the response does not always produce all the changes described. You should, however, have a general idea of the kind of physiological change pattern that goes on. You should also be aware that all of these changes reflect one central purpose: to prepare for muscular activity to survive a physical threat. Here is a summary of the physiological changes that can be elicited by Cannon's fight or flight response:

1. Increased heart rate
2. Increased force of myocardial contraction
3. Increased cardiac stroke volume
4. Increased cardiac output
5. Vasodilation of deep muscle and coronary arteries
6. Vasoconstriction of superficial and abdominal arteries
7. Increased arterial blood pressure
8. Increased blood coagulation and decreased clotting time
9. Increased serum glucose
10. Increased respiration rate
11. Increased respiration depth
12. Increased oxygen consumption
13. Increased carbon dioxide production
14. Bronchodilation
15. Increased skeletal muscle strength
16. Pupillary dilation
17. Perspiration
18. Piloerection
19. Decreased gastric movement
20. Decreased intestinal peristalsis
21. Decreased abdominal blood flow
22. Sphincter contraction
23. Stimulation of adrenal medulla secretion

How We Respond Today

As stated previously, the fight or flight response is the initial phase of the psychogenic stress response. Even though the response pattern was programmed into our bodies during a time when humans had to struggle for physical survival, that response is still part of us today. From a biological, or physiological, perspective, we are the same as our primitive ancestors who had to meet constant physical challenges just to stay alive.

Consider how we live now in this culture. Our technological and social development has insulated us from nearly all physical threats to survival. Our elaborate, thermostatically controlled dwellings protect us from wind, rain, temperature extremes, and predators. Threats to our physical survival are rare indeed. When the fight or flight response evolved into the human organism, it afforded us a great survival advantage. Now we rarely need it. Think back over your lifetime. How many times have you actually needed the fight or flight response to survive a dangerous situation?

An important question arises. If we rarely need this response mechanism, does its presence do us any harm? To answer this question, look at how the response fits in with our contemporary life-style.

Look over the list of effects of the fight or flight response once again. How often have you felt those changes occurring in your own body? Daily? Probably. Even though we rarely need the response, it is often triggered. Remember that this response happens whenever you perceive something that you interpret as threatening to your survival; remember that physical contact or damage is not required (this is a preparatory response); and remember that these physiological changes occur whether the threat is real or imaginary. Since we do not really need it, why is the response triggered so frequently?

As we evolved culturally, we expanded our concept of survival. Our contemporary notion of survival encompasses far more than physical survival. We now talk about economic survival, academic survival, social survival, and survival of self-esteem. Anytime we feel our survival being threatened in any way, we react as if our physical survival were being threatened. We become emotionally aroused. Our body interprets this arousal as an indication that a physical threat is present. That is the way it was designed. Hence, whenever we get upset or feel threatened for whatever reason, a fight or flight reaction is triggered. The body was designed to assume that any threat requires a physical reaction.

Think about the times when this response has been triggered in you. Maybe it was the last time you took a tough examination, or just walked into the room to take a tough examination, or when you got lost on an unfamiliar highway late at night and miles from home. Situations like these can trigger fight or flight responses, yet they are not physically threatening. Our mind takes a simple event and interprets it as a threat. Emotional arousal occurs, and the biological response is triggered. The body does not know the difference; it reacts to meet a physical challenge even though the threat is imaginary. This is the first step in converting what was once a highly beneficial biological response mechanism into a life-threatening condition of stress.

What difference could it possibly make to the long-term functioning or health of the human body to have this response turned on when it is not needed? To answer this question, we must look a little further into how we behave once the fight or flight response has been triggered.

We are striving to be a civilized culture composed of rational human beings. Part of this effort means that when we are presented with a nonphysical threat, we should respond in a nonphysical way. When you feel threatened over failing an important examination, for example, it is not appropriate, or polite, to punch the instructor. Most of the threats that we encounter daily are nonphysical, so we do not respond to them in an overt physical way. The body is prepared to fight or flee, but we cannot reasonably do that;

so we sit and sweat. Is this going to hurt us? Another of Cannon's fundamental discoveries helps us answer this question.

Besides outlining the fight or flight response, Cannon made a discovery that is crucial to physiology. It is called **homeostasis**. Literally translated, homeostasis means to remain the same (Greek homoios: like or similar; stasis: position or standing). Homeostasis refers to the efforts of the body to maintain steady internal conditions in the face of an ever-changing environment. Homeostatic processes keep the body functions in balance and within the delicate tolerance limits necessary to sustain life. For example, if blood pressure begins to rise too high, homeostatic mechanisms bring it back down to normal again. The typical example used to illustrate homeostasis is the thermostat. Just as a thermostat directs furnace and air conditioning systems to keep internal temperatures comfortable, so does homeostasis keep the vital functions of the body operating within a healthy range. The body has at its disposal many tools to regulate the activity of every internal organ. Some of these mechanisms of homeostasis are internal and others are behavioral.

Behavioral mechanisms of homeostasis are of great importance to the normal recovery of the body from the arousal elicited by the fight or flight response. The fight or flight response generally elevates internal organ activity. It prepares the body for vigorous muscular activity; it is designed to be followed by that activity. In other words, the body is designed to first turn on internally and then to act physically. There is good evidence to suggest that this subsequent physical activity is the principal homeostatic mechanism necessary to bring the body back to normal within a reasonable time period. Once fight or flight elicits internal arousal, the body needs the subsequent physical activity to burn off that arousal and return to a resting state. If that physical activity does not occur, the internal organs will stay at an elevated arousal level for a long time, keeping blood pressure high, heart rate elevated, blood flow to the hands restricted, and so forth.

We can now see the difficult position in which our body is being placed. The fight or flight response is being triggered often when physical threats are not present and physical responses are inappropriate. The body is internally aroused, but does nothing to burn up that arousal. Physical arousal lingers. Internal organs are operating at an increased work load unnecessarily and for a longer time than is biologically appropriate. The changes produced by the fight or flight response present no problem to the human body. If they linger as a result of a failure to act physically, however, the pathogenic stress response begins.

We could say that the fight or flight response is now an "evolutionary anachronism." Our technical, cultural, and social evolution has outpaced our biological evolution. The conditions under which we live have changed but our bodies have not. Randal (1977) says:

> The "fight or flight" response was appropriate for early man in his struggle to survive in a primitive world populated with wild beasts and other physical dangers. But in modern situations, the "fight or flight" response is inappropriate. We can neither fight or run. We can only suffer the wear and tear that stress inflicts on our bodies.

Can We Change?

The preparatory response was so advantageous to survival during our distant history that those few individuals who had it had a greater probability of surviving the daily challenges of predation, finding food, and so forth. They therefore had a greater chance of surviving to reproductive age, and their offspring in turn inherited the response. Gradually, the mechanism became a part of nearly every member of the species. It now exists in nearly every mammal on earth. It does not appear that the response will now begin to evolve out of our systems with future generations. It is a prime contributor to and initiator of the psychogenic stress response, but stress takes decades to kill. It does not remove individuals from the species before they are old enough to reproduce. The response pattern that initiates stress in our bodies is therefore something that we are born with and that is probably here to stay. We must now learn to use it to our advantage.

Be aware that the fight or flight response by itself is not stress. By itself, fight or flight represents no biological threat to the healthy organism. The psychogenic stress process begins when we experience the internal arousal of the fight or flight response and then fail to act on it in a vigorous, physical fashion.

If fight or flight is the beginning of the stress response, what is the nature of the rest of it? To answer this, we return now to Selye.

GENERAL ADAPTATION SYNDROME

As emphasized previously, the experience of Cannon's fight or flight response is not problematic in and of itself. It represents the physiological onset of psychogenic stress. Selye first discovered, investigated, and outlined the stress response in its totality.

According to Selye, the discovery of the human stress phenomenon began around 1925. At this time, Selye was a medical student at the University of Prague. He was observing ill patients in an effort to learn how diverse symptomatology was related to specific disease states. During the course of this empirical training, he made a simple observation that launched the investigation of human stress.

Selye noticed that individuals suffering from a wide variety of physical disorders all seemed to share a common cluster of overt symptoms. He observed that regardless of what physical problem or bug had caused the illness, nearly everyone "felt and looked ill, had a coated tongue, complained of more or less diffuse aches and pains in the joints, and of intestinal disturbances with loss of appetite" (Selye 1976). He also commonly noted a loss of muscular strength, elevated body temperature, and a depressed psychological affect in physically ill people. He saw diverse physical conditions eliciting the same symptoms. Whenever a definable constellation of symptoms is repeatedly observed, it is medically labeled a syndrome. Selye labeled his observed collection of general illness symptoms the **syndrome of just being sick**. This syndrome is our earliest reference to what was later to evolve into the stress concept.

Selye first believed that he was observing the effects of a hormone that had yet to be discovered. Experimentation in pursuit of this idea forced him to abandon this theory.

In the decade and a half that followed his initial observation, Selye investigated the phenomenon and determined that illness was not the only thing capable of eliciting this syndrome. He realized that this pattern of bodily responses was manifested whenever the internal or external environment of an organism was altered in some significant way. He reasoned that when environmental conditions change, the organism must adapt (remember homeostasis). Adaptation requires effort. He further hypothesized that the work of the adaptation mechanisms and efforts strains the body and produces degrees of wear and tear over time. He thus concluded that the syndrome of just being sick represented the symptoms of an adaptation response. His syndrome, and the processes that lead up to its appearance, received a new name to reflect this adaptation concept. We now call this complete process the **general adaptation syndrome** (GAS), a long-term physiological response pattern to adaptation. We now equate the stages of GAS with the processes and development of human stress. Selye outlined the following three phases of the syndrome:

1. Alarm reaction
2. Stage of resistance
3. Stage of exhaustion

The **alarm reaction** is analogous to Cannon's fight or flight response. It is the onset of the stress process. During the alarm reaction, the body reacts to a change in circumstances. It is as though a physiological alarm went off somewhere inside the body, suddenly mobilizing internal activity. Imagine an alarm going off at a military base. Hundreds of people and machines suddenly spring to life, like an ant farm falling off a bookshelf. In this phase, the body notes the environmental change and reacts by initiating its adaptive defenses. An environmental change could mean anything internal or external—a change in outside air temperature, or a change in chemical balance within the body, or standing in the shower when the hot water runs out, or tripping on a sidewalk and breaking your ankle. The alarm reaction is the body's first response to begin adapting to the new set of circumstances. Homeostasis is called into action.

The **stage of resistance** is a plateau phase of the response. During this stage the body continues to adapt by actively using its homeostatic resources to maintain its physiological integrity and resist the changes imposed on it. This is the longest phase of the GAS. It may last for months, years, or even decades.

The **stage of exhaustion** occurs when one or more organ systems can no longer hold up under the increased work load of the adaptation effort and something breaks. In this last phase, some facet of the functioning of the human body fails. When one or more organ systems fail or become exhausted under the stress of adaptation, the organism has a **disease of adaptation**. Diseases of adaptation are the end result of GAS. At this point, stress manifests itself as a definable medical problem such as a heart attack, gastric ulcer, stroke, breakdown of the immune system, or diabetes. Such diseases of adaptation are also referred to as **stress-related diseases**. Exactly how stress physiologically results in some of these specific disease states is discussed in Chapters 5 and 6.

Selye performed the first studies of the physiological and pathogenic effects of GAS on laboratory rats. He "stressed" the animals by injecting various ovarian and placental extracts into their bodies as well as the highly toxic substance Formalin. He observed three basic pathological changes in the animals: enlargement of the adrenal cortex (the tremendous importance of this finding is explored in Chapters 5 and 6); atrophy (shrinkage) of the thymus gland, spleen, lymph nodes, and all other lymphatic structures of the body (a phenomenon called thymicolymphatic involution); and deep, bleeding ulcers in the linings of the stomach and duodenum. Selye called this pattern of pathogenic changes "the typical triad of the alarm reaction." Subsequent research has confirmed that nearly any significant alteration in internal or external environment will produce this pattern of effect. Stimuli capable of eliciting this dramatic triad range from exposure to cold, overcrowding, and bacterial invasion to anticipation of electric shock, reinforcing the nonspecific nature of the stress response.

Medical science identifies distinct physical disease conditions when observable damage is present in the body. In many instances, the manifestation or observation of damage occurs long after the actual onset of the disease process. Disease is the end result of a long-term process of adaptation or stress. What medicine now considers to be distinct disease categories may actually be no more than the severe, long-term symptoms of stress. When, then, do physical diseases begin? The pathogenic process certainly starts long before symptoms appear. It begins as our bodies initiate and sustain ineffective adaptation efforts. We could say that all of us are diseased now; we are all under stress. It will merely take some time before the organs begin to fail under the load and each of us manifests our particular diseases of adaptation. Selye (1976) made this point in his early observations:

> Why is it, I asked myself, that such widely different disease-producing agents as those which cause measles, scarlet fever, or the flu, share with a number of drugs, allergens, etc., the property of evoking the nonspecific manifestations which have been mentioned? Yet evidently they do share them to such an extent that, at an early stage, it might be quite impossible, even for our eminent professor, to distinguish between various diseases.

For the purposes of this text, we will consider many discrete physical disease conditions to be merely the severe, long-term symptoms of a more globally debilitating disorder—human stress. The physiological mechanisms and evidence to support this idea, which is somewhat contrary to traditional medical thinking, are presented in Chapter 6.

With all this information about adaptation now clearly in mind, let us review Selye's (1946) definition of stress: "Stress is the nonspecific response of the body to any demand made upon it to adapt, whether that demand produces pleasure or pain." Since stress is an adaptation response, we equate it with the general adaptation syndrome. It is important to reemphasize that stress is a physical reaction of the body and to remember that the body does not differentiate between pleasure and pain. Anytime the mechanisms of adaptation are called into play, stress becomes a part of our system.

Since the body does not distinguish pleasure from pain in terms of stress reactivity, we may ask whether all stress conditions are damaging. Should all stress be avoided? Is some stress good for us? Is stress always life threatening, or can it be growth promoting, or both? To address these issues, let us expand and refine our understanding of stress and examine a critical distinction between its two forms.

DISTRESS VERSUS EUSTRESS

Remember that Selye (1976) once defined stress as "essentially the rate of wear and tear in the body." This definition assumes that all stress is damaging to the body, but that is not the case. In fact, a certain amount of stress is essential for life and growth. Selye has stated many times that the complete absence of stress would be death. Stress is not something that is to be avoided absolutely. We need to ask what the difference is between damaging, pathogenic stress and essential, growth-promoting stress. Selye distinguished damaging from growth-promoting stress with the labels **distress** and **eustress**.

We most often conceptualize stress as distress. Distress is damaging stress—the pathogenic kind. When stress is defined in terms of wear and tear, or in its capacity to foster disease, the reference is to distress.

Eustress is the other side of the issue. Whereas distress represents an agent of damage, eustress represents a challenge, a stimulus for growth and positive development. Eustress is the spice of life, the effort that serves as an invigorating challenge. Distress breaks down a living system; eustress is essential for its growth and survival.

The distress-eustress dichotomy can be understood further in quantitative terms. The **Yerkes-Dodson law**, outlined in 1908, illustrates the relationship between the quantity of induced stress and resulting performance.

To explain this law, let us look at the effects of ever-increasing stress on performance. Performance can mean anything such as running speed, examination scores, mental recall, Thursday night bowling agility, target shooting accuracy, reading comprehension, and so forth. To a point, performance of any kind tends to increase as you increase the amount of stress associated with the task. This makes sense. It takes a little incentive to get results. We seem to do our best under a little pressure or when there is a challenge to be met. For every performance activity and each person, there is a given amount of stress that will produce optimal performance. If we increase the stress associated with a given task beyond that optimal point, performance declines. If you push someone too far, he gradually shuts down.

The Yerkes-Dodson law can be illustrated graphically as an inverted U. If we place stress on a horizontal axis and performance on a vertical axis, the interaction we have discussed takes on the visual character shown in Figure 1.1.

The dashed line in the center of the curve indicates the optimal stress level at which performance is at its best. Clearly, the region of this curve on the left hand side of the optimal stress line represents levels of stress that serve a positive, challenging function. From a quantitative perspective, this region of the curve is the domain of eustress—challenging, growth-promoting stress (Figure 1.2). The area to the right represents distress, where stress is so excessive that performance or growth or both are impaired and is now damaging the system and detracting from optimal functioning.

This quantitative distress-eustress dichotomy also relates to biological and cognitive growth and development. Consider the example of the development of the skeletal muscles. If the muscles are to grow and develop, you must place a demand on them through such activities as lifting weights and exercising. Clearly, the proper amount of

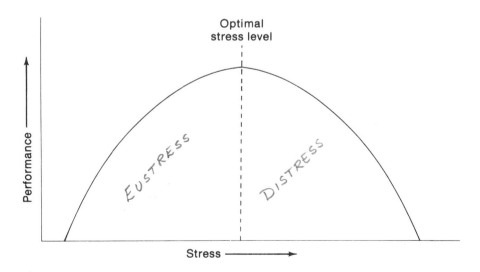

Figure 1.1. Yerkes-Dodson law—stress and performance relationship.

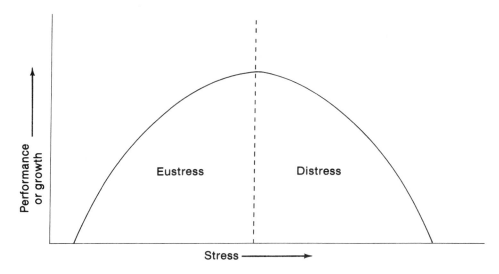

Figure 1.2. Quantitative eustress-distress relationship.

activity will develop the musculature, but too much will damage it. If you wish to condition the heart, running will help. When you begin, you may run about 2 km three days a week; you do not start by trying to run 40 km on the first day of training. On the other hand, no stress at all leads to muscular atrophy. When a person stops all physical exertion for an extended time, the body softens and strength diminishes. Thus, some stress is essential and healthy, the optimal amount is ideal, and too much is damaging.

We all understand too well the reality of damage from too much stress, yet the need for eustress is a novel concept. An excellent example of the critical need for eustress comes from a surprising physiological change in the Skylab 4 astronauts, who had been in space for 84 days. X-ray analysis of the bone structure of the astronauts revealed marked evidence of osteoporosis, or decalcification of bone tissue. Osteoporosis, which makes the bones highly susceptible to fractures, usually occurs in the elderly. In only 84 days, young healthy men experienced a 0.3 to 0.4 percent reduction in body calcium and the appearance of a bone disease that normally affects elderly people. The absence of gravitational stress caused the problem. The weightless environment removed the eustress that is necessary for maintaining the basic bone structure of the human body. In weightless states, normal healthy bone tissue rapidly deteriorates. Based on this finding, medical treatment for osteoporosis now involves not removing physical stress from the body of the afflicted patient, but rather adding weight to stimulate recalcification of the long bone tissues.

The quantitative approach is one way to distinguish eustress from distress. They also can be differentiated by qualitative characteristics. In other words, the same amount of stress may serve as eustress or distress, depending on how one interprets events triggering it. According to Selye, the critical difference is whether one interprets stressors as challenge or threat. He believes that if we consider life's stressors to be threats, then damaging results occur. If, however, we look at the same events as challenges, they foster growth. Selye's personal strategy for stress management does not involve a reduction of stress. Rather, he views stressors as challenges—healthy, growth-promoting opportunities. This idea is explored further in Chapter 8.

Recent investigations into the personal characteristics of "stress-resistant people" support Selye's attitude about the healthy consequences of a qualitative approach to the distress-eustress distinction. In a study on 670 middle- and upper-level utility managers, Kobasa, Hilker, and Maddi (1979) compared people who experienced high stress and low illness rates with those who experienced low stress and high illness rates. They uncovered clear personality distinctions between the two groups. In this comparison, the high-stress, low-illness individuals displayed three basic tendencies: "They were much more actively involved in their work and social lives than those who became sick under stress, they were more oriented to challenge, and they felt more in control of events" (Pines 1980). This triad of involvement, challenge, and perceived control was labeled "psychological hardiness"—a model for the eustress attitude. Disease-resistant people may be successful with their personal health because of the attitude they have toward the experience of change and stress in life. Therefore, one way to control stress is not through a reduction in quantity or avoidance but through a qualitative attitude shift. The importance and impact of the elements of psychological hardiness are discussed in Chapter 4.

SUMMARY

Stress is "the nonspecific response of the body to any demand made upon it to adapt, whether that demand produces pleasure or pain" (Selye 1946). Most stress that individuals encounter in our culture is psychogenic; a state of mind triggers the adaptation process. Psychogenic stress is a physiological phenomenon that begins with the eliciting of Cannon's **fight or flight response**. In this culture, we trigger and react to the fight or flight response in ways that are biologically inappropriate. We have redefined the construct of survival and what constitutes a survival threat. The response is therefore initiated on a daily basis, throughout our lives, when it is biologically unnecessary. Further, when this physical arousal occurs, we fail to act on it in an overt physical way. Thus, the physiological arousal lingers. This maladaptive stimulation of the fight or flight response represents the first phase of Selye's **general adaptation syndrome**, a long-term physiological response pattern that we equate with the concept of stress. The end result of the three stages of the general adaptation syndrome is exhaustion and breakdown of one or more organ systems. At this point the stress process manifests itself as a disease of adaptation. It is important to reemphasize that not all stress is physically damaging; some stress is growth promoting and essential for the continuance and development of living systems.

In conclusion, the physiological phenomenon of human stress owes its existence in our current culture to the following three factors:

1. *Environment*—This includes external conditions that provide stressors, as well as the sociocultural set and setting that establish the guidelines of appropriate interpretation and conduct that make the fight or flight response a maladaptive, evolutionary anachronism.
2. *Mind*—This refers to our psychological preprogramming, the way we have been taught to interpret nonphysically threatening stimuli, as well as our dominant mode of consciousness that tends to label and judge observations (see also Chapter 11).
3. *Body*—This is our biological preprogramming, referring to our inborn, physiological response patterns to threat and adaptation—the fight or flight response and general adaptation syndrome, respectively.

REFERENCES

Benson, H., and Allen, R. E. "How Much Stress Is Too Much," *Harvard Business Review*, 86-92, Sept.-Oct. 1980.

Cannon, W. B. *Bodily Changes in Pain, Hunger, Fear, and Rage*, C. T. Branford, Boston, 1953.

———. "The Emergency Function of the Adrenal Medulla in Pain and in the Major Emotions," *American Journal of Physiology*, v. 33, 356-372, 1914.

———. *The Wisdom of the Body*, Norton, New York, 1931.

Cannon, W. B., and Paz, D. "Emotional Stimulation of Adrenal Secretion," *American Journal of Physiology*, v. 28, 64-70, 1911.

Cox, T. *Stress*, University Park Press, Baltimore, 1978.

Dixon, B. "Space Aging," *Omni*, v. 31, 28, Oct. 1980.

Dubos, R. *Man, Medicine, and Environment*, Mentor Books, New York, 1968.

Kobasa, S. C., Hilker, R. R. J., and Maddi, S. R. "Psychological Hardiness: A Model for the Stress-Resistant Personality," *Journal of Occupational Medicine*, v. 21, 595-598, 1979.

Pelletier, K. *Mind as Healer, Mind as Slayer*, Delta, New York, 1977.

Pines, M. "Psychological Hardiness: The Role of Challenge in Health," *Psychology Today*, 34-44, Dec. 1980.

Randal, J. E. "Stress: The Ticking Bomb," *Science Year*, 26-39, 1977.

Selye, H. "Confusion and Controversy in the Stress Field," *Journal of Human Stress*, v. 1 (2), 37-44, 1975.

———. "General Adaptation Syndrome and Diseases of Adaptation," *Journal of Clinical Endocrinology*, v. 6, 117-230, 1946.

———. *The Stress of Life*, McGraw-Hill, New York, 1976.

———. *Stress Without Distress*, Lippincott, New York, 1974.

Yerkes, R. M., and Dodson, J. D. "The Relation of Strength of Stimulus to Rapidity of Habit Formation," *Journal of Comparative Neurology and Psychology*, 459, 1908.

CHAPTER 2

Psychosomatic Theory: A Model for the Mind-Body Interaction

For this is the great error of our day, that physicians separate mind from body.

Socrates

For a millennium, medical science has considered and treated the mind and the body as two separate entities. Are they indeed separate? Do they interact with each other? Will a change in the state of one alter the state of the other? Is it even functionally valid to recognize a distinction? Are the mind and body merely monads—separately ticking clocks that just happen to display the same time because at some moment in the past their hands were set in similar positions? Or are they two interrelated movements of a singular, exquisite, biological clock?

We learned in the preceding chapter that the most common manifestation of stress is psychogenic stress, a physiological stress reaction triggered by mental states. Implicit in this assertion is the assumption that the mind and body are in some way related, capable of influencing each other. In the following exploration of the mind-body relationship, we will outline a theoretical model for the psychosomatic interaction that will outline the basic steps and sequence of events from stressor to disease. This model will serve to identify the critical factors involved in the development of psychogenic stress and the etiology of stress-related disease. It will also serve as an intervention model to aid us in designing effective stress management techniques.

Recognition of the tangible, physically effective interaction between the mind and body is essential to understanding human stress and learning to control it effectively.

IS IT REALLY ALL IN YOUR HEAD?

Psychosomatic means mind and body (psyche: mind; soma: body). The term refers to an interaction between the two. Most people, even many physicians, interpret the term

17

psychosomatic to mean imaginary illness. We think that a psychosomatic condition is only in the person's mind, that no real physical damage exists and no real medical problem can be found. This is *not* an accurate definition. Imaginary illness involves conditions called hypochondria or hysterical neurosis. These are not the same as psychosomatic states.

David Graham (1979), past president of the Society for Psychosomatic Medicine, has noted that even medical professionals routinely err by equating psychosomatic illness with hypochondria or neurosis. He states that when "psychosomatic consultations" are requested by attending physicians, it is "for one or more of the following characteristics: (1) his (the patient's) behavior disturbs nurses, physicians, or other persons, (2) x-rays and laboratory tests show no abnormalities, (3) he reports symptoms that medical students have long been taught to call 'emotional' or 'psychological.' " He further states that " 'psychosomatic' is used as synonymous with 'neurotic,' " a clear misunderstanding of the concept.

A psychosomatic disease is one in which a state of mind triggers or mediates real physical damage to the body. Medical tests reveal positive results and measurable damage when psychosomatic disease is present. A person with a psychosomatic disease is really sick, yet the mind has played a major role in the problem.

Psychosomatic diseases are perhaps the most dramatic (and painful) examples of the physical interplay between mind and body. Examples of psychosomatic diseases include ulcers, migraine headaches, hypertension, and even cancer. The precise mechanisms by which the mind can produce these profound changes in bodily functioning will be discussed in the chapters on physiology and disease.

In fact, the mind plays a critical role in nearly all physical disease. It is hard to imagine any somatic disease that cannot be potentially influenced by states of mind, given what we know about the ubiquitous nature of the psychogenic, physiological stress response. In this light, Graham (1979) has asserted that "the distinction between psychiatric and medical disease is arbitrary, artificial, and useless."

There are several different types of mind-body interactions. The first important distinction lies between diseases that are **psychosomatic** and those that are **psychogenic**. A psychosomatic disease is a condition in which the mind influences a physical state in any way. Psychosomatic conditions are those in which the mind is either the principal *cause* of the disease problem or those in which it merely influences or exacerbates an existing disease that was caused by something else. Psychosomatic is a comprehensive label. Psychogenic is a more specific label. A psychogenic disorder is one in which the mind is a possible cause of the physical problem. A psychogenic disease is one that can be initiated in the body merely through a change in mental state. Psychogenic conditions are a subcategory of psychosomatic conditions. A psychosomatic disorder is one in which the mind either caused or influenced the state of bodily dysfunction, whereas psychogenic disorders are those in which the mind could be a cause of the physical problem.

Almost all physical problems are psychosomatic. Examples include ulcers, asthma, high blood pressure, influenza, and even broken bones. The mind does not cause such conditions as fractures and infectious disease or allergies, but it certainly influences the progress of the condition or the body's rate of recovery. Psychogenic disorders are those in which the mind may serve as a cause of the problem, such as high blood pressure, migraine headaches, or constipation. These conditions could (and often do) have other causes or multiple causes, but the mind is theoretically capable of being the principal agent initiating the problem.

The mind and body may interact in ways that are **psychosomatic** or **somato-psychic**. The distinction lies between the direction of effect, or whether the change started in the mind or in the body. When a change in mental state influences the body, it is a psychosomatic interaction. When a change in the state of the body influences the state of mind, it is said to be somatopsychic. Figure 2.1 illustrates this difference. When physical pain makes you anxious or irritable, for example, this is a somatopsychic effect. The distinction between these two ideas will acquire greater significance when we discuss different stress management schemes.

THE PSYCHOSOMATIC MODEL

How can the mind's interpretation of external events trigger a somatic change? What are the theoretical components, or steps, in the psychogenic stress process? What elements connect the environment, mind, and body in a way that results in physical disease? To gain insight into this process, we can create a theoretical model, a psychosomatic model, that illustrates the sequence of theoretical components going from stressor to disease. The psychosomatic model gives us insight into the factors involved in the etiology of stress-related disease. It serves to identify and develop an understanding of areas associated with psychosomatic disease and factors that affect human health through psychosomatic interactions. Finally, it identifies critical points of intervention to guide us in developing and understanding effective stress control strategies. If the model is a valid interpretation of the sequence of events going from stressor to disease, interrupting the model at one or more points should allow us to manage stress. This model is only one of an infinite variety of ways that the stress process can be conceptualized.

The discussion that follows outlines the theoretical steps of the psychosomatic model. Subsequent chapters discuss each step of the model in detail.

Sensory Stimulus

The first step in this psychosomatic model is the **sensory stimulus**, or an environmental agent that triggers the stress response. We could also call the sensory stimulus the **stressor**. It is the initial, external cause of the resultant stress reaction.

Sensory stimuli capable of eliciting a stress response can present themselves in several different forms. In the stress context, the sensory stimulus can be anything capable of triggering an adaptation response, any event capable of being interpreted as a threat, or any sudden, unexpected, high-magnitude stimulus (e.g., a gunshot). This last

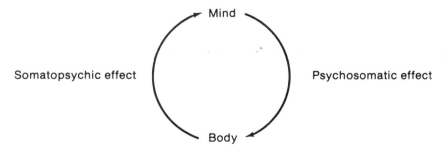

Figure 2.1. Psychosomatic-somatopsychic pathways.

category refers to a specific kind of stimulus called the rapid-onset stressor. Rapid-onset stressors and the nature of all other stimuli evoking stress are discussed in Chapter 3.

Perception

Since the sensory stimulus is an external or environmental agent, it must enter the mind-body system before it can exert any influence on psychosomatic functioning. We will call the entry of the stimulus **perception**. Perception is the sensory intake of the potential stressor. Do not confuse perception with appraisal. We commonly use the word perception when we are referring to cognitive processes (e.g., "Things aren't all that bad, it depends on how you perceive them"). This is a misuse of the term. Perception does not involve thought, cognition, or interpretation; these processes involve appraisal. When we perceive something, we attach no label to it, we form no opinion; we merely see it, hear it, smell it, taste it, or touch it. Perception involves only the senses picking up and delivering the stimulus to the brain. Thought comes later. Since no interpretation goes on at the perceptual stage of the model, it may seem unnecessary even to include it. We will learn, however, that some stress management activities operate by altering our sensory perception. Therefore, as a theoretical point of intervention, it is an important component of the model.

Cognitive Appraisal

Once the stimulus has been perceived, the next step is **cognitive appraisal**, which involves interpreting, categorizing, and labeling the stimulus. This is an important step. Cognitive appraisal represents a fork in the road of the psychosomatic model. For many stimuli, our cognitive appraisal determines whether we perceive the event as a stressor. Cognitive appraisal is the stage at which thought enters the model. Here, we interpret the event as either red or yellow, good or bad, threatening or nonthreatening. Our appraisal of events often determines whether psychosomatic arousal occurs. If we interpret an event as some sort of threat, for example, then we will proceed along the remaining steps of the model. If we attach no significance to it, it dies off in a benign direction with no harm done.

Many factors influence our cognitive appraisal. Some of these include our personal histories, cultural upbringing and attitudes, innate or learned fears, personal stereotypes and prejudices, value systems, morals, religious training, and daily moods. Since we all have different personal histories and infinitely diverse appraisal strategies, we may all interpret the same event differently. Therefore, a serious stressor for one individual may have no effect at all on someone else. From a psychogenic perspective, events are rarely (if ever) inherently stressful; most situations require appraisal to be considered stressors.

Emotional Arousal

If we appraise a given situation as a stressor, the next step of the model—**emotional arousal**—is triggered. No one knows what emotion is. It was once thought of as simply the awareness of physical or vasomotor responses to arousal. That idea was shot down effectively by Cannon in 1927. He then supplied another theory that located emotion exclusively in the brain, independent of somatic factors. He still was at a loss to define the construct, however. If you consult 12 different psychology texts, you will find 5 different definitions of emotion and the other 7 books will not even try to define it. Emotion is an affective state. It is intangible, yet it is clearly part of our inner experience. For our purposes, we will equate emotion with increased cerebral arousal. Although this is a weak way of looking at it, it will serve our simple needs. When we appraise something as stressful, emotion comes into play. This increase in mental activity could be exhibited as, for example, anger, fear, ecstasy, joy, hatred, euphoria, or anxiety. Even though we cannot define it well on paper, you have a subjective idea of what an emotion is. Whenever any emotion is evoked, psychosomatic arousal carries us to the next level of the model. The basis of psychosomatic theory is the assertion that the mind and body are in some way connected. We will consider the steps of perception, cognitive appraisal, and emotional arousal to be within the domain of the mind.

The Mind-Body Connection

A **mind-body connection** is the next step in our model. This theoretical element links the mind and body so that changes manifested in one elicit a parallel alteration in the other. Our theoretical mind-body connection is a transducer of emotional arousal into physical arousal. This link is critical to the validity of the entire model. Without it, the mind and body would be autonomous, unrelated entities. For now, we must merely assume that such a connection exists and that it is a physically tangible one. It has an actual anatomical identity and a well outlined physiological operation that we will soon discuss in detail.

Physical Arousal

The mind-body connection converts emotional arousal into the next element of the model, **physical arousal**, or the mobilization of the body. During this phase, messages are sent throughout the body to get it ready for action. This stage of the model does not yet include changes in internal organ activity. Physical arousal simply means that messages are being sent, through physiological pathways, to direct the organs to alter their level of functioning. Physical arousal involves an increase in the activity of specific branches of the peripheral nervous system and the release of several specific hormones. These two changes will direct the activity of the internal organs and cue their adaptation response. We will go into detail on the specific physiological nature of physical arousal in Chapter 5.

Physical Effects

When the physical arousal messages reach the organs, we can observe the appearance of **physical effects**, which are measurable changes in the activity of the internal organs. Physical effects occur at body structures called end organs. Examples of end organs are the heart, liver, arteries, bronchioles, skeletal muscles, and intestines. These are the structures that perform the work of the body. They are, in a sense, the end of the line for physical arousal; hence the label end organ. The changes occurring at the physical effects stage include the effects of the fight or flight response discussed in the first chapter. Other long-term changes are part of this physical effects level also. These are discussed at length in Chapter 5.

Disease

The last step of the psychosomatic model is **disease**. If the physical effects of psychogenic arousal persist long enough, the resultant somatic imbalance finally breaks an organ system. The organ has spent too much time near its tolerance limit and it breaks, producing disease. Selye would call this a disease of adaptation. Due to the nature of this model, we can say that the person who develops a disease of adaptation has a psychosomatic disease. Examples include ulcers, infarctions, and strokes. The body is in a state in which real, observable, physical damage is present. This damage was initiated or mediated by the person's state of mind.

The complete sequence of steps in the psychosomatic model is illustrated in Figure 2.2.

The model has thus far been presented as a linear pathway, a chain of events. Think of each stage as a domino in a series. Imagine that if the last domino falls, disease results. The significance of this analogy is that each step of the model is essential for the manifestation of disease; each successive step depends on the occurrence of the one preceding it. The implication for stress management is that all we need to do to minimize the occurrence of stress-related disease is interrupt the chain of events. We need only remove or modify one step in the model to prevent the events of the next stage from occurring. This theoretical approach will serve as our model for exploring stress control in the latter half of this text.

SOMATOPSYCHIC INTERRELATIONSHIPS

At this stage of our discussion, the psychosomatic model appears to be a linear, terminal pathway. It looks as though a single stressor will send a person down the psychosomatic path to arrive at some physical effects that either fade in time or perhaps produce a disease. The term end organ, used to describe the organs in which the physical effects appear, reinforces the idea that the model is a terminal pathway that ends at the organs. This is not, however, quite the way the mind-body system operates. Recall that in addition to psychosomatic influences (mind affecting body), there are also somatopsychic interactions (body affecting mind). Physical effects and disease in the body can serve as stressors via feedback to the mind. Suppose, as an extreme example, that your life of distress has resulted in a psychosomatic disorder, say cancer. Imagine your reaction when your physician tells you. Knowing that you have cancer will be a new stressor for you. The whole sequence of events will be triggered again, probably further exacerbating the disease.

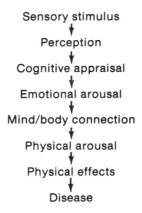

Figure 2.2. Sequential steps of psychosomatic model.

It has long been known that visceral changes are fed back to the brain and can influence levels of cerebral arousal. The most influential organ system in this regard is the musculature. Muscle tension signals that result from psychogenic arousal are returned to the brain. The brain, because it is being bombarded with sensations from the body, then increases its level of general arousal. "Tension breeds tension," we say. If the muscles tense because of an original psychosomatic reaction, those tension sensations return to the brain. The brain becomes more aroused, and is thus more reactive to any new stimulus or potential stressor. This new cerebral arousal may elevate muscle tension further, sending more signals to the brain. This type of condition is called a positive feedback loop or an exacerbation cycle. The system of maladaptive arousal perpetuates itself through its cyclic behavior. The psychosomatic model represents a vicious cycle in which the effects of psychogenic stress perpetuate themselves until disease or death results.

These somatopsychic influences can involve the entry of an arousal message at many points along the model. Some of these influences we are aware of; others occur at a nonconscious, physical level. Figure 2.3 illustrates the complete scheme of psychosomatic interrelations by indicating several lines of somatopsychic influence in the psychosomatic model. The returning lines to the left and right are the possibilities for somatopsychic influence. They all mean one thing: Psychogenic stress can feed itself and build in intensity within the mind-body system.

This cyclic facet of the model also explains how the mind-body system operates to produce the "bad day phenomenon." An initial stressor can begin a sequence of exacerbating arousal in which one little event builds on the next, making you more and more tense, anxious, and pathogenically aroused as each moment goes by, until something snaps. You oversleep on the morning of an important examination. You have no clean socks. You cannot find your car keys. You miss every light on the drive to campus. All the parking lots are full. You make it to the examination but find you have studied the wrong material. When you run out of gas on the trip home, you explode in a fury. This example

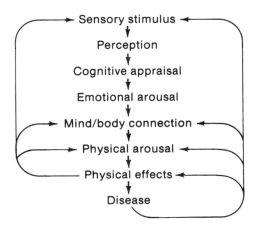

Figure 2.3. Psychosomatic model.

illustrates a common phenomenon. Since psychosomatic effects are cyclic and exacerbating, events that produce relatively small amounts of arousal by themselves can add up. The result is that by the end of the day your system is so aroused that an insignificant thing is enough to push you to the breaking point, producing emotional explosions, physical pain, or even, eventually, disease and death. According to Nix (1981), "It's like wearing a hair shirt over a sunburn; that's just about all you can stand and any little thing will set you off."

Consider a graphic representation. We can illustrate level of arousal against time by using one line to represent our basal, or resting, arousal level and another line to indicate tolerance, or the breaking point for a given system. Level of arousal can include such measures as blood pressure, heart rate, emotional state, or muscular tension. Figure 2.4 illustrates these factors; it also indicates the magnitude of arousal produced by one average, daily stressor. Notice that the increase in arousal due to a single event is far from being great enough to push you to the breaking point if you begin at a resting state. If we allow sufficient time and perform appropriate activities after each stressor we experience, we return to our normal resting level of arousal. If we always do so, we will be nowhere near our emotional or physical breaking point. The trouble is that we do not allow ourselves to return to normal. We let one stressor build on the one before it, so that as the day goes on we get progressively closer and closer to our breaking point. Our deadline-oriented life-styles, nonphysical behavior, and the cyclic nature of the psychosomatic model all contribute to this stairstep building of arousal. This idea is depicted in Figure 2.5.

The fact that we do not allow ourselves to recover appropriately from each simple stressor means that arousal will build to the point that an insignificant event can push us over the edge. Think about all those days when you feel tension, intolerance, and maybe even pain slowly growing, until you explode (or collapse) from an insignificant occurrence.

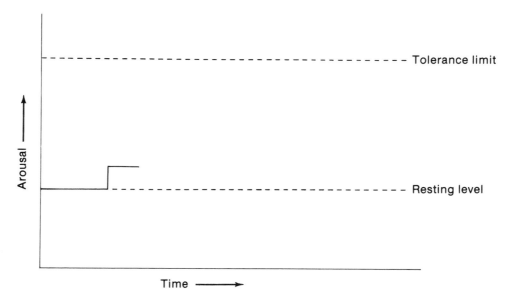

Figure 2.4. Single stressor arousal.

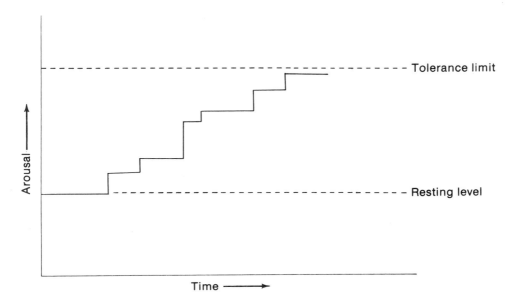

Figure 2.5. Additive arousal.

SUMMARY

The psychosomatic model, which represents the theoretical sequence of events in the mind-body interplay that result in diseases associated with psychogenic stress, identifies the basic, theoretical components in the etiology of psychosomatic disease. The model is an exacerbating, vicious cycle of psychosomatic and somatopsychic interactions that can allow physical and cognitive arousal to grow violently in the mind-body system. Since it operates in a sequential (dominolike) fashion, however, we can learn to control stress by simply interrupting the chain of events. Since the model is a cycle, we can even curtail disease by intervening at the late, physical effects stage. An attitude shift, in which one considers events to be challenging rather than threatening is an example of intervening in the psychosomatic model at the level of cognitive appraisal. Clearly, the model has some use for conceptualizing the mechanisms of effectiveness for theoretical stress control schemes. If we assume that the psychosomatic model is a valid sequence of cascading events leading from stressor to disease, interrupting the process is all that is necessary to control stress.

REFERENCES

Allen R., and Hyde, D. *Investigations in Stress Control*, Burgess, Minneapolis, Minn., 1980.

Cannon, W. B. "The James-Lange Theory of Emotions: A Critical Examination and Alternative Theory," *American Journal of Psychology*, v. 39, 106-124, 1927.

Engel, G. L. "The Need for a New Medical Model: A Challenge for Biomedicine," *Science*, v. 196, 129-136, 1977.

Girdano, D. A. "Preventive Treatment: An Intermediate Step," *Health Education*, 8-10, July/Aug. 1977.

Graham, D. T. "Health, Disease, and the Mind-Body Problem: Linguistic Parallelism," *Psychosomatic Medicine*, v. 29, 52-71, 1967.

————. "What Place in Medicine for Psychosomatic Medicine," *Psychosomatic Medicine*, v. 41(5), 357-367, 1979.

James, W. "What Is an Emotion?" *Mind*, v. 9, 188-205, 1884.

Jenkins, C. D. "Psychosocial Modifiers of Response to Stress," *Journal of Human Stress*, 5(4), 3-15, 1979.

Nix, D. "It's like wearing a hair shirt," Personal conversation, Alexandria, Va., May 27, 1981.

Simeons, A. T. W. *Man's Presumptuous Brain: An Evolutionary Interpretaton of Psychosomatic Disease*, Dutton and Co., New York, 1961.

PART II

The Causes
and Effects of Stress

What specific factors trigger the stress response in our contemporary society? Which elements determine why people react differently to stress and why some of us are more susceptible to it than others? What does stress really do to the body? Can it kill you? If so, how? Does stress really have any effect on the mind, the personality, or performance?

The next three chapters elaborate on the basic segments of the psychosomatic model. Through discussions of stressors, personality, and the psychophysiology of the stress response, we will continue exploring the way the environment, the mind, and the body contribute to our experience of stress and produce in individuals a vast array of causes, responses, and manifestations. We will also examine the effects of stress on the body by physiologically linking the experience of stress to somatic diseases.

CHAPTER 3

Stressors and Life Events

If you find a path with no obstacles, it probably doesn't lead anywhere.

Frank A. Clark

Stress is a physical phenomenon. It is a physiological reaction of the body. Stress is not an environmental event, an adverse situation, mental frustration, or anxiety; it is a somatic reaction to these things. The agent that triggers a stress response within the body is called a **stressor**. The stressor is a stimulus and stress is a response. The stressor is the cause and stress the effect.

THE NATURE OF STRESSORS

A stressor is any stimulus capable of eliciting a somatic adaptation response. We can place stimuli of this type into three broad categories. First, any event or agent that changes the external or internal physical environment of an organism can be a stressor. A stressor can also be any sudden, unexpected, high-magnitude stimulus. Finally, any event or situation that is capable of triggering a cognitively elicited emotional response in an individual is a potential stressor.

We will call these physical, rapid onset, and cognitive stressors, respectively. A physical stressor is any change in the physical environment (internal or external) that requires physical adaptation and hence calls the somatic mechanisms of stress into play. Rapid onset stressors are sudden stimuli. Our reactions to them are almost reflexive in character. Examples of rapid onset stressors include things such as gunshots, slamming doors, headlights suddenly flashing in your face as you walk down a deserted street, or someone sneaking up behind you and dropping an ice cube down your shirt. Both physical and rapid onset stressors can elicit a somatic response in the absence of immediate awareness. They produce a stress reaction regardless of your cognitive processes, state of mind, or interpretation of the event. The classic psychosomatic stressors are cognitive. Cognitive stressors are events that require your interpretation before they affect your body. They are not inherently physically damaging or threatening situations. Your interpretation of an event determines whether it affects your body. Cognitive stressors represent our most common source of stress and they are the type of stressor over which we can potentially exert the most immediate control. The cognitive stressor is conceptually parallel to our expanded definition of what constitutes a threat to survival as discussed in Chapter 1.

PHYSICAL STRESSORS

Physical stressors were the first type of stressors studied. When research into the biological stress phenomenon began, stress was assumed to be a physiological adaptation reaction to physical demands or changes. Selye's early work with stress in rats used Formalin injections to change physically the internal environment of the animal's body. He soon discovered that changes in the physical environment, such as temperature variations, also could elicit the internal adaptation response. Even in his current writing, he places a heavy emphasis on physical stressors. Selye (1976) has provided the following list of events capable of eliciting the somatic adaptation response:

1. Trauma
2. Drugs
3. Hormones and hormonelike substances
4. Diet
5. Physical agents
6. Microorganisms and their toxins
7. Immunity
8. Hypoxia, decreased barometric pressure, including hyperbaric oxygenation
9. Hemorrhage
10. Muscular exercise
11. Restraint
12. Athletics
13. Neuropsychologic stimuli
14. Climate, environment
15. Biorhythms
16. Occupation
17. Physiologic states
18. Genetics, race, constitution
19. Tumors
20. Combined effects of various agents

This list indicates the broad range of general conditions that have been established as being capable of eliciting a stress response. Although many of these are highly nonspecific (physical agents, physiologic states, combined effects of various agents), the list indicates the significant impact of physical conditions in triggering stress reactions. Only two entries in Selye's list, occupation and neuropsychologic stimuli, are from a genre fundamentally different from the physical stressors. We will discuss these agents later in this chapter.

A physical stressor is any change in the body's internal or immediate external environment that is capable of eliciting an adaptation response. Technical advances have eliminated much of the impact that physical stressors have on our daily existence. We live in climate-controlled environments that insulate us from most physically traumatic conditions. Yet we are regularly exposed to two physical stressors that merit some discussion. The two are **pseudostressors** or **sympathomimetics**, and **noise**; both are environmental pollutants that place a physical stress demand on the body.

Pseudostressors are chemicals capable of eliciting a nervous stress reaction through artificial nervous stimulation. Specifically, pseudostressors stimulate the branch of the nervous system that activates the body during the fight or flight response. This major division of the peripheral nervous system is called the **sympathetic nervous system**. Sympathomimetic refers to substances that get into the body and mimic the effects of sympathetic stimulation. These chemicals produce a response in the organs that is identical to the fight or flight response, yet you may never be directly aware of it. That is the reason for the label pseudostressor, or false stressor.

The caffeine in coffee, Coke, and chocolate is a sympathomimetic. So is the theobromine in tea. So is the nicotine from tobacco. Any stimulant, such as amphetamine, triggers a physiological stress response as well. These pseudostressors are potentially avoidable.

Noise, another physical stressor, is a by-product of our contemporary life-style. There is a vast body of research documenting the physiological arousal effects of excessive noise. Not all sources of perceived noise trigger a somatic stress reaction, however. In fact, not all loud noises adversely affect the body. Very loud noise that is constant and stable actually seems to relax the body. People who work around loud industrial fans and machinery, for example, display decreases in blood pressure and muscular tension. The type of noise capable of producing a stress reaction is transient noise. Any sound that changes constantly in intensity, pitch, or frequency of presentation can be a stressor. The explanation for the difference in somatic reactivity to stable versus dynamic noise is simple. A stressor is an agent that changes the environment, and hence requires continued adaptation and somatic adjustments. Even if noise is loud, we become accustomed to it when it is constant and steady. Selye's conceptualization of stress is a response to adaptation. Transient sounds seem to bother our bodies, whereas steady noise seems to dissolve perceptually from our environment and helps us relax physiologically.

We have created our own noise stressors. The U.S. Environmental Protection Agency has ranked noise sources considered "highly annoying." According to the agency's surveys and research, motorcycles create the most stress-fostering noise for most people. Second in line are large trucks and automobiles, followed by construction noise, sports cars, traffic, small trucks, and buses. What we consider essential modes of transportation contribute to our experience of the effects of physical noise stress.

Where you choose to live also helps determine the amount of noise stress to which you are exposed. Figure 3.1 lists examples of outdoor day-night average sound levels measured at various locations.

In many of our attempts to make life more comfortable, we clearly have created physical stressors that damage our quality of life and help to kill us.

RAPID ONSET STRESSORS

A rapid onset stressor is any sudden, unexpected, high-magnitude stimulus. Any time you hear a loud, unexpected noise, experience a sudden bright flash of light or visual movement, or feel a sharp pain, you have experienced a rapid onset stressor. We experience them frequently, and since we cannot avoid them, all we can do is learn to condition our nervous reactivity so they produce only minimal disruption within our bodies. Ways to accomplish this conditioning will be explored in the latter half of this text.

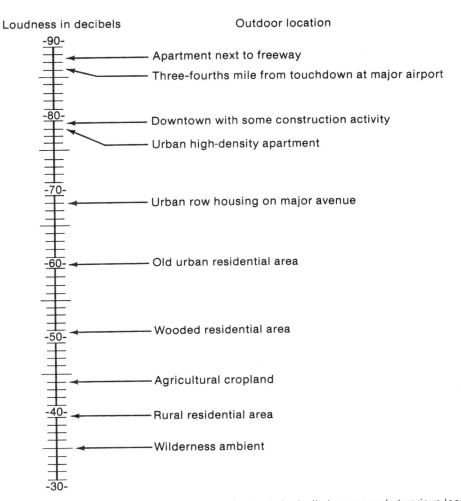

Figure 3.1. Examples of outdoor day-night average sound levels in decibels measured at various locations. (U.S. Environmental Protection Agency, *Protective Noise Levels*, EPA 550/9-79-100, Nov. 1978).

Rapid onset stressors do not generally represent a threat to our overall health because their effect does not last long. The contribution of a given stressor to the development of a stress-related disease is a function of the duration of the body's reaction. Rapid onset stressors, by definition, are usually unpredictable. They can trigger a psychophysiological reaction without our going through cognitive processes. In the psychosomatic model from the previous chapter, the pathway of the rapid onset stressor can be indicated as an arrow from perception to the mind-body link, bypassing appraisal and emotion. Rapid onset stressors trigger a response via psychophysiological pathways; they do not require either interpretation or emotional arousal to elicit the nervous, somatic stress response. Unless your organs are in a fragile, deteriorated, weak, or "close to the edge" condition, rapid onset stressors will have only minor impact on the probability that a psychosomatic disease will develop later. These stressors can, however, take you through the psychosomatic model twice. First you will experience the immediate, almost reflexive, reaction to the sudden stimulus. Then, you may react cognitively to the event and trigger an emotion, sustaining the psychosomatic response and elevated physical arousal. An example might be sitting down on a hot wood-burning stove. Without the necessity (or delay) of cognitive effort, you will leap up and go through some temporary autonomic arousal. Then you think about what just happened and suddenly realize you may have burned yourself. This triggers a second nervous stress reaction and prolongs your state of elevated psychosomatic arousal.

COGNITIVE STRESSORS

Most of the stressors that affect biological integrity are in the cognitive domain. These are events that require interpretation to trigger stress response. A cognitive stressor can be any situation that stimulates emotional arousal. These may include events that we misinterpret as threats to our survival or any situation requiring cognitive adaptation. An infinite variety of cognitive stressors commonly affect us; we will focus on just a few.

Crowding and Violation of Personal Space

Crowding is one of the first cognitive stressors to be researched in a significant way. Nearly all higher animals are territorial by nature. They stake out and defend a certain amount of physical space. Several early investigations assessed the behavior of and physiological effects on laboratory animals subjected to chronic overcrowding.

Classically, these studies involve placing animals in a closed environment and taking care of all their physical needs (food, water, waste removal) except the need for space. Marked behavioral change occurs as population density rises. (Keep in mind that there is no necessity for competition for food or water. The animals have plenty of everything except space.) At a low population density, laboratory animals exhibit a lot of positive physical behavior, such as grooming, playing, and sleeping together in piles. As population numbers rise in this closed container, the animals soon become aggressive and even violent toward each other. Positive grooming behavior ceases and is replaced by physical aggression, violence, and increased mortality. Even though food and water for all the animals is plentiful, as population density rises, so does the mortality rate. During high population densities, many animals are killed due to this aggressive and violent behavior. In some early studies, many seemingly young and healthy animals died in the absence of any overt signs of physical damage.

Autopsy of these animals revealed: (1) atrophy of the thymus and lymph glands, (2) severe ulcerations in the linings of the gastrointestinal system, and (3) hypertrophy or severe enlargement of the adrenal glands—the same pattern as Selye's alarm reaction! In Selye's original work, he noted that these pathogenic changes accompany the onset of the long-term physiological response to stress. In fact, overcrowding represents such a severe stressor that it is capable of killing young healthy animals due to the pattern of physiological changes induced by a cognitive response.

Overcrowding seems to be a universal stressor for most animals, including human beings. People who live in urban areas are no doubt familiar with the kind of mental arousal that overcrowding can produce. Waiting in lines, dealing with traffic jams, or being shoved together in crowded elevators triggers a cognitive stress response. Even though we are not being deprived of food, water, or oxygen, we react adversely when our living space is invaded.

One manifestation of this territoriality that contributes to adverse cognitive reaction occurs when our personal space is violated. Most Americans walk around surrounded by an invisible shell or boundary. We get anxious and uncomfortable when people come too close. Imagine that you arrive early for a movie and sit down somewhere off to one side. You are the only person in the theater. A second patron enters the theater and chooses the seat right next to you. Your reaction will probably trigger a psychosomatic stress response.

Social Stressors

Interactions with other people are another source of stress. Most of these interpersonal stressors are related to one central phenomenon: expectations. When we expect others to behave in a certain way, or when others expect certain standards of performance or behavior from us, we set the stage for cognitive stressors. Expectations represent an image that we create in our minds of how we think the world is or how we want it to be. We may have little pictures in our minds (like doll houses) of exactly how the rooms in our house should appear. We might imagine exactly how our friends and relatives should behave. Sometimes we are comfortable in our expectations; we settle into this cognitive picture of how we think the world is or should be. When someone comes along and violates our expectations, we have to change our image of what we think the world ought to be to fit the way reality is presenting itself. In line with our classical definition of what stress is, this process of cognitive adaptation will serve as a stressor. You may have expectations of the standard of cleanliness or tidiness of each room in your house. If your roommate violates your expectations, problems arise. If you expect to live in clean fresh air, a roommate who smokes is going to be a stressor for you. When the real world does not fit our expectations, our mind has to adapt to the difference. We must adjust our image of reality to fit its presentation to us. If we choose not to adjust our image, we will be forced to experience chronic stressors as our expectations are continually violated.

Our families can be a great source of support, but just as often they can be sources of stress. Again, these stressors originate because of expectations. Have you met all the expectations your parents have for you? Do you know anybody who has? Do you expect your parents to leave you alone and let you lead your own life? Parents tend to expect things from us, and we expect that they will not expect things at all. Such a cycle can be the source of many social stressors.

Social stressors generally occur when the mind set of the individual must change or adapt to external conditions that in some way deviate from what that person thinks is correct, just, reasonable, or expected. Job stress probably represents the most universal and intense kind of stress. According to Pelletier (1977), job stress can result from factors including conflict with co-workers, conflict with supervisors, job dissatisfaction, an overload of on-the-job responsibilities, lack of support, unclear job expectations, and time pressures. Other authors have sited boredom and inappropriate demands as sources of job stress as well. Some people think they are not adequately trained for the jobs they are expected to perform; others think they are placed in job situations in which they are not allowed to use their skills. Anytime conflict or disharmony exists between the individual and the working environment, severe stress can result. Results of numerous studies have shown that under conditions such as stimulus overload and excessive time pressure, significant stress-related blood chemistry changes occur in response to the working environment. These changes have included elevations in serum cholesterol levels and increases in the production and release of catecholamines. The significance of these changes will be defined and discussed in Chapter 5.

Levels of job stress and the resultant physiological reaction tend to be totally independent of social and economic factors. It does not seem to matter how much money you make. Your relationship to the job you have and the tasks you are required to perform are independent determinants of your probability of encountering a psychosomatic disease. Job stress, however, often accompanies two other predisposing factors in the experience of stress-related disease. These are life change, discussed later in this chapter, and the Type A pattern of behavior, discussed in Chapter 4.

Personal Stressors

We are also subject to many personal cognitive stressors. Pelletier calls one such stressor ego maintenance. Ego maintenance stressors manifest themselves when a gap exists between an individual's ideal self and the perceived real self. We all have an image of what we would like to be, in an ideal fashion, and we can all see something of our real selves. For most of us, there is some distance between the two. Quite often, our ideal self is not a good fit. Our physical characteristics or the real goals we have in life may be in conflict with our fantasy image. We go to a lot of trouble to try to bridge the gap between our real and ideal self. We curl our hair (or we straighten it). We lift weights. We buy fashionable clothes. We look for new friends. Think about yourself, not just in terms of physical appearance, but in terms of your daily behavior and life-style. Think about all the times you tried to fit your real self into a style that was not your own. Such attempts require a bit of effort and perhaps expense, and they sometimes waste a lot of time and energy. Ego maintenance is a manifestation of a basic dissatisfaction that we have with ourselves and the resultant efforts we make to overcome our perceived inadequacies. The result is that we never get better, just different, and in the process we raise the probability of experiencing psychosomatic disease.

Life Changes

One of the most extensively researched sources of stress is the construct of life change, or how much the normal events of a person's life are changing. The study of life change has resulted in the first quantification of stressors that we experience in life. The first measures of the degree to which we are exposed to stressors have come from attempts to assess the impact of life change on physical health.

The first evidence to suggest that life change might be related to disease came in 1942. During the 1940-1941 blitz attacks on London, 16 London hospitals reported unusually high rates of duodenal ulcers. After a bombing attack, the hospitals would be filled with patients suffering from broken bones, flash burns, and other physical traumas. About ten days after an attack, the hospital would be filled with patients complaining of gastrointestinal pains and discomfort. Hospital staffs soon adapted to this situation by preparing for traumatic injuries while the bombing attacks were going on and then, about ten days later, they would prepare for the flood of ulcer patients. The bombing was a significant stressor, in terms of fear and anguish during the event. It also disrupted the daily routine of peoples' life to such a significant extent that psychosomatic diseases would manifest themselves quickly after each attack. The specific reason for this ten-day delay will be discussed in Chapter 5. Peacetime calamities such as earthquakes, floods, hurricanes, tornadoes, and maritime disasters all seem to produce similar results.

According to Selye's stress model, this reaction makes perfect sense. Life change can result in psychosomatic disorders. Any change in the routine of life or its regular events will call the body's mechanisms of adaptation into play, thereby releasing the stress response. Clearly, life change has the capacity to increase our susceptibility to psychosomatic disease.

The first individual to make an attempt to quantify the degree of life change that an individual experiences was Adolf Meyer. Meyer developed a clinical tool that he called the Life Chart. This chart consisted of a detailed account of a patient's personal, social, and physical history. Based on these accounts, Meyer noted that significant numbers of social and personal changes seemed to precipitate both psychiatric and somatic complaints in his patients.

The first standardized instrument to quantify the kind of events that were addressed in Meyer's life chart was developed in 1957 by Hawkins and Holmes. The first draft of this instrument was called the **Schedule of Recent Experiences** (SRE). This checklist allowed subjects and patients to indicate which of various life change events they had experienced over the past ten years. This instrument was later revised by Holmes and Rahe. The revised SRE consisted of a 42-item checklist. Each item represented a life change, such as marriage, pregnancy, change in financial status, vacations, trouble with in-laws, or changing place of residence. Individuals simply checked off the changes they had experienced during the previous year. This SRE was designed to estimate quantitatively varying degrees of life change and readjustment secondary to experiencing life events. Scores on this scale were simply a tally of the number of items checked.

The next modification of the measure of life change came with the addition of the social readjustment rating questionnaire. The design of this questionnaire incorporated the realization that different kinds of events have different degrees of impact on a person's life. For example, losing one's spouse will change a person's life and produce the need for a greater degree of adaptation than getting a parking ticket will. Each of the 42 items on the scale has a weight or point value that represents the amount of life change it elicits. A 100-point scale is used in weighing each of the 42 items. A 100-point change represents the maximum degree of life change that a person could experience as a result of a single event. Initially, a sample of 394 ordinary, or healthy, people was used to assign weights to the 42 items. To give them all a common framework as to how to rate each other on this 1 to 100 scale, the participants were told to assume that marriage represented the average amount of life change and would therefore arbitrarily be assigned a value of 50. The subjects then rated each item in relation to this average value. The final draft of the scale obtained is shown in Table 3.1.

Several subsequent efforts have been made to test the validity of the weighting assigned to each item on the scale. Most subsequent investigations have been in close agreement with the original point values. Cross-cultural studies have also indicated significant agreement with the nature of the events contained in the scale and their relative weights.

The units of measure for this construct are called **life change units** (LCU). The point value assigned to each of the 42 items is in terms of LCUs. The number of LCUs a person accumulates during a year seems to be a significant factor in determining a person's probability of encountering illness. Try filling out the scale yourself. Go back to Table 3.1 and check off each event that has occurred in your life within the last 12 months. Then total up the LCU values for all the items you have checked. This total life change score is related to your probability of encountering physical illness during the coming year.

Persons who score 150 or below on this scale have roughly a 30 percent chance of experiencing significant illness during the coming year. Those who score 300 and above face roughly an 80 percent chance of experiencing some significant illness within the next

Table 3.1. The Social Readjustment Rating Scale

Event	Value (LCU)*
Death of spouse	100
Divorce	73
Marital separation	65
Jail term	63
Death of close family member	63
Personal injury or illness	53
Marriage	50
Fired from work	47
Marital reconciliation	45
Retirement	45
Change in family member's health	44
Pregnancy	40
Sex difficulties	39
Addition to family	39
Business readjustment	39
Change in financial status	38
Death of close friend	37
Change to different line of work	36
Change in number of marital arguments	35
Mortgage or loan over $10,000	31
Foreclosure of mortgage or loan	30
Change in work responsibilities	29
Son or daughter leaving home	29
Trouble with in-laws	29
Outstanding personal achievement	28
Spouse begins or stops work	26
Starting or finishing school	26
Change in living conditions	25
Revisions of personal habits	24
Trouble with boss	23
Change in work hours, conditions	20
Change in residence	20
Change in schools	20
Change in recreational habits	19
Change in church activities	19
Change in social activities	18
Mortgage or loan under $10,000	17
Change in sleeping habits	16
Change in number of family gatherings	15
Change in eating habits	15
Vacation	13
Christmas season	12
Minor violation of the law	11

*Life change units.

Reprinted with permission from T. H. Holmes and R. H. Rahe, "The Social Readjustment Rating Scale," *Journal of Psychosomatic Research*, v. 11, 213–218, 1967.

12 months. Life change is certainly not the only factor predisposing an individual to organic disease, but a reasonable amount of attributable risk seems to be associated with the experience of excessive adaptation.

Two points deserve mention. First, several items on the list appear to be positive events. Examples include an outstanding personal achievement, a vacation, or Christmas. Remember that both positive and negative events contribute to our experience of stress. Anytime you must change or adapt to different circumstances, you trigger the stress response, regardless of whether that change is positive or negative. Marriage, for example, is usually thought of as a positive life event, but it can trigger some of the same biological adaptation responses as the death of someone close to you and thus carries a similar probability of stimulating a disease.

A second point is that although most of the items are fairly absolute, others are ambiguous. What does it mean, for example, to have a change in the number of marital arguments? What is meant by an outstanding personal achievement? If you decide to paint your bathroom, does that mean you have had a change in living conditions? Go back and look at some of the ambiguous items again. Notice which ones you decided to check and which you left blank. What decision-making process guided you? Usually people will check off one of these ambiguous items if they feel it has had a significant impact on their life. They will leave it blank if it seems to be of minor importance. Superficially, this seems like a deficiency in the instrument. Remember, however, that stressors are determined not necessarily by the nature of the external event itself but by how we choose to interpret it. A given event may occur in the lives of two different persons. It will have a significant impact on one and not affect the other. Most of the stressors that touch our lives in a significant way are a matter of personal appraisal. It is not so much the event itself but how you choose to think about it that determines what its biological impact is going to be and what role it is going to play in your health or potential for disease.

Stressors of Subgroups

Certain segments of the human population may be predisposed to the experience of specific stressors. Workers who are exposed to toxic chemicals or hazardous situations would be one example. In our culture, two significant segments of the population—women and the elderly—are often overlooked in discussions of unique stressors.

Over the past two decades the role that women play in this culture has changed significantly. Increasingly more options and opportunities are now available to women in terms of career choices, recreational pursuits, and life-style options. Along with the increased opportunities available to women have come increased demands and expectations. Due to the increased availability of new life-style options, many women face a significant stressor called role ambiguity. A woman must decide whether to play the traditional role of the housewife, or pursue a career, or do both. She must decide which of these choices is most appropriate for her. The availability of new options and opportunities makes it difficult for many women to decide which life course to take.

Another source of stress that is not restricted to women yet affects them almost universally is called multiple-role stress. Women may now be expected to play an essential role in taking care of the family and developing a career at the same time. Multiple-role stress is experienced when one person is expected to meet many major diverse responsibilities. Women are now given more roles to perform, and they must face expectations regarding their performance in settings where much ambiguity over the appropriate role for a woman exists. The evolving status of women in this culture has clearly created many stressors of social adaptation.

Other segments of the population do not share to the same degree many of the stressors that are common in the life experience of an older person. Perhaps the most significant of these is social isolation. A common facet of growing old in this culture is a progressive, yet often unnecessary, withdrawal from contact with other people. As we grow older, death, migration, and neglect gradually begin to reduce our circle of friends and acquaintances. Many older adults are left with little opportunity for meeting other people in their later years. Consider how we treat people as they get old and begin to experience medical problems. Often they are institutionalized and locked away from the social mainstream. Contact with friends is minimized or eliminated, and visits from family members are often infrequent. As we will discuss in the next chapter, social isolation is one of the most profound stressors a human being can experience. Of all stress experiences, the denial of social contact with other human beings can have the most serious of all biological consequences. It is quite possible that the social isolation we subject older adults to is a factor that precipitates early death and significantly impairs quality of life.

Many other subgroups in our culture have their own unique stress experiences. Certainly groups of people with varying ethnic backgrounds, children, and bereaved individuals all experience particular kinds of stressors. By identifying such groups, we can learn better how to cope with stress from many diverse perspectives.

SUMMARY

A stressor is any agent capable of eliciting a somatic adaptation response. Three different types of stressors are physical stressors, rapid onset stressors, and cognitive stressors. Cognitive stressors, which are the most common type of stress-induced experience, are events that require interpretation to produce a subsequent stress response. They represent the redefined threats to survival discussed in Chapter 1.

One of the most thoroughly researched sources of stress is the construct of life change. The degree to which a person experiences disruption in daily life routine has been found to be a significant predictor of physical illness.

Many subgroups of the population can identify specific sources of stress that they commonly experience. Examples include the role ambiguity and multiple-role stress experienced by women and the social isolation that is a common facet of the living conditions of the elderly in this culture.

Before proceeding, take a minute to identify the stressors you experience in your own life. Try to identify the significant events that cause emotional upset or maladaptive arousal for you. Gaining an awareness of the factors that predispose you to stress is the first step in learning how to control stress effectively.

REFERENCES

Allen, R. J. "Development and Application of Psychophysiological Testing Protocol for Evaluating the Efficacy of Diverse Stress Control Strategies," University of Oregon Microforms, Eugene, 1980.

Anderson, G. "College Schedule of Recent Experiences," Unpublished Master's Thesis, North Dakota State University, Fargo, 1972.

Cobb, S. "Social Support as a Moderator of Life Stress," *Psychosomatic Medicine*, v. 120, 71-82, 1976.

Cochrane, R., and Robertson, A. "The Life Events Inventory: A Measure of the Relative Severity of Psycho-social Stressors," *Journal of Psychosomatic Research*, v. 17, 135-139, 1973.

Coddington, R. D. "The Significance of Life Events as Etiological Factors in Diseases of Children," *Journal of Psychosomatic Research*, v. 16, 205-213, 1972.

Cooper, C. L., and Crump, J. "Prevention and Coping With Occupational Stress," *Journal of Occupational Medicine,* v. 20, 420-425, 1978.

Cooper, C. L., and Marshall, J. "Occupational Sources of Stress: A Review of the Literature Relating to Coronary Heart Disease and Mental Ill Health," *Journal of Occupational Psychology,* v. 49, 11-28, 1976.

Dohrenwend, B. S. "Life Events as Stressors: A Methodological Inquiry," *Journal of Health and Social Behavior,* v. 14, 167-178, 1973.

Dohrenwend, B. S., and Dohrenwend, B. A. *Stressful Life Events: Their Nature and Effects,* John Wiley and Sons, New York, 1974.

Hinkle, L. E., and Wolf, S. "A Summary of Experimental Evidence Relating Life Stress to Diabetes Mellitus," *Mount Sinai Journal of Medicine New York,* v. 19, 537-570, 1952.

Holmes, T. H., and Masuda, M. "Life Change and Illness Susceptibility," in Dohrenwend, B. S., and Dohrenwend, B. A., *Stressful Life Events: Their Nature and Effects,* John Wiley and Sons, New York, 1974.

Holmes, T. H., and Rahe, R. H. "The Social Readjustment Rating Scale," *Journal of Psychosomatic Research,* v. 11, 213-218, 1967.

House, J. S. "Occupational Stress and Coronary Heart Disease: A Review and Theoretical Integration," *Journal of Health and Social Behavior,* v. 15, 12-27, 1974.

Kobasa, S. C., et al. "Who Stays Healthy Under Stress?" *Journal of Occupational Medicine,* v. 21 (9), 595-598, 1979.

Krueger, D. W. "Stressful Life Events and Return to Heroin Use," *Journal of Human Stress,* v. 7, 3-8, 1981.

Levi, L. "Occupational Mental Health: Its Monitoring, Protection, and Promotion," *Journal of Occupational Medicine,* v. 21, 26-32, 1979.

Lief, A. *The Common Sense Psychiatry of Dr. Adolf Meyer,* McGraw-Hill, New York, 1948.

Marx, M. T., et al. "The Influence of Recent Life Experiences on the Health of College Freshmen," *Journal of Psychosomatic Research,* v. 19, 87, 1975.

Mechanic, D. "Some Problems in the Measurement of Stress and Social Readjustment," *Journal of Human Stress,* v. 1, 43-48, 1975.

O'hara, N. M. "The Relationships Among Life Change, Social Support and Health Status in a College Population," Unpublished Master's Thesis, University of Maryland, College Park, 1980.

Rabkin, J. C., and Strueing, E. L. "Life Events, Stress, and Illness," *Science,* v. 194, 1013-1020, 1976.

Rahe, R. H., et al. "Cluster Analysis of Life Changes, I., Consistency of Clusters Across Large Navy Samples," *Archives of General Psychiatry,* v. 25, 330-332, 1971.

———. "The Epidemiology of Illness in Navy Environments, Parts I and II," *Military Medicine,* v. 135, 443-458, 1970.

———. "A Longitudinal Study of Life Change and Illness Patterns," *Journal of Psychosomatic Research,* v. 10, 335-366, 1967.

———. "Simplified Scaling for Life Events," *Journal of Human Stress,* v. 6, 22-27, 1980.

———. "Social Stress and Illness Onset," *Journal of Psychosomatic Research,* v. 8, 35-44, 1964.

Rahe, R. H., and Arthur, R. "Life Change and Illness Studies: Past History and Future Directions," *Journal of Human Stress,* v. 4, 3-15, 1978.

Rahe, R. H., and Lind, E. "Psychosocial Factors and Sudden Cardiac Death: A Pilot Study," *Journal of Psychosomatic Research,* v. 15, 19-24, 1971.

Ruch, L., and Holmes, T. "Scaling of Life Change: Comparison of Direct and Indirect Networks," *Journal of Psychosomatic Research,* v. 15, 221-227, 1971.

Selye, H. "Confusion and Controversy in the Stress Field," *Journal of Human Stress,* v. 1, 37, 1975.

———. *Stress in Health and Disease,* Butterworth, Boston, 1976.

Suedfeld, P. "Stressful Levels of Environmental Stimulation," in Sarason, I. G., and Spielberger, C. D., *Stress and Anxiety,* v. 6, John Wiley and Sons, New York, 1979.

U.S. Environmental Protection Agency, *Protective Noise Levels,* EPA 550/9-79-100, 1978.

Woon, T. H., et. al. "The Social Readjustment Rating Scale: A Cross Cultural Study of Malaysians and Americans," *Journal of Cross Cultural Psychology,* v. 2, 373-386, 1971.

CHAPTER 4

The Stress-Prone Personality

Well, everybody's different.

Roger Allen

Most of the stressors we encounter in life require our appraisal. In our contemporary culture, few of the stressors that adversely affect our health are inherently stressful. The way we choose to think about, or interpret, events largely determines whether they will trigger a stress response and present a health threat.

Many factors influence how we appraise a given event. Some of them are personal history, religious ideologies, cultural values, parental attitudes, daily moods, immediate setting and environment, innate or learned fears, and prejudices. Personality is a dominant element. Definable facets of personality color our personal interpretations of life's events, making us generally more prone or more resistant to stress. We can assert, therefore, that some personality styles make a person more suceptible to encountering stress and disease, whereas other definable styles are valuable in helping a person minimize stress and the probability of illness. In this chapter, we will theoretically define elements of the stress-prone and stress-resistant personalities.

Personality can be related to stress and disease in a variety of ways. First, personality can predispose a person to experience unnecessary stress. An example would be the type of person who sees the negative or threatening side of every issue. Such people tend to see everything in life as a problem, no matter what the characteristics or outcomes of a situation may be. They are the kind of people who get upset when they get a raise because now they will have to pay more taxes. Persons with this style of personality create unnecessary stressors for themselves. They see life as a negative experience or threat.

The second way personality can influence stress is that some personality types tend to seek out stressful or competitive situations. Personality factors seem to place such individuals in stressful situations continually. They may set tight or unrealistic deadlines for themselves, and they may work under time pressures constantly. They may choose competitive rather than noncompetitive activities, and they may be highly aggressive or dogmatic in business life or personal affairs. Such people seem to enjoy the experience of stress, for they work hard to get into it.

Finally, personality can determine the course of an already stressful situation. Once a person's responses to given stressors are manifesting themselves, personality variables can determine the duration and magnitude of further reactivity. Think about an extreme example. Suppose you are ill and have to be hospitalized, clearly a stressful situation, regardless of whether your illness is related to a prior experience of stress. Your personality is going to help determine whether the stress of hospitalization exacerbates your illness or helps your systems to heal. Your personality can make an existing stress situation worse, thereby exacerbating or continuing the problem, or it can act as a buffer against stress, helping you adopt an attitude that facilitates the resolution of the problem.

SPECIFIC VERSUS NONSPECIFIC PERSONALITY-ILLNESS THEORY

Researchers have focused on the relationship between personality and stress in two basic ways. We can characterize these two approaches as the specific and nonspecific theories of personality influence on psychosomatic disease. The specific orientation basically asserts that a specific pattern of personality characteristics can result in a specific organic disease state. This would mean that there is a cancer-prone personality, a migraine-prone personality, or a coronary-prone personality. The thinking here is that a cluster of personality variables influences psychophysiological activity throughout life in a specific way, so that ultimately a specific disease state results. So far, however, no one has been able to identify the physiological mechanism whereby a specific kind of personality can result in a specific kind of physical problem.

The nonspecific approach to personality is a somewhat more defensible view. This theory asserts that there is a general stress-prone personality and a general stress-resistant personality. The nonspecific theory supposes that we can glean a host of personality factors that are related, or seem related, to many different disease states and combine them to get a picture of the type of personality variables that can contribute to the experience of stress. Conversely, a similar cluster of personality variables can be identified that would make one resistant, in a general way, to the experience of stress and its related diseases. The nonspecific theory is more in line with Selye's concept of stress as a nonspecific response. Your personality, it states, can make you more or less reactive to stress and thereby increase or decrease your probability of encountering some disease state. Using the nonspecific theory, it would be impossible to predict with any certainty exactly what particular disease a person might encounter.

Evidence linking specific personality facets to specific disease states is not yet sufficient to establish causal connections. Evidence is inadequate to suggest that particular personality patterns can cause highly specific patterns of physiological changes that will result in a specific organic disease. Realize that the specific theory does not mean that everyone who has a particular disease has the same personality pattern, or that everyone who manifests a particular personality will undoubtedly get sick in a specific way. Even with this understanding, however, current knowledge and evidence are not yet adequate to support the specific theory.

In this chapter, we are going to emphasize the nonspecific theory between personality and stress. We will discuss components of personality and behavior that have been found to be predisposing factors, or associated factors, in the development of several different disease states. From this information, we will create a picture of what the stress-prone individual looks like. Conversely, we can identify a stress-prone personality type, and then we can identify opposing characteristics as part of the stress-resistant personality.

Researchers have identified a number of different personality traits that seem to contribute to susceptibility to stress-related disease. Examples include low self-esteem; lack of assertiveness; inability to express anger, hostility, or aggression in one's own defense; external locus of control; and feelings of helplessness. Some of the behavioral manifestations of these traits have been found to be highly associated with stress-related disease. Examples of personality-based stress-prone behaviors include self-sacrificing behavior and the Type A behavior pattern.

SELF-ESTEEM

Some authors link cancer to **low self-esteem** and self-sacrificing behavior. Researchers have noted that people afflicted with cancer are often described as being "almost too good to be true." Their friends or relatives often view them as overly warm, kind, or generous persons who would do "anything for anyone." In some cases, this kind of behavior can be indicative of low self-esteem or low self-worth. If people think that they have little value as individuals, they may view their own needs and interests as secondary to the interests and needs of others. Such individuals may sacrifice their own interests, comfort, and energies in the service of people who they think perform more valuable tasks than they do. Such persons may think that their needs do not matter, and that other people are always more important. Consequently, they may strive to do things for other people, while being forced to make severe sacrifices of their own needs.

We think it is nice if someone will "give you the shirt off their back." We do not stop to think that while we are wearing their shirt, they are getting cold. A friend of mine recently loaned me her car to drive to work while mine was being repaired. I was pleased at not having to worry about transportation, but I did not realize until I got home that she had ended up taking the bus to work that day. Altruistic behavior is a wonderful thing and far too scarce in most human beings. If, however, the source of this behavior is a belief that other people's needs and interests and values are of greater importance than your own, you may be creating a host of unnecessary stressors for yourself. If it becomes a part of your permanent life-style, self-sacrificing behavior can gradually wear down your organ systems through the frequent experience of the stressors and difficulties you have created for yourself. Although low self-esteem and self-sacrificing behavior have been observed in some instances to be associated with cancer, it is not at all clear how this style of thinking and acting could result in this particular disease. Rather, it seems clear that this style of behavior could elevate one's general susceptibility to stress.

LOCUS OF CONTROL

Locus of control means location of control. As a personality construct, it refers to where you believe the point of control for your life's circumstances and outcomes is located. Locus of control is a critical determinant of our reactivity to stressful situations. The locus of control construct is related to several other dimensions of stress associated with personality patterns, such as helplessness and social autonomy versus social identification. This collection of personality facets, which all center around the idea of control, has been found to be associated with the most severe of all psychophysiological reactions. Under appropriate cognitive circumstances, these variables can precipitate a reaction called **psychosomatic death**. In such cases, the principal stimulus that triggers death is state of mind. Locus of control may be the most important cognitive factor that determines the nature and magnitude of the effects of psychogenic stress on our minds and bodies.

Locus of control is generally referred to as either internal or external. Persons with an internal locus of control tend to believe that control over their life is located within themselves. They may believe that the amount of money they make, the kind of job they have, the kind of grades they get in school, and their physical health are all factors within the realm of their control. Internally controlled persons tend to believe that if they are dissatisfied with any aspect of their life, they can change it through their own efforts. Internally controlled persons also tend to feel responsible for the way their life is going at the moment and feel a sense of personal responsibility for both the negative and positive events that occur in their life.

In contrast, externally controlled individuals tend to believe that control over their life is located outside themselves. External persons may believe that luck or chance, or other people, or governmental forces, or the CIA play a greater role in determining what happens to them than their own actions do. Externally controlled persons tend to feel helpless in directing their life. External persons may believe that the job they have is simply a matter of good or bad luck. The amount of money they make has nothing to do with how hard they work. Getting good breaks in life may simply be a matter of being in the right place at the right time—it does not have any relationship to personal effort. Thinking of people as being totally internally or totally externally controlled is inappropriate. In reality, locus of control is a continuum. In some situations, we believe we have some control; in others, we believe we are being manipulated.

Locus of control has nothing to do with objective reality. None of us can know, in an objective way, whether we have influence over what happens. Locus of control does not refer to how much control you have over life, but to whether you *believe* you have control. The personality construct is only concerned with whether you *think* you are in control or out of control of events in your life. Internally controlled people believe they can exert an influence over things that happen in life; externally controlled people believe they cannot. In a general sense, internal locus of control is part of the stress-resistant style of personality, whereas external control is in the stress-prone direction. If we believe we have some control over life's events, then life's stressors seem to exert less negative impact on us than if we believe we are out of control and are being victimized by life.

Helplessness

Helplessness is a cognitive phenomenon associated with an extreme external locus of control. Helplessness can precipitate the most severe of all psychophysiological reactions: sudden death.

Evidence linking helplessness to the sudden death response in animals was provided in a 1957 study by Richter, who was interested in studying wild rats. Richter first wanted to know how long a rat could swim. He placed wild rats in large vats of warm water that afforded no possibility of escape. He found that the average wild rat could swim for about 60-70 hours before drowning in complete exhaustion. Richter was interested in more than just how long a rat could swim, however. He thought that if he took a wild rat and created in it a state of helplessness, he could induce death quickly. He believed that if the rats were restrained in human hands with their whiskers trimmed, they would learn a sense of helplessness and be unable to swim very long. The whiskers on a rat are its primary sense organs, analogous to our eyes, so a whiskerless rat is much like a blinded human being. By removing the rat's whiskers and then restraining it in the hand of a human being, Richter thought he could teach the animal a profound sense of helplessness. He took rats that had been "blinded" and restrained and tossed them into the same tank of water in which he had observed rats swimming for about 60 hours. Upon hitting the water, the rats swam around, splashing and struggling frantically. Most of them sank to the bottom and drowned within a few minutes. Richter devised a way to test whether the induced helplessness could have been the cause of death. It was particularly important to continue the investigation at this point, because many of the restrained rats never saw the water at all. Quite a number of them died in the experimenter's hand.

With his next group of rats, Richter again trimmed off their whiskers and held them in the same restrained fashion, but, before throwing them in the water, he let them go. After letting them go once, he held them again; after they stopped struggling, he let them go again. The rats were restrained and released, restrained and released several times. Richter thought that this might immunize the rats against the feelings of helplessness induced by restraint. When placed in the water, these rats swam as long as the original ones had, about 60 hours. To further test his hypothesis, Richter took another group of whiskerless rats, exposed them to the same restraint procedure, and then immediately tossed them into the water. Before they drowned, however, he lifted them out and then tossed them in again several times in another attempt to immunize them against their feelings of helplessness. These rats were also able to swim for about 60 hours. Essentially, the results of Richter's experiment indicated that feelings of helplessness can precipitate sudden death in an animal.

An interesting question was why some of the rats who had been trimmed and restrained died before even entering the water. Autopsy of these animals revealed something unusual. We usually associate sudden death with a hypermetabolic state, a condition associated with such reactions as elevated blood pressure, increases in heart rate, and muscular tension. These rats, however, did not die from this kind of physiological state. Their hearts were found to be engorged with blood, a state indicative of the opposite kind of physiological response; we call it a parasympathetic response. (This response will be explained further in Chapter 5.) A parasympathetic response is much like the body giving up completely. All the vital functions slow way down. The direct cause of death was probably a decrease in arterial blood pressure, meaning there no longer was enough hydrostatic pressure to help deliver the oxygen from the blood into the cells and vital organs such as the brain. To establish this fully, Richter treated a number of the rats with atropine, a substance that blocks parasympathetic activity. A significant number of rats treated with atropine did not show the sudden death response when exposed to whisker trimming, restraint, and then the water. This result further reinforces the notion that helplessness may have been the prime trigger contributing to the sudden death of Richter's rats.

Seligman (1976) reported a further study that lends even more support to the importance of helplessness in the psychosomatic death response:

> Bennet Galef and I wondered whether inescapable shock in learned helplessness experiments works upon the same mechanisms that Richter activated by restraining wild rats. So, we built a Skinner box, bought chain mail gloves and started a colony of wild rats. We used two groups of adult females. One received immunization, with escapable shock (of mild intensity). The second group was yoked. They received the same sequence of shocks, but all of them were inescapable. We had intended to put both groups in the vat of water, expecting that the escapable shock group would swim for 60 hours and the yoked group might show sudden death. To our surprise, however, six of the twelve in the yoked group laid down paws splayed beneath the grids and died in the box during mild long duration shock. Their hearts were engorged with blood. None of the other group died.

Psychosomatic death resulting from feelings of helplessness is not limited to laboratory animals. The phenomenon is unusually common in human beings as well. Walter Cannon first mentioned psychosomatic death of humans in 1942. He reported in a journal called *American Anthropologist* on the phenomenon of "voodoo death." In this paper, he cited many examples of sudden death occurring in human beings as a result of the cognitive state of helplessness:

A Brazilian Indian condemned and sentenced by a so called medicine man is helpless against his own emotional response to this phenomenon and dies within hours. In Africa, a young Negro unknowingly eats the inviolable banned Wild Hen. On discovery of his "crime" he trembles, is overcome by fear, and dies within 24 hours. In New Zealand, a Maori woman eats fruit that she only later learns has come from a tabooed place. Her chief has been profaned. By noon of the next day, she is dead. In Australia, a witch doctor points a bone at a man. Believing that nothing can save him, the man rapidly sinks in spirits and prepares to die. He is saved only at the last moment, when the witch doctor is forced to remove the charm.

The man who discovers that he is being boned by an enemy is indeed a pitiable sight. He stands aghast, with his eyes staring at the treacherous pointer and with his hands lifted to ward off the lethal medium, which he imagines is pouring into his body. His cheeks blanch and his eyes become glassy and the expression of his face becomes horribly distorted. He attempts to shriek, but usually the sounds choke in his throat and all that one might see is froth at his mouth. His body begins to tremble and his muscles twitch involuntarily. He sways backward and falls to the ground and after a short time appears to be in a swoon. He finally composes himself, goes to his hut and there frets to death.

The phenomenon of voodoo death requires two elements to manifest itself. The first is that an individual must encounter a situation that he or she believes to be lethal. In primitive cultures, this could involve breaking tribal laws or being "attacked" by a person who the victim believes has special supernatural powers. The second requirement is that the victim believes that death is totally inescapable and that the situation is indeed hopeless. Under these cognitive conditions, death often results within 24 hours in normal, young, healthy human beings.

Sudden psychosomatic death is by no means limited to primitive cultures, however. A profound sense of helplessness can have the most serious psychosomatic consequences and even result in the death of human beings in any culture. Seligman (1976) cited a report by H. M. Lefcourt of a case involving sudden death, thought to be due to cognitive states, that occurred in an institution in this country:

This writer witnessed one such case of death due to a loss of will within a psychiatric hospital. A female patient, who had remained in a mute state for nearly ten years, was shifted to a different floor of her building along with her floor mates, while her unit was being redecorated. The third floor of this psychiatric unit, where the patient in question had been living, was known among the patients as the "chronic hopeless floor." In contrast the first floor was most commonly occupied by patients who held privileges, including the freedom to come and go on the hospital grounds and to the surrounding streets. In short, the first floor was an exit ward from which patients could anticipate discharge rather rapidly. All patients who are temporarily moved from the third floor were given medical examinations prior to the move and the patient in question was judged to be in excellent medical health though still mute and withdrawn. Shortly after moving to the first floor, this chronic psychiatric patient surprised the ward staff by becoming socially responsive, such that within a two week period she ceased being mute and was actually becoming gregarious. As fate would have it, the redecoration of the third floor unit was soon completed and all previous residents were returned to it. Within a week after she had been returned to the "hopeless unit" this patient, who like the legendary Snow White had been aroused from the living torpor, collapsed and died. The subsequent autopsy revealed no pathology of note and it was whimsically suggested at the time that the patient had died of despair.

Although it may not be as obvious or dramatic as it is in primitive cultures, psychosomatic death may be common in this country. Consider the elderly. Quite often, as people in this culture get older and begin to require external support and care, they are institutionalized. They feel they will never be able to leave. Their friends and life acquaintances begin to die. Their families tend to ignore them, visiting them less and less frequently. Conditions such as these can easily foster hopelessness and despair. Our treatment of the elderly, besides reducing the quality of their lives dramatically, may be precipitating the early death of many people.

External locus of control is highly related to the construct of helplessness. Externally controlled individuals often believe they are victims of life rather than co-creators of their own future. Their resulting sense of helplessness can have disastrous consequences for their health. In contrast, internally controlled individuals may avoid the catastrophic health consequences of hopelessness through the belief that no matter what happens in life they will always have some say in the outcome. The construct of control seems to be essentially important in the degree to which external events affect our biological integrity, as filtered through personality.

Autonomy Versus Social Identity

Two dichotomies are closely related to the idea of helplessness and to internally versus externally controlled personality types. The first of these involves the notion of the **autonomous** versus the **socially identified** individual. Socially identified people are those who behave according to the standards, behavior, and fashions of their immediate cultural and social environment. Basically such people let the social structure affect all their decision-making. They choose their clothes, their neighborhood, even their value systems and code of ethics according to what those around them do. Socially identified individuals are a bit like externally controlled individuals. They purposely place much of the control over their life outside themselves. Such people are generally okay as long as the social structure stays intact. If the structure that they trust collapses or cracks, however, they too suffer a catastrophic collapse. Autonomous persons, on the other hand, make their own decisions, regardless of the behavior of the larger social group. Sometimes they conform and sometimes they do not. Fashions of the social order do not influence autonomous individuals; they merely provide options for consideration. Such persons must often meet challenges and face critical decisions almost alone, but they view this situation as a challenge. As challenge becomes a way of life for autonomous individuals, they acquire strength that shields them from any collapse or shift in the social order. They are strong and robust in the face of change. The autonomous individual is somewhat analogous to the internally controlled individual and represents, in a general sense, the most healthy or stress-resistant pattern of personality.

Distress Versus Eustress

Distress versus eustress represents the second dichotomy that is closely related to internal versus external locus of control. As you may recall from Chapter 1, the distinctions between these two types of stress can be made along either quantitative or qualitative lines. From a qualitative perspective, the difference between distress and eustress seems to lie in how one chooses to interpret potential stressors. If people view stressors as threats, thereby seeing themselves as victims, they are in distress or pathogenic situations. If, however, they view life's events as challenges, they are in a eustress situation, capable of promoting growth. When we feel helpless or out of control in relation to the events of our lives, when we feel like victims, we are in a potential distress situation. When we view life's occurrences as challenges to be met, we place ourselves (simply through our cognitive processes) in a positive, growth-promoting situation. In most instances of psychogenic stress, our physiological reactions are determined not by the events we experience, but by how we choose to interpret them. We will discuss this idea in greater detail in Chapter 8.

Exceptions to the Rules

In the general sense, external locus of control is part of the stress-prone personality pattern and internal locus of control helps make us more resistant to the diseases or problems associated with stress. There are exceptions, however. In some instances, an external locus of control can be beneficial in helping us cope with the stress of life. When externally oriented individuals place faith or trust in a power greater than themselves, they believe they will always be taken care of. Religion is probably the best example. Individuals who believe they are not in control of their life, that some higher power pulls all the strings and that this higher power will always take care of them and ensure their ultimate well-being, may be quite healthy through life. Even though it is externally oriented, faith in positive outcomes can be an adaptive cognitive attitude.

An internal locus of control can be damaging when a person feels completely responsible for negative outcomes in life. Such a feeling can produce significant guilt reactions. A student of mine recently came to me complaining of a host of serious psychosomatic problems. She was young, normal, healthy and had no previous history of problems of this nature. The psychometric instruments that we routinely administer in class revealed that she had a strongly developed internal locus of control. While discussing recent events in her life that may have contributed to her physical state, I found out that her parents had just been involved in a serious earthquake in the Dominican Republic. It turned out that she was to have visited them during the week the earthquake occurred. She had had an offer to go skiing in New Hampshire and had called her parents with the explanation that she had a heavy examination schedule and wanted to postpone the trip for a few weeks. While she was skiing, the earthquake hit. As she described the situation, she looked at the floor, shook her head, and said, "How could I have allowed that to happen?" I thought she meant the trip to New Hampshire. "No," she said, "I mean the earthquake." She had such a strongly developed internal locus of control that she felt personally responsible for serious external events. The extreme guilt that this created manifested itself as serious psychosomatic problems.

Exceptions to the general ideas we have presented do exist, so individuals must evaluate their own personality, take a look at their own sense of control, and determine whether their belief system is an adaptive one.

TYPE A BEHAVIOR

To date, the most thoroughly researched behavioral risk factor in the etiology of psychosomatic disorders is the **Type A behavior pattern**. Type A behavior was first noted and described by Rosenman and Friedman, two cardiologists. They noted that this style of behavior was highly associated with the incidence of coronary disease. The term Type A behavior is often used synonymously with coronary-prone behavior. Type A behavior is not specifically a personality style, however; it is a style of behavior. Underlying personality factors certainly may precipitate this behavioral style, but Type A is actually defined as a way of acting, not a way of thinking.

According to legend, it was not Rosenman and Friedman who discovered this highly significant and pathogenic behavioral pattern, it was their upholsterer. As the story goes, the occupants of the building in which Rosenman and Friedman had their offices decided as a group to have their furniture reupholstered. The upholsterer they hired dutifully noted the unique upholstery needs of the furniture in each physician's office. He went to a dentist's office and noticed the characteristic clawing marks on the armrests of the chairs, he visited the pediatrician's office and examined tiny chairs for wear, he went to the urologist's office and pondered what he could do to remove all those nasty stains; but he could not understand what he saw in the office of the two heart specialists. The waiting room chairs were not worn where a waiting room chair should be—in the seat or the back or the middle of the armrests. The centers of the seats were almost perfect; the backrests looked brand new. Instead the chairs were worn out, and in a very pronounced fashion, right across the front edge of the seat. The front edges of the armrests were also worn and so was the lower front portion of the chair as though people had been bracing their heels against it. The upholsterer called in Rosenman and Friedman to discuss his unusual findings. What kind of patients wore out waiting room chairs in such an unusual fashion, he wanted to know.

Picking up on the upholsterer's findings, Rosenman and Friedman started watching. The first thing they observed was, in fact, how their patients sat in their chairs. They looked like horses lined up at the gate before the start of a big race. They all seemed to be in a tremendous hurry. The doctors began to notice other interesting characteristics common to most of their patients. They all seemed to know what time it was, all the time. Most of them wore watches. They were impatient people, always aware of time, deadlines, and getting things done quickly. If someone spoke too slowly, they usually finished their sentences for them. They tried to perform several tasks at the same time. They just sat still in the waiting room; they brought work and tried to get something accomplished while they waited. The doctors also noticed a profound quantity orientation in their patients. Rather than describing things in terms of quality, they converted everything in life into numbers.

This unique behavioral style was so striking to the two physicians that they decided to give it a label: Type A behavior. Type As are characterized by a chronic sense of time urgency, an orientation toward numbers, and, often, by a strong competitive drive. Rosenman and Friedman identified persons who do not manifest Type A characteristics as exhibiting the Type B behavior pattern. Type Bs are considered to have a far lower susceptibility to coronary disease.

The accompanying chart outlines some of the characteristics of Type A behavior that Rosenman and Friedman identified. Reading this list may call to mind people you know who manifest Type A tendencies. Use them as examples to facilitate your understanding of this coronary-prone behavioral style.

We all know people who behave like this. Through teaching classes on how to control stress, I have encountered many. I recall one woman who did not like to waste time in the morning. She would get up, get dressed, grab her makeup bag, and hop into the car for the drive to work. She looked awful. She was believed to be a major cause of early morning traffic accidents. She had figured out that of the 14 stop lights along her route, she would have to stop for 6 of them on any given morning. At the first red light, she would take half the curlers out of her hair. At the next one, she would undo the other half. She would start brushing it out at the next light. At the next, she would make up one eye. At the next,

CHARACTERISTICS OF TYPE A BEHAVIOR

Time Urgency

If you always move, walk, and eat rapidly.

If you almost always feel vaguely guilty when you relax and do absolutely nothing for several hours to several days.

If you attempt to schedule more and more in less and less time, and in doing so make fewer and fewer allowances for unforeseen contingencies. A concomitant of this is a *chronic sense of time urgency*.

If you believe that whatever success you have enjoyed has been due in good part to your ability to get things done faster than your fellow men.

If you are afraid to stop doing everything faster and faster.

Impatience

If you feel (particularly if you openly exhibit your feelings to others) an impatience with the rate at which most events take place.

If you find it difficult to restrain yourself from hurrying the speech of others.

If you attempt to finish the sentences of persons speaking to you before they can.

If you find it intolerable to watch others perform tasks you know you can do faster.

If you become impatient with yourself when you are obliged to perform repetitious duties.

Polyphasia

If you indulge in polyphasic thought or performance, frequently striving to think of or do two or more things simultaneously.

Quantitative Attitude

If you find yourself increasingly and uncontrollably committed to translating and evaluating not only your own but also the activities of others in terms of numbers.

Egocentricity

If you find it *always* difficult to refrain from talking about or bringing the theme of any conversation around to those subjects that especially interest and intrigue you.

Competitiveness

If, on meeting another severely afflicted Type A person, instead of feeling compassion for his affliction, you find yourself compelled to outdo him.

Existential Dysfunction

If you do not have any time to spare to become the things worth *being* because you are so preoccupied with getting things worth *having*.

Weird Speech

If you have (1) a habit of explosively accentuating various key words in your ordinary speech, even when there is no real need for such accentuation, and (2) a tendency to utter the last few words of your sentences far more rapidly than the opening words.

Unconscious Tension

If you resort to certain characteristic gestures or nervous tics. If in conversation, for example, you frequently clench your fist, or bang your hand on a table, or pound one fist into the palm of your hand in order to emphasize a point.

If the corners of your mouth spasmodically, in ticlike fashion, jerk backward slightly, exposing your teeth.

If you habitually clench your jaw, or even grind your teeth. Such muscular phenomena suggest the presence of a continuous *struggle*.

Dulled Senses

If you no longer observe important or interesting or lovely objects that you encounter.

If you enter a strange office, store, or home, and, after leaving, you cannot recall what was in them. This inability indicates you no longer are observing well or, for that matter, enjoying life very much.

she did the remaining eye. By the time she drove through that last traffic light, she looked great. This sounds frantic. It is. But that is the way Type As like to operate. They do not like to waste time. They get nervous when they have to sit and relax. It is easy to imagine how rushing around at such a pace could produce some profound stress problems.

Type A is a common behavioral style among Americans. It is also clearly associated with the incidence of coronary disease. Type As do not live as long as Type Bs. They tend to suffer heart attacks at early ages. Why then is this behavioral style so common? The answer is implicit in the mind set of most Americans: We assume that Type A behavior is required for success in this culture. The characteristics of the Type A pattern of behavior look like the characteristics of a successful, productive, and accomplished individual. We assume that if we are always on time, if we are polyphasic, if we are competitive and quantitative, we will rise to a level of success far above our Type B counterparts who find it more valuable to allow space to relax in life and who tend to take things one at a time. Most Americans, I think, would accept this assumption without question.

To date, more than two dozen studies have been done to assess whether Type A individuals are more productive or more successful than their Type B counterparts. Surprise; only one recent study has found a difference. In all the rest, no significant differences have been observed between Type As and Type Bs on many dimensions of performance and success. Issues looked at have included such things as yearly income, level of job status, speed at which factory workers can screw on rearview mirrors, and many other measures of job success and work productivity. In most of the instances studied, Type As did *not* outperform Type Bs. In fact, it was noted on at least one occasion, in a study of corporate executives, that Type A individuals occupied the lower levels of the corporate ladder, whereas the top positions were usually held by Type Bs. The explanation seems to be that Type As are often so concerned with the trivial details of a project, with hurrying and getting it done by a certain time, that they ignore the overall goals and purpose of the activity. Type Bs, with their more holistic and qualitative attitude, tend to be better equipped to meet the overall goal of a project. Is it worth shaving years off your life just to be more productive? That apparently is not the question. The issue is whether it is worth shaving years off your life just to think you are being more productive and just to absorb yourself in the frantic management of trivia.

Type A behavior is not always a pathogenic condition. Type A is a behavioral style, not a dimension of personality. Many Type A individuals stay perfectly healthy and live long lives, whereas others suffer coronary disease and an early death. Why does Type A behavior foster a stress-related disease in some individuals and not in others? Evidence suggests that when Type A individuals think that the way they are performing genuinely helps them get things done, they are okay. If they think that they have chosen to behave in this style and that it is productive for them, they do not tend to suffer the psychosomatic disease consequences. If, however, they think they *must* behave in this style in order to get things done, they have serious problems. If they think that even though they are rushing and hurried and polyphasic, they are always behind, they will suffer the coronary consequences of Type A behavior.

Imagine that there could be such a thing as a Type A and a Type B personality to go along with behavior. Type A personalities and Type A behavior would seem to be a combination that does not pose a threat to health. Such people behave in a way they believe enhances their productivity. They may in fact thrive on the experience of stress. This style of behavior for these individuals may represent a eustress situation rather than distress. People who seem to have trouble—and this is the majority of people in this culture—are Type B personalities who feel forced into Type A behavior in order to get done all the things that are forced on them. The type of individuals who are likely to suffer physical health difficulty are the ones who do not choose to behave in this way, but think they have to. It goes back to the issue of control. If Type As believe that their behavior keeps them in control of their life's situation and their level of productivity, they seem to be fine. If people behave in a Type A fashion because they think that they must and that control is really out of their hands, they are in a dangerous situation.

A lot of this personality information sounds highly subjective. Usually it is. Yet, in the case of the Type A pattern of behavior, there now exists complete and strong evidence suggesting that, under the right cognitive circumstances, this style of behavior can actually play a causal role in the development and manifestation of coronary disease. It has even been noticed that there are significant differences in serum cholesterol levels between Type As and Type Bs.

Can We Change Our Personality?

Take a close look at yourself. Think about the instances in which you display Type A behavior. Most of us do in one circumstance or another. When you act in a hurried and polyphasic fashion, do you think that it is helping you get things done and that you are doing it as a matter of choice, or do you think that you have to in order to meet demands that have been thrust on you? Let yourself become aware of the serious consequences of this style of behavior.

Realize, though, that in the interest of controlling stress, it is probably not a good idea to try to change your personality. You may identify certain facets of the stress-prone personality within yourself, but you may run into great difficulty if you try to avoid the experience of stress-related disease by altering cognitive patterns.

One clinical effort did try to alter individual personality in the hopes of reducing disease incidence. The project was done with a number of Type A patients who had a history of at least one myocardial infarction and a good probability of having another. These people were obviously serious cardiovascular risks. The clinicians thought that if they could change a Type A's style of behavior, then they could perhaps lower the person's risk of having further heart attacks. The Type A people were asked to perform many Type B tasks. They did things like sort marbles and read long Victorian novels. The clinicians thought these kinds of activities would change behavior, lowering susceptibility to heart attacks. In fact, all it did was make the Type As extremely anxious; it actually increased the incidence of heart attacks in the clinical sample. There are even rumors that the experimenters lost a few subjects in the effort.

For the purposes of this textbook, we are going to assume that personality is a given factor. When you use the techniques presented in the second half of this book to try to control stress, do not assume that you necessarily have to change your personality. Just become aware of its facets. Then learn to apply the stress management technique that will be a good fit.

SUMMARY

There are two theories that link personality to stress-related disease. The specific theory asserts that specific personality patterns predispose one to encounter particular diseases. The nonspecific theory asserts that several personality facets combine to form a stress-prone personality, which can contribute to the manifestation of any stress-related disease problem.

Low self-esteem, external locus of control, and the Type A behavior pattern are elements of personality and behavior that can be related to the development of stress-related disease. Low self-esteem has been associated with the experience of cancer, extreme external locus of control has been associated with psychosomatic death, and Type A behavior seems to be highly related to coronary disease.

For each trait of the stress-prone personality, a complementary trait exists that generally makes one stress-resistant. Stress-resistant personality facets include positive self-esteem, internal locus of control, and Type B behavior.

REFERENCES

Barber, T. X. "Death by Suggestion: A Critical Note," *Psychosomatic Medicine*, v. 23, 153-155, 1961.

Blumenthal, J. A., et al., "Type A Behavior Pattern and Coronary Atherosclerosis," *Circulation*, v. 59, 269-279, 1974.

Bowers, K. S. "Pain, Anxiety, and Perceived Control," *Journal of Consulting and Clinical Psychology*, v. 32, 596-602, 1968.

Cannon, W. B. "Voodoo Death," *American Anthropologist*, v. 44, 169-181, Apr. 1942.

Chaisson, E. D. "A Psychological Study of Tension Headaches as a Psychophysiological Disorder and Their Relationship to Locus of Control," *Dissertation Abstracts International*, v. 38, 4576A-4577A, 1978.

Clune, F. J. "A Comment on Voodoo Deaths," *American Anthropologist*, v. 75, 312, 1973.

Coolidge, J. C. "Unexpected Death in a Patient Who Wished to Die," *Journal of the American Psychoanalyst Association*, v. 17, 2, 1969.

Corah, N. L., and Boffa, J. "Perceived Control, Self-Observation, and Response to Aversive Stimulation," *Journal of Personality and Social Psychology*, v. 16, 1-4, 1970.

DeGood, D. E. "Cognitive Control Factors in Vascular Stress Responses," *Psychophysiology*, v. 12, 399-401, 1975.

Dynes, J. B. "Sudden Death," *Disease of the Nervous System*, v. 30, 24-28, 1969.

Eliot, R. S., and Todd, G. L. "Sudden Coronary Death and Acute Myocardial Infarction," *Primary Cardiology*, May 1977.

Engle, G. L. "Sudden and Rapid Death During Psychological Stress," *Annals of Internal Medicine*, v. 74, 771-782, 1971.

Friedman, M. "Type A Behavior Pattern," *Bulletin of the New York Academy of Medicine*, v. 53, 593-603, 1977.

Friedman, M., et al. "Serum Lipids and Conjunctival Circulation After Fat Ingestion in Men Exhibiting Type A Behavior Pattern," *Circulation*, v. 29, 874-886, 1964.

———. "Coronary-Prone Individuals: Some Bio-chemical Characteristics," *Journal of the American Medical Association*, v. 212. 1030-1037, 1970.

———. "The Relationship of Behavior Pattern A to the State of the Coronary Vasculature: A Study of 51 Autopsy Subjects," *American Journal of Medicine*, v. 44, 525-537, 1968.

———. "Instantaneous and Sudden Deaths, Clinical and Pathological Differentiation in Coronary Artery Disease," *Journal of the American Medical Association*, v. 22, 1319-1328, 1973.

Friedman, M., and Rosenman, R. H. "Association of Specific Overt Behavior Pattern With Blood and Cardiovascular Findings," *Journal of the American Medical Association*, v. 169, 1286-1296, 1959.

Greene, W., et al. "Psychosocial Aspects of Sudden Coronary Death," *Archives of Internal Medicine*, v. 129, 725-731, 1972.

Greer, J. H., et al. "Reduction of Stress in Humans Through Nonverdical Perceived Control of Aversive Stimulation," *Journal of Personality and Social Psychology*, v. 16, 731-738, 1970.

Holt, W. C. "Death by Suggestion," *Canadian Psychiatry Association*, v. 14, 81-82, 1969.

Houston, B. K. "Control Over Stress, Locus of Control, and Response to Stress," *Journal of Personality and Social Psychology*, v. 21, 249-255, 1972.

Jenkins, C. D. "Recent Evidence Supporting Psychologic and Social Risk Factors for Coronary Disease," *New England Journal of Disease*, v. 294, 987-994, 1976.

Jenkins, C. D., et al. "Prediction of Clinical Coronary Heart Disease by a Test for Coronary-Prone Behavior Pattern," *New England Journal of Medicine*, v. 290, 1271-1275, 1974.

Lefcourt, H. M. "The Function and the Illusions of Control and Freedom," *American Psychologist*, v. 28, 417-425, 1973.

Lester, D. "Voodoo Death: Some New Thoughts on an Old Phenomenon," *American Anthropologist*, v. 74, 386-390, 1972.

Levi, L. "Occupational Mental Health: Its Monitoring, Protection and Promotion," *Journal of Occupational Medicine*, v. 21(1), 23-32, Jan. 1979.

Lex, B. W. "Voodoo Death: New Thoughts on an Old Explanation," *American Anthropologist*, v. 76, 818-823, 1974.

Lundberg, V., and Frankenhaeuser, M. "Psychophysiological Reactions to Noise as Modified by Personal Control Over Noise Intensity," *Biological Psychology*, v. 6, 51-59, 1978.

Mathias, J. L. "A Sophisticated Version of Voodoo Death," *Psychosomatic Medicine*, v. 26, 104-107, 1964.

Monat, A., and Lazarus, R. S. "The Key Cause—Type A Behavior Pattern," *Stress and Coping*, Columbia University Press, New York, 1977.

Monitz, A. P., and Zamcheck, S. "Sudden and Unexplained Deaths of Young Soldiers," *American Medical Association Archives of Pathology*, v. 42, 459-494, 1946.

Pervin, L. "The Need to Predict and Control Under Conditions of Threat," *Journal of Personality*, v. 31, 570-587, 1963.

Pines, M. "Psychological Hardiness," *Psychology Today*, 34-98, Dec. 1980.

Rahe, R. H., and Lind, E. "Psychosocial Factors and Sudden Cardiac Death: Pilot Study," *Journal of Psychosomatic Research*, v. 15, 19-24, 1971.

Richter, C. P. "On the Phenomenon of Sudden Death in Animals and Man," *Psychosomatic Medicine*, v. 19, 191-198, 1957.

Rosenman, R. H., and Friedman, M. "Association of Specific Behavior Pattern in Women with Blood and Cardiovascular Findings," *Circulation*, v. 24, 1173-1184, 1961.

Rosenman, R. H., et al. "Coronary Heart Disease in the Western Collaborative Group Study: A Follow-up Experience of 4.5 Years," *Journal of Chronic Disease*, v. 233, 872-877, 1975.

———. "Coronary Heart Disease in the Western Collaborative Group Study," *Journal of the American Medical Association*, v. 196, 130-136, 1966.

Rotter, J. B. "Generalized Expectancies for Internal vs. External Control of Reinforcements," *Psychological Monograms*, v. 80, 1966.

Seligman, M. E. P. *Helplessness: On Depression, Development and Death*, W. H. Freeman, San Francisco, 1975.

Seligman, M. E. P., and Maier, S. F. "Failure to Escape Traumatic Shock," *Journal of Experimental Psychology*, v. 74, 1-9, 1967.

Seligman, M. E. P., et al. "Learned Helplessness in the Rat," *Journal of Comparative and Physiological Psychology*, in press.

Staub, E., et al. "Self-Control and Predictability: Their Effects on Reactions to Aversive Stimulation," *Journal of Personality and Social Psychology*, v. 18, 157-162, 1971.

Stotland, E., and Blumenthal, A. L. "The Reduction of Anxiety as a Result of the Expectation of Making a Choice," *Canadian Journal of Psychology*, v. 18, 139-145, 1964.

Thornton, J. W., and Jacobs, P. D. "Learned Helplessness in Human Subjects," *Journal of Experimental Psychology*, v. 87, 369-372, 1971.

Voth, H. M. "Choice of Illness," *Archives of General Psychiatry*, v. 6, 151-157, 1962.

Watson, A. A. "Death by Cursing: A Problem for Forensic Psychiatry," *Medicine, Science and the Law*, v. 13(3), 192-194, 1973.

Watson, D. "Relationship Between Locus of Control and Anxiety," *Journal of Personality and Social Psychology*, v. 6, 91-92, 1967.

Wolf, S. "The End of the Rope: The Role of the Brain in Cardiac Death," *Canadian Medical Association*, v. 97, 1022-1025, 1967.

CHAPTER 5

Psychophysiology of the Stress Response

It is highly dishonorable for a reasonable soul to live in so divinely built a mansion as the body she resides in, altogether unacquainted with the exquisite structure of it.

Robert Boyle

Human stress is a physical phenomenon. We have thus far discussed it in theoretical terms and presented factors that elicit it. In this chapter, we will outline the psychophysiology of the stress response as it evolves from cerebral activity to somatic change. Specifically, we will discuss three linked facets of stress psychophysiology: the functional organization of the human brain, the physiological workings of the mind-body link and the physiological pathways and somatic effects of stress.

There are several important reasons for covering the psychophysiology of stress in such detail. First, the study of human stress management is a new field. It has yet to establish fully its credibility, so it is important to present the medical model of stress, thereby pointing out its basic relationship to established scientific disciplines in their own terms. Second, understanding the psychophysiology of stress will help you understand the first step in psychosomatic disease etiology. It will also bring the mind-body linkage out of the theoretical realm and into the concrete field of physiology. Your grasp of the following material will enhance your ability to manage stress effectively. The better you understand how your body operates, the greater will be your capacity to gain control over your own health.

As you study this chapter, strive for an *understanding* of how the body works in relation to stress. Do not simply memorize terminology. Being able to recall the labels that humans have attached to phenomena is unimportant compared to understanding the function, rationale, and significance of those events.

Our goal is not to confuse, impress, or snow you with physiological trivia; we want you to understand. We will start with the basics of physiology and move on to describing the complex details of some of the body's most intricate structures and outlining its most comprehensive physiological response pattern. Try to understand each step clearly before you move on to the next.

BASIC NATURE OF THE RESPONSE

Stress is a **neuroendocrine** physiological response; it operates through both the nervous and endocrine systems. It is often described as a **double-barreled** response. The nervous and endocrine systems are the two regulatory systems by which the body controls its internal activity. The reason that stress can be so globally damaging is that it does not focus on individual organ systems; it alters the activity at the centers of somatic control.

The nervous system is responsible for immediate, short-term adjustments in bodily activity such as pupillary dilation in response to changes in light intensity, or a quick increase in cardiac output when you go from a seated to a standing position. It can operate quickly because it is based on a type of electrochemical communication. Think of nervous innervation to the organs as telephone wires. When a message to adjust a function goes out to the body, delivery is almost immediate. It is almost as though a phone wire went from the brain to the organ. Anatomically, this is nearly the case. The functional unit of the nervous system is a cell called a neuron. The largest part of the neuron is a long fiber called the axon. The cell bodies of all neurons are located in the brain or spinal cord. The long axons then extend out to the various organs to form direct lines of electrical communication between the brain and the body. When a fast adjustment is needed, such as a change in finger position, the nervous message is instantly delivered. When the brain stops sending the message, somatic response ceases immediately.

Long-term regulation of somatic balance is controlled by the endocrine system. This system ensures the prolonged normality of internal activity. When your blood pressure quickly rises from sudden emotional arousal, the nervous system elicited the change; the fact that your average arterial blood pressure may hover around a value of 120/80 for years is due to endocrine regulation. Whereas nervous messages are delivered almost instantly, endocrine messages can take minutes, hours, or even days to produce a measurable change in the organs. Rather than sending messages from control centers to the organs via electrochemical wires, the endocrine system uses mechanical delivery of chemical messengers. Whereas nervous regulation is analogous to delivering instructions to someone over the phone, endocrine regulation is more like mailing someone a letter.

The endocrine system comprises four functional structures: glands, hormones, circulation, and the target organs. Glands manufacture and release hormones, which are chemicals capable of altering the activity of one or more end organs. They serve as chemical messengers that communicate necessary changes to internal organs. Blood flow, or circulation, is the medium of delivery for the hormonal message. Unlike electrochemical, immediate message delivery by axons of the nervous system, hormones must be carried mechanically to their target organs through the bloodstream. This will take a minimum of 20 to 30 seconds.

Sending out a regulatory message via the endocrine system is more like mailing a letter than making a phone call. The message must be carried mechanically to its destination. When you write and mail a letter, you are like a gland producing and releasing the message. The letter itself is like the hormone. Our reliable postal service is analogous to the body's circulation. It will physically carry the message to its destination. The recipient of your message is the target organ.

Because of their functional modes of operation and structure, the nervous and endocrine systems have several effective differences that allow them to meet different regulatory needs in the body. As mentioned, the nervous system acts immediately, whereas there is a mechanical delay built into the endocrine system. When the nervous message terminates in the brain, the organ quickly returns to its original state. When hormonal release ceases, it may be some time before the target organs return to normal activity because the hormones are still floating around in the circulatory system. In many cases, a hormonal effect will linger for hours and, in one pathway of the stress response, it can last for two months following original glandular release of the hormone. Finally, the nervous system regulates acute adjustments in somatic activity and the endocrine system takes care of long-term regulation.

The neuroendocrine stress response is one of the most comprehensive and globally damaging physiological response patterns because stress functions by altering the activity of the body's only two regulatory systems. No organ system can avoid being affected in some way by the experience of stress.

As we have discussed in earlier chapters, most of the stress we experience is psychogenic—it originates in the mind. Our first step in understanding the pathways of stress will be to analyze the functional structure of the brain, the primary control center.

CEREBRAL ORGANIZATION

We do not understand the function or organization of the brain very well. All we can provide are theories. We will discuss two dominant theories regarding cerebral function: the **reductionist model** and the **integral model**.

Reductionist Model of Organization

The reductionist interpretation began with a man named Franz Gall (1758-1828), who founded the pseudoscience of phrenology. Phrenology was based on the idea that the brain was functionally divided into regions (26 or 27), each of which was the domain of a separate human function or virtue. Gall divided up the brain like a butcher's chart and ascribed a different attribute to each region. He had areas for such attributes as hope, cautiousness, veneration, self-esteem, friendship, parental love, combativeness, mirthfulness, and order. He further postulated that the size of each area in an individual brain determined the degree of development of each trait. If the area for agreeableness was large, for example, the person would be easy to get along with. Phrenology soon led to the practice of reading the bumps on the head as a means of assessing character. If a person's skull bulged over the ears, for example, it meant the person was highly secretive, due to the underlying cerebral development of that region.

Another of Gall's postulates was that overall cerebral mass was a measure of intellect. For example, the weight of Byron's brain was 2,000 grams, significantly higher than normal. Alas, this notion was the end of phrenology. When Gall died, his students decided to dissect the master's skull. Among other observations, they found that Gall's brain weighed a mere 1,100 grams, a grossly subnormal mass. Apparently the man had no head for science.

Although Gall's theories had no basis in scientific observation, he originated the reductionist model for cerebral organization that many scientists feel is still valid. This model has two postulates: that the brain is functionally and anatomically divisible into discrete regions and that each region performs a distinct, definable function. In other words, the brain has many parts and each part has a separate purpose. Although this way of conceptualizing how the brain functions is not completely valid, it does give us an idea of what role each of the various parts of the brain performs. The description of the function of each cerebral structure is no more accurate than a reasonable guess. In reality, the holistic functioning of the overall organ makes many of the distinctions we draw invalid.

Several of the major structures of the brain and related structures are shown in Figure 5.1. Descriptions of each area follow.

Spinal Cord. The spinal cord is a comprehensive bundle of nerve fibers that connect the brain to the body. **Efferent** fiber tracts carry messages from the brain to the body and **afferent** tracts carry sensory information from the body to the brain. Do not confuse the spine with the vertebrae. The spinal cord is simply the nerve fibers; the vertebral column is the protective, bony sheath that encases the spine.

Medulla Oblongata, Mesencephalon, and Pons. No one understands the individual function of these three structures. Together they make up the **brainstem**. Besides physically connecting the brain and spinal cord, the brainstem initiates a number of basic, vital functions. Brainstem stimulation triggers respiratory, cardiac, and vasomotor activity. Note that the brainstem does not regulate these functions; it merely triggers their occurrence.

Cerebellum. The cerebellum receives constant kinesthetic information regarding the orientation of the body and the position of its various appendages. We think the cerebellum coordinates posture, balance, and movement without necessarily involving awareness. When you perform a well-learned activity such as walking, you do not have to think about it; the cerebellum takes care of movement integration for you. The cerebellum may also be the brain structure that allows you to reach out and pick up an object. It anticipates, integrates, and coordinates many muscles, allowing the smooth performance of highly complex motor tasks. The cerebellum does not initiate movement or muscular activity; it coordinates it and liberates awareness and thought. That is why most of us can walk and speak at the same time.

Pituitary Gland. Although it is not part of the brain, the pituitary gland is a closely related structure, both functionally and anatomically. It is often called the **master gland** because it regulates the activity of most other glands in the body. It is the center of endocrine regulation. Like other glands, the pituitary manufactures and releases hormones. Its hormones do not operate on the end organs, however; they operate on other glands. For this reason, the pituitary hormones are called **trophic** (regulatory) hormones. The anatomical and functional proximity of the pituitary to the hypothalamus allows this master gland to mediate long-term homeostasis.

Hypothalamus. The hypothalamus has no clear anatomical boundaries within the cerebral mass. It is a general region near the brainstem that is composed of several nuclei. These nuclei appear to be regulatory centers for vital functions. The hypothalamus is the brain center for overall homeostasis. It is thought to be responsible for regulating the **vegetative functions**—those activities necessary to keep the body alive. It regulates the basic life functions of the organism, including blood pressure, internal temperature, pupillary dilation, gastrointestinal movement and secretion, hunger, feeding behavior, satiety sensations, rage and fear responses, water balance, heart rate regulation, sex drive, and bladder contraction. Biological drives and pleasure and pain sensations all seem to originate from the hypothalamus. Later in this chapter, we will discuss the hypothalamus as the hub of the mind-body link.

Thalamus. This structure is often called the roundhouse or switchboard of the brain. It is believed to be the central unit that relays all cerebral intracommunication to the appropriate areas. It facilitates proper communication among the various areas of the

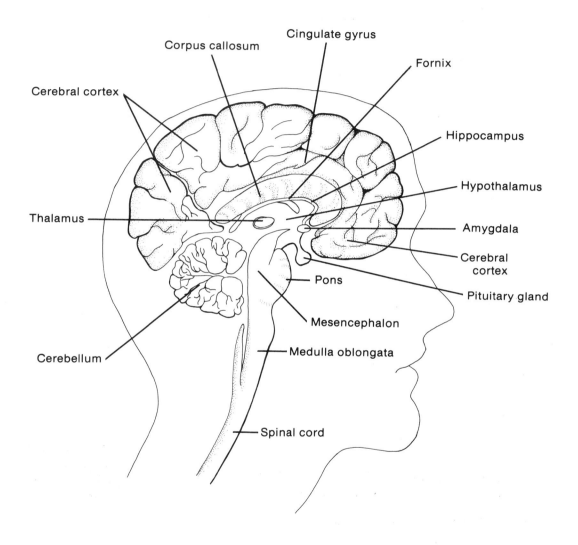

Figure 5.1. Major cerebral structures.

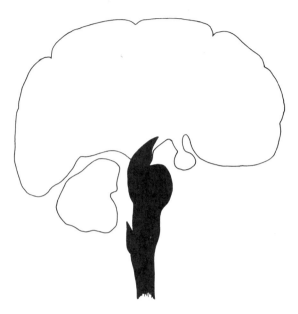

Figure 5.2. Level one: brainstem.

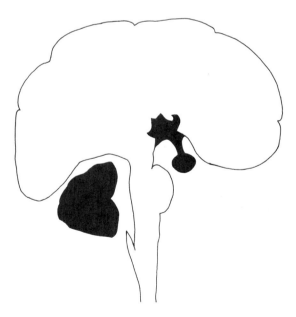

Figure 5.3. Level two: regulatory structures.

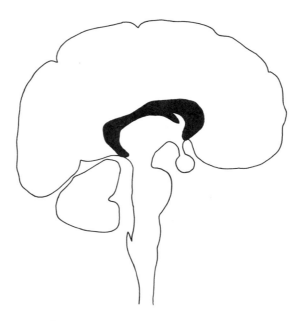

Figure 5.4. Level three: limbic system.

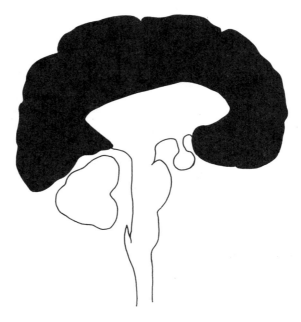

Figure 5.5. Level four: cerebral cortex.

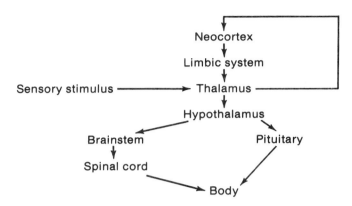

Figure 5.6. Cerebral stress response pathway.

brainstem and the pituitary? Second, what are the somatic pathways and effects of the physiological stress response itself?

THE MIND-BODY LINK

How can thought result in physical change? How can emotion result in visceral arousal? How are the psyche and soma connected? What are the tangible links between the brain and the body? Is this connection merely a nebulous theoretical construct, or can we outline the psychosomatic link physiologically?

The mind-body link is real. It is composed of several structures that are tangible and easily definable from both anatomical and physiological viewpoints. In this section we will outline several of the mind-body bridges that are involved in the psychogenic stress response.

In terms of stress reactivity, we will consider all psychosomatic connections to begin with the hypothalamus. The hypothalamus is the brain structure that facilitates somatic regulation and directly affects somatic processes. There are three basic pathways by which the hypothalamus can influence somatic activity. These include direct organ innervation via the brainstem, spinal column, and efferent peripheral nerves; communication with the anterior pituitary gland via the hypohypophyseal portal system (explained below); and additional stimulation of posterior pituitary secretion via direct innervation from neurosecretory cells. In short, the hypothalamus can innervate the visceral organs directly or through the pituitary. These two methods represent the nervous and endocrine halves of the stress response, respectively.

The most direct communication pathway between the hypothalamus and the internal organs is by way of **direct organ innervation**. In such an instance, the hypothalamic nuclei increase their activity and send a neural arousal message down the brainstem and into the spinal cord. The peripheral nerve tracts that branch out from the spine carry the message to the visceral organs.

The peripheral nervous system is divided into efferent and afferent nerve tracts. Efferent nerves carry effector messages from the brain out to the body; they represent the psychosomatic nerve tract. Afferent nerves carry sensory information from the body to the brain; they represent the somatopsychic nerve tract.

The efferent branch of the peripheral, autonomic nervous system is further divided into two parts: the **sympathetic nervous system** and the **parasympathetic nervous system**. Nearly every organ in the body is innervated by a sympathetic fiber and a parasympathetic fiber. These two nerve tracts have complementary effects on each organ. Generally, sympathetic activity increases the level of activity of the organ, whereas parasympathetic activity reduces or stabilizes organ activity. The sympathetics are mainly responsible for dynamic changes and adaptation; the parasympathetics are responsible for low arousal, stability, and restoration.

Think of these systems as akin to the accelerator and brake pedal in a car. In most instances, the sympathetics act like an accelerator and the parasympathetics are the brake. The activity of any organ is a function of the balance between sympathetic and parasympathetic stimulation. If there is relatively more sympathetic activity, the organ increases whatever it is doing. If there is relatively more parasympathetic activity, the organ generally slows down. The analogy holds: The speed of a car is related to the balance between the amount of pressure you apply to the accelerator and the brake pedal.

Sympathetic stimulation generally arouses the organ and parasympathetic stimulation generally calms it down, but there are some notable exceptions. The exceptions arise because overall sympathetic activity elicits the visceral changes of the fight or flight response. Organ systems not needed for muscular activity are suppressed by sympathetic stimulation and aroused by parasympathetic stimulation. This reaction primarily refers to regulation of gastrointestinal activity.

Table 5.1 lists the effects on various organs of sympathetic and parasympathetic stimulation. Note the direct relationship between the effects of sympathetic stimulation and the correlates of the fight or flight response listed in Chapter 1.

By skimming through this list, you can readily see that in most cases the sympathetics and parasympathetics are complementary systems. Although the list is long, it is easy to recall if you understand the concept. Sympathetic activity gets the body ready for muscular activity and parasympathetic activity produces the opposite effects, resulting in decreased arousal and facilitation of restoration processes (such as digestion).

This psychosomatic link is not theoretical. It exists from both functional and anatomical perspectives. To help establish this point, Figure 5.7 illustrates the major pathways of the sympathetic and parasympathetic nervous systems. This wiring diagram is biological reality. It shows how the brain connects to the various internal organs via the peripheral efferent nerve tracts.

The principal psychosomatic link in the endocrine system is the **hypohypophyseal portal system**. This is a tiny circulatory structure that connects the hypothalamus and the pituitary gland. It serves as the primary mind-body link in the endocrine system.

This structure is called a portal system because it is a tiny, almost independent circulatory system within the body. You have portal systems at several sites, notably in the kidneys. A portal system allows adjacent structures to communicate directly with each other via the blood. Direct circulatory communication between adjacent structures could not take place without some kind of special structure because all blood that leaves an organ, and any hormones or circulatory messages that it may be carrying, travels through the veins to the heart, then to the lungs (to pick up oxygen), then back to the heart, and finally out into the systemic arteries before it encounters another organ. Without a portal system, the hypothalamus would release chemical messages and then wait until they had traveled through the entire body before reaching the pituitary, even

Table 5.1. Sympathetic-parasympathetic effects

Organ	Sympathetic Effect	Parasympathetic Effect
Heart muscle	Increased rate	Decreased rate
	Increased contractile force	Decreased contractile force
Blood vessels		
Coronary	Vasodilation	Vasoconstriction
Skin surface	Vasoconstriction	Vasodilation
Deep muscle	Vasodilation	———*
Superficial muscle	Vasoconstriction	———
Abdomen	Vasoconstriction	———
Blood coagulation	Increased	———
Blood glucose	Increased	———
Arterial blood pressure	Increased	Decreased
Bronchioles (in lungs)	Dilated	Constricted
Skeletal muscles	Increased strength	———
Gut	Increased glycogenolysis	———
Lumen	Decreased motility	Increased motility
Sphincter	Contraction	Decreased tone
Gallbladder	Inhibited	Excited
Bile ducts	Inhibited	Excited
Pupil of eye	Dilated	Contracted
Piloerectors	Excited	———
Adrenal medulla secretion	Increased	———

*No effect.

though the pituitary gland is only about half an inch away. The term hypohypophyseal portal system simply refers to a functionally independent circulatory system connecting the hypothalamus (hypo) to the pituitary (hypophyseal, referring to an older name for the pituitary gland—hypophysis). The major components of this portal system are illustrated in Figure 5.8.

The functioning of the portal system is not difficult to understand. When the hypothalamus becomes aroused (as a result of higher limbic activity), several of its nuclei are activated and their nerve endings release chemicals called **releasing factors** into the top of the portal system. The portal system itself is the tiny pathway of blood flow going down from the hypothalamus to the pituitary inside a structural tube called the infundibulum. After the releasing factors enter the portal system, blood flow carries them down to the anterior pituitary. At this point, the blood from the portal system, which is carrying the releasing factors, bathes the cells of the anterior pituitary. These cells have been manufacturing and storing **trophic hormones**. The cells of the anterior pituitary are sensitive to the presence of the releasing factors. When the portal blood flow delivers releasing factors to the anterior pituitary, its cells release their trophic hormones into the systemic circulation of the body. Trophic hormones do not directly alter the end organs. They stimulate other glands in the body to release the hormones that will produce the measurable, long-term, physical effects of stress.

There are three hypothalamic nuclei that direct pituitary activity via the portal system. Each nucleus releases its own specific releasing factor. Also, the anterior pituitary contains three kinds of cells. Each kind of cell manufactures and stores a different trophic hormone and is sensitive to a different one of the three releasing factors. This gives the

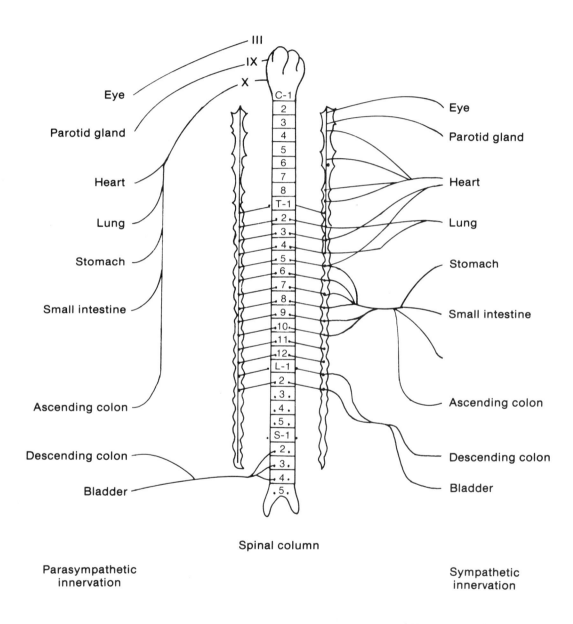

Figure 5.7. Anatomy of sympathetic-parasympathetic nerve tracts.

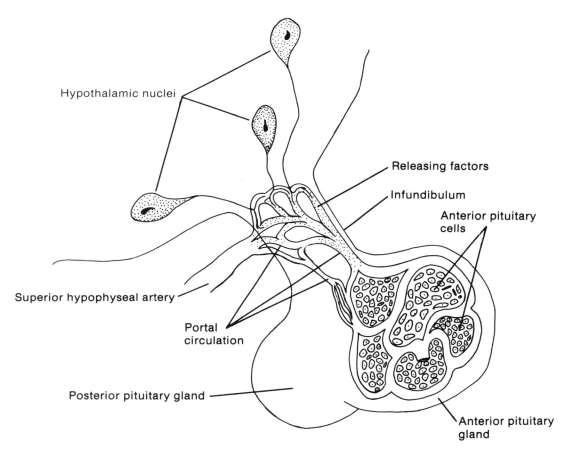

Figure 5.8. Hypohypophyseal portal system.

system a high degree of specificity, allowing a single nucleus of the hypothalamus to regulate the release of one specific trophic hormone from the pituitary.

Now that we have discussed the general operation of the nervous and endocrine bridges linking thought to somatic activity, we can present the details of the psychophysiological stress response pathways and their somatic effects.

THE NEUROENDOCRINE RESPONSE

There are basically three facets to the stress response. They are illustrated in Figure 5.9.

Immediate Effects

The sympathetic nervous system is the pathway for the immediate effects of stress. These effects, which are listed in Table 5.1, are triggered by **direct organ innervation**.

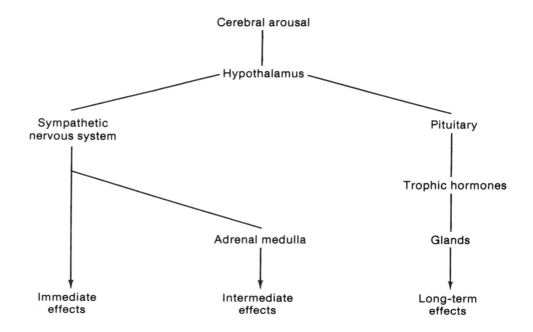

Figure 5.9. Basic neuroendocrine stress response.

The sympathetic nerve fibers plug directly into a sensitive site at each organ. When stimulated, these fibers release chemicals that alter the activity of the organ.

Most sympathetic nerve endings release **epinephrine** and **norepinephrine** to effect change at the end organs. These two chemicals, called **catecholamines**, are similar, and they elicit the same basic changes in each organ. The primary functional difference between them is the way they act on the cardiovascular system. Epinephrine exerts a greater influence on the myocardium (heart muscle) than norepinephrine does. When you feel your heart pounding during a stressful situation, epinephrine is mainly responsible. Norepinephrine elevates heart rate and stroke volume as well, but it is only about a fourth as effective as epinephrine. Norepinephrine affects cardiovascular functioning through vasoconstriction. It is the substance that makes your hands feel cold when you are nervous. It has about four times more vasoconstrictive power than epinephrine does. The two catecholamines produce a synergistic effect to raise blood pressure; epinephrine acts on the heart and norepinephrine on the vascular system. On most other visceral sites, the catecholamines both produce the same effects.

The immediate effects of stress are generally the result of catecholamine release by the sympathetic nerve endings at the end organs. These effects are qualitatively the same as those previously mentioned for both the fight or flight response and the sympathetic nervous system. They are:

1. Increased heart rate
2. Increased force of myocardial contraction
3. Increased cardiac stroke volume

 4. Increased cardiac output
 5. Vasodilation of deep muscle and coronary arteries
 6. Vasoconstriction of superficial and abdominal arteries
 7. Increased arterial blood pressure
 8. Increased blood coagulation and decreased clotting time
 9. Increased serum glucose
10. Increased respiration rate
11. Increased respiration depth
12. Increased oxygen consumption
13. Increased carbon dioxide production
14. Bronchodilation
15. Increased skeletal muscle strength
16. Pupillary dilation
17. Perspiration
18. Piloerection
19. Decreased gastric movement
20. Decreased intestinal peristalsis
21. Decreased abdominal blood flow
22. Sphincter contraction
23. Stimulation of adrenal medulla secretion

These effects are observable on the surface of the body within two to three seconds following perception of a stimulus. All but two are triggered by epinephrine and norepinephrine. The two exceptions are perspiration and secretion of the adrenal medulla, which are elicited by acetylcholine release from sympathetic nerve endings. You will understand the reason for these exceptions after reading about the intermediate effects of the stress response.

Remember, the catecholamines are released directly onto the organ site from the sympathetic nerve endings. These nerve endings are tiny and cannot store a large quantity of catecholamines. Further, after they have been released and have produced their effect, the catecholamines are immediately broken down by enzymes. Therefore, the effects of direct organ innervation cannot last very long. Under conditions of mass sympathetic discharge, you may be able to sustain autonomic arousal for 5 or 10 minutes. There are many instances in which animals, including humans, need to maintain a high level of arousal for much longer than this. If you are being chased at midnight by a nasty looking assailant, you may need to sustain a fight or flight response for a longer period of time than allowed by the small supply of catecholamines at your nerve endings. Luckily, the human body has neatly anticipated such situations. It has provided a beautifully orchestrated mechanism to perpetuate the fight or flight arousal response—the response of the adrenal medulla.

Intermediate Effects

In the list of the immediate effects of stress, note that the last one is stimulation of secretion from the **adrenal medulla**. The adrenal medulla is a gland whose hormonal secretions are triggered by acetylcholine release from sympathetic nerve fibers T5 through T10 (see Figure 5.7).

The adrenal medulla is the central portion of the adrenal gland. Humans have two adrenals. They are relatively small, triangular shaped structures located immediately on top of the kidneys. Each adrenal is composed of two parts, a cortex (or crust) and a medulla. Think of the adrenal as a slightly squashed peach. The exterior cortex of the adrenal is like the soft edible portion of the peach; the medulla is like the pit. Although they are fused, the adrenal cortex and medulla are functionally independent glands.

Figure 5.10 illustrates the location, relative size, and shape of the adrenals. Early anatomists labeled the adrenals the suprarenal capsules, meaning capsules above the kidneys. They labeled them capsules because they thought the adrenals merely took up space. We now know that each "capsule" is actually at least two glands wrapped in one, each with a separate physiological function.

The adrenal medulla is a gland, so it manufactures, stores, and releases hormones. It produces the catecholamines epinephrine and norepinephrine, the same hormones as those released from the sympathetic nerve endings. The sympathetics can store and release only minute quantities of catecholamines, so part of the nervous stress response triggers the release of additional catecholamines into the bloodstream from some more plentiful source, the adrenal medulla. The result? Sympathetic response—fight or flight arousal—is sustained. Isn't the body wonderful?

The intermediate effects of medullary release of catecholamines are qualitatively the same as the immediate effects. The catecholamines from the medulla simply perpetuate sympathetic arousal. There is, however, a quantitative difference. It takes about ten times as long for medullary effects to be observed at the end organs, and they last about ten times longer than the effects of direct innervation. Medullary catecholamine effects take 20 to 30 seconds to appear following perception of a stimulus because the catecholamines must be delivered through the blood. Their effects may last one to two hours because they are released in relatively large quantities and linger awhile in the blood instead of being broken down directly at the organ sites.

There are a few other points of interest regarding the adrenal medulla. First, remember that in two places the sympathetic nerve endings release acetylcholine instead of epinephrine and norepinephrine. One of these places is the sweat glands. This means that perspiration only lasts as long as direct sympathetic arousal. The sweat glands are not sensitive to catecholamines, so their activity is not perpetuated by medullary secretion. Response to medullary secretion explains why your muscles may tremble uncontrollably for half an hour after a near-miss car accident, yet perspiration only occurs while you are actually under nervous arousal. Sweating is the most transient of all organ effects during stress.

The second site of sympathetic acetylcholine release is in the adrenal medulla itself. Clearly, if catecholamines were used by the nerves to stimulate medullary secretion, catecholamines from the medulla could do this as well. To avoid maladaptive, perpetual self-stimulation, the medulla releases its hormones in response to the presence of acetylcholine.

You have no doubt heard of adrenaline. When we hear about people who perform miraculous feats of physical strength when they are frightened or enraged, we say that adrenaline did it. Adrenaline is a common name for epinephrine. Noradrenaline is another label for norepinephrine. Next time you see a toddler lift a refrigerator off of his dog's tail, you can astound everyone by saying that epinephrine did it.

Epinephrine (or adrenaline) and norepinephrine are not forms of energy for the body. The popular conception of adrenaline is that it gives us increased energy to perform miraculous physical feats during times of alarm and high emotion, but technically this is not quite the case. The catecholamines do stimulate gluconeogenesis, which will provide the body with extra fuel, but they themselves are not actually fuel sources. The catechol-

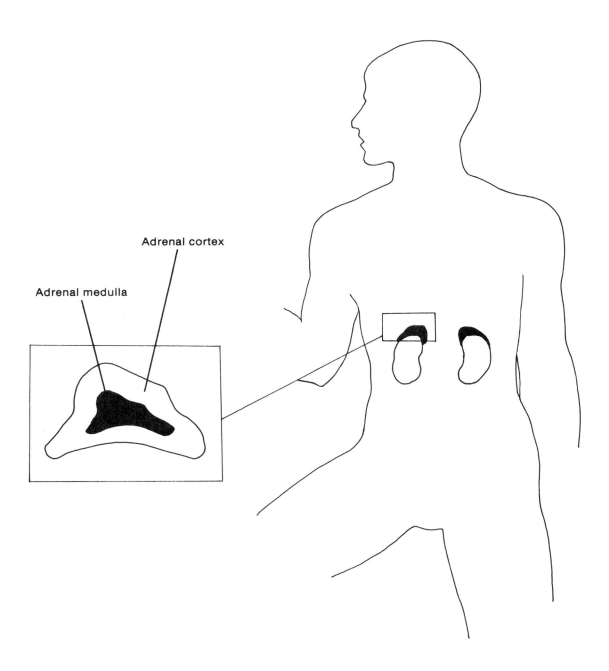

Figure 5.10. Location of adrenal glands.

amines merely orchestrate a change in internal physiology that gives the body a greater physical capacity to act. The feeling of increased energy is mainly due to an overall change in somatic functioning that is directed at facilitating muscular action, not simply to a fresh shot of fuel. The catecholamines are not a fuel source; they are psychosomatic messengers. Yet, for sustained fighting or fleeing, the body needed to develop some way of providing increased available energy. Biologically, that is where the long-term effects of stress take the stage.

The immediate and intermediate effects of stress represent Cannon's fight or flight response. The long-term effects represent the pathogenic response, the endocrine domain of the general adaptation syndrome.

Long-Term Effects

The immediate and intermediate effects of stress are not pathogenic in themselves. They do not last long enough to foster the long-term somatic imbalances that precipitate a physical disease. There are three principal axes, or pathways, to the long-term stress response: the ACTH axis, the thyroxine axis, and the vasopressin axis. The first two of these pathways follow the general scheme involving the hypohypophyseal portal system and trophic hormone release from the pituitary. The third, the vasopressin axis, is a simpler pathway.

The ACTH Axis

The **ACTH axis** was the focus of most of Selye's initial investigation into the physiology of the general adaptation syndrome. In fact, Selye considered ACTH, the central trophic hormone of the pathway, to be the most important hormone of the entire stress response.

The ACTH axis begins in the hypothalamus. Specifically, the neurosecretory cells of a hypothalamic region called the **median eminence** inject **corticotrophin releasing factor** (CRF) into the hypohypophyseal portal system. The CRF then floats down the infundibulum via the portal circulation to the **anterior pituitary**. Chemophobes, one type of cell in the anterior pituitary, are sensitive to CRF. When the CRF reaches the anterior pituitary, it stimulates the release of the trophic hormone that the chemophobes have been manufacturing and storing. This trophic hormone is ACTH. It is released from the pituitary into systemic circulation.

ACTH stands for **adrenocorticotrophic hormone**. The name is easy to remember because it tells you exactly what this chemical does. First, it is a trophic hormone, meaning that it will not directly affect end organs, but it will stimulate a gland. Which gland? The adrenal gland (adreno). Which part will ACTH operate on? Clearly, on the cortex (cortico). ACTH, then, is a trophic hormone that will stimulate the cortex of the adrenal glands.

When ACTH has floated through the body's circulatory system and found the adrenals, it will stimulate the **adrenal cortex** to release its hormones. These hormones are called **corticoids** (hormones from the cortex).

Figure 5.11 shows the sequence of steps and structures involved in the ACTH axis.

The five corticoids that are released fall into two categories: the mineralocorticoids and the glucocorticoids.

Release of Mineralocorticoids. The mineralocorticoids, as the name implies, are hormones from the cortex that have something to do with minerals. The mineralocorti-

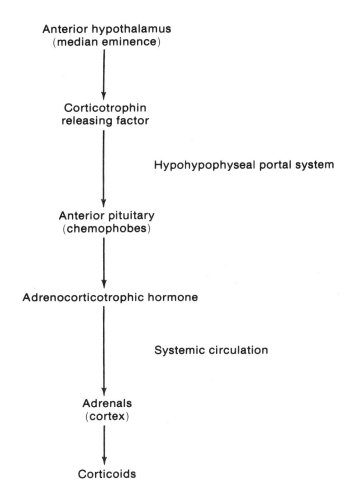

Figure 5.11. ACTH axis.

coids act on the kidneys to help regulate salt balance within the body. There are two mineralocorticoids, aldosterone and deoxycorticosterone. We will discuss the principal one, **aldosterone**, because both do basically the same thing and deoxycorticosterone is released only in minute quantities.

The mineralocorticoids, specifically aldosterone, operate on the salt absorption of the kidneys to raise blood pressure. The presence of aldosterone causes the kidneys to retain salt, principally sodium. The body must maintain the proper concentration of salt (balance between fluid and salts), so when the kidneys start retaining salt, aldosterone will increase water retention. Water retention is a passive process caused by the osmotic pressure gradient that is established as the body begins to get saltier. The water has to go somewhere, so it goes into the blood, resulting in increased blood volume. Increased blood volume means increased blood pressure, because there is now more fluid flowing through a container that has not increased in size. Aldosterone thus increases blood pressure in four easy steps:

1. Salt retention in the kidney
2. Resultant water retention
3. Resultant increase in blood volume
4. Resultant increase in blood pressure

The presence of ACTH is required for the release of the mineralocorticoids from the adrenal cortex, but increases in ACTH levels do not seem to increase mineralocorticoid secretion. ACTH is therefore said to have merely a permissive effect on mineralocorticoid release. It is like opening a gate. A minimum quantity of ACTH is required for release, but beyond that amount, nothing more happens because the gate is already unlatched. Other somatic and endocrine factors then actually regulate the rate of mineralocorticoid secretion. For this reason, the mineralocorticoids are not generally considered a central part of the stress response. Evidence so far has not indicated that stress is the central factor mediating mineralocorticoid release.

Release of Glucocorticoids. The presence of ACTH is the principal factor regulating the release of the glucocorticoids from the adrenal cortex. There are three: cortisol, corticosterone, and cortisone. The principal one (and the one we will discuss) is **cortisol**. The other two glucocorticoids are functionally the same as cortisol, but they are released in only small quantities. The effects of cortisol represent the glucocorticoids collectively.

The glucocorticoids are hormones from the cortex that have some relationship to the level of available glucose (fuel) in the body. When readily available fuel supplies are needed for prolonged fighting or fleeing, cortisol steps in to help meet the new energy demand. Cortisol itself is not a fuel source, but its actions provide the glucose (fuel for the nervous system) and glycogen (fuel for the muscles) that the body believes it now needs. The main effect of cortisol is called gluconeogenesis, or the creation (genesis) of new (neo) somatic fuel (gluco).

In the process of gluconeogenesis, cortisol mobilizes the energy reserves of the body. It makes this new fuel by breaking down fat and protein and converting them into immediately usable energy. Cortisol starts working on both fat and protein at the same time, but since protein mobilization is a more complex biochemical process, the fat begins disappearing from the body first. At first, this sounds okay; most of us would not mind losing a little fat. The mobilization of protein, however, is another matter. This effect alone may make cortisol the most dangerous hormone of the entire stress response.

The mobilization of protein by cortisol means that it is being broken down from its many forms in the body and converted to readily usable fuel. So what? The reason this is so damaging is that protein plays many vital roles in the raw material that makes up most of the body. Protein is to the body what lumber is to a house. The biological reasoning behind protein mobilization by cortisol is that right now you need energy or you will not survive. Cortisol will sacrifice, or burn up, some of the body's structure to help you live through the present situation. It assumes that this threat, even though it may be life-threatening, is only temporary. Part of the body will be burned up now, but you can rebuild later.

The logic of cortisol is something like being snowbound in a mountain cabin with little wood to keep a fire going. When you run out of fuel, the first stuff to go will be the "fat" in the house—old magazines, decorative fringe around the curtains, games you never play, and so on. You know that if you do not keep burning something you will die, so next you start chopping up the cabin itself. You burn up floorboards, closet doors, stair planks, and ceiling beams to stay alive. You assume that a spring thaw will come and you can rebuild, but you keep chopping and burning as long as the cold persists. Cortisol operates on the body in exactly this way. The body thinks you need energy to survive, so it will burn itself up and hope for spring.

Cortisol provides new somatic fuel by mobilizing fatty acids from adipose tissue (fat), increasing cellular oxidation of fatty acids, mobilizing amino acids (the basic building blocks of protein) from the tissues, increasing deaminization of amino acids by the liver, and elevating by six to ten times the normal rate of amino acid conversion to glucose in the liver. The immediate result of all this is a rise in serum glucose levels.

Protein plays diverse roles in the body, so protein-based gluconeogenesis can produce many negative effects. Muscle wasting occurs. Protein is not available for manufacturing new cells to replace those that die, so the body deteriorates faster and cellular immunity is significantly impaired. Particularly affected are the white blood cells, or lymphocytes, a human's principal line of defense against infection. Lymphocytes do not live long, so, to maintain immunity, new ones must be manufactured continuously. By mobilizing proteins, cortisol decreases production of lymphocytes, resulting in a condition called lymphocytopenia.

Vitamins and enzymes are made of protein. They are an easy target for cortisol, resulting in significant vitamin depletion due to stress. The B complex vitamins seem particularly susceptible to cortisol mobilization. Like vitamins and enzymes, antibodies are also victims of the cortisol ax. Antibodies are merely strands of protein that float throughout the circulatory system. Their specific shapes allow them to attach themselves to foreign toxins that have invaded the body and detoxify them. Antibodies play a significant role in the body's immune response. By converting the antibodies to fuel and mobilizing protein that was to be used to build new white blood cells, cortisol severely impairs immunity and provides easy access for infectious disease.

As a further immunosuppressive measure, cortisol release results in thymicolymphatic involution. This is an atrophy (shrinkage) of the thymus gland, lymph glands, and spleen. It is harmful to the immune system because the atrophied structures are some of the sites where the components of cellular immunity are formed and mature.

The overall aim and result of the increased presence of cortisol is elevation of blood glucose levels, which can create problems if it happens often. The elevation of serum glucose stimulates production of insulin by the beta cells, which are located in the islets of Langerhans. Under stress conditions, the beta cells are required to produce vastly greater quantities of insulin than normal. Unlike many tissue structures, beta cells burn out when they are overworked. This is called degranulation of islets of Langerhans cells, or simply beta cell depletion. When insulin-producing cells burn out, they are not replaced, and the body's insulin production capacity is impaired. As you have probably guessed, the ACTH axis is a significant factor in the exacerbation or precipitation of blood sugar disorders such as diabetes.

Cortisol has two effects that operate directly to increase blood pressure. The first is called stress polycythemia. Polycythemia is an increase in red blood cells. Remember that cortisol's job is to provide energy for prolonged physical demands. Providing fuel is only half the task. If fuel is to be burned, oxygen is essential. Oxygen is delivered from the lungs to the tissues, where it is consumed via the red blood cells. Red blood cells contain an iron-based chemical called hemoglobin, which attaches to oxygen in the lungs and delivers it to the cells of the body. If all the new fuel that cortisol has created is to be burned, oxygen delivery to the cells must be increased, so the density of red cells in the blood goes up. The indirect result of stress polycythemia is that a higher percentage of the blood will be formed cells as opposed to fluid, making the blood thicker, more viscous, and hence more resistant to flow. The result is an increase in arterial pressure. As a second mechanism of blood pressure elevation, the presence of cortisol perpetuates the vaso-constrictive effects of norepinephrine.

The following list summarizes the effects of the glucocorticoids:

1. Fat mobilization
2. Protein mobilization
3. Amino acid mobilization
4. Deaminization of amino acids
5. Gluconeogenesis
6. Increased serum glucose levels
7. Decreased body weight
8. Muscle wasting
9. Lymphocytopenia
10. Breakdown of antibodies
11. Thymicolymphatic involution
12. Impaired immunity
13. Vitamin depletion
14. Beta cell depletion
15. Decreased insulin production
16. Polycythemia
17. Perpetuation of catecholamine vasoconstriction
18. Increased arterial blood pressure

The real danger from cortisol is not related to its initial effects on the body. Problems arise when frequent and prolonged cortisol secretion occurs. Disease-free functioning of the organism requires that the protein mobilization of cortisol be temporary and that it be followed by a significant recovery period to restore the body. The problem is that most of us are inappropriately in a state of arousal so often that our bodies behave as though a constant, perpetual state of emergency existed. We rarely allow ourselves the necessary recovery periods, so our bodies are continually degraded. Cortisol may indeed be the most dangerous product of the entire stress reponse.

The Thyroxine Axis

The longest acting of all pathways in the human stress response is the **thyroxine axis**. One release of thyroxine, triggered by a single stimulus, requires two to three days to produce an observable effect, and its effects can linger in the body for six to eight weeks. The somatic effects of thyroxine are most noticeable when they peak, approximately ten days to two weeks following the original stimulus.

The thyroxine axis is a parallel physiological tract to the ACTH axis. The same steps are involved, but the structures and hormones are different.

This axis begins in the **paraventricular nucleus** of the anterior hypothalamus. The neurosecretory cells of this nucleus release **thyrotrophic hormone releasing factor** (TRF) into the hypohypophyseal portal system. The TRF floats down the portal system to the **anterior pituitary**, where it stimulates the basophils. Basophils manufacture and store **thyrotrophic hormone** (TTH). The presence of TRF stimulates the basophils to release TTH into the systemic circulation. The **thyroid gland**, of course, is their target.

TTH stimulates the thyroid to release two hormones, thyroxine and triiodothyronine. Triiodothyronine is released in tiny quantities and behaves just like thyroxine, so we will center our discussion around **thyroxine**. (The thyroid gland also manufactures and releases a hormone called calcitonin, but there is no current evidence to suggest that stress can trigger the release of calcitonin.)

Figure 5.12 illustrates the steps in the thyroxine axis.

The main effect of thyroxine is an increase in overall metabolic rate, the rate at which chemical processes take place and fuel is burned within the body. It can elevate metabolism as much as 60 to 100 percent. The results of elevated metabolic activity are increased

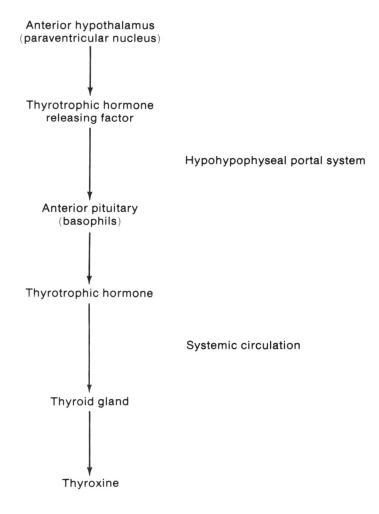

Figure 5.12. Thyroxine axis.

oxygen consumption, increased rate and depth of respiration (up to 50 to 60 breaths per minute), cardioacceleration, increased cardiac output (up to 50 percent), local vasodilation, and elevated core temperature.

The cardiac changes are of particular concern because previous protein mobilization has resulted in decreased myocardial strength. Thyroxine places increased output demands on a weakened muscle, inviting the possibility of cardiac failure. Cardiac failure is not a heart attack (although one may soon follow); it is a condition in which the heart's activity fails to meet the demands of the body for blood flow.

Thyroxine changes gastrointestinal activity in precisely the opposite fashion of the alterations produced by the catecholamines. Thyroxine stimulates digestive activity. It results in increased gastric and intestinal motility (diarrhea often results), increased rate of digestive juice secretion, and increased rate of absorption from the tract. This pattern of changes, along with the biological timing of their appearance, suggests that the thyroxine pathway may be designed to rebuild the body as a followup to the mobilizations of cortisol.

Thyroxine also acts on the nervous system by increasing the rate of cerebration. This is a difficult concept to explain, but basically it refers to the level of excitability or activity within the nervous system. Specific symptoms of increased cerebration rate include fine muscle tremors, worry, anxiety, paranoia, and insomnia. This condition is characterized by racing thoughts. Not being able to shut off your mind can lead to anxiety, worry, paranoia, or difficulty in falling asleep. Such difficulty may be caused by thyroxine release due to stress.

We can summarize the effects of the thyroxine axis as follows:

1. Increased metabolic rate (60-100 percent)
2. Increased oxygen consumption
3. Increased respiration rate (up to 50-60 breaths per minute)
4. Increased respiratory depth
5. Cardioacceleration
6. Increased cardiac output (up to 50 percent)
7. Decreased myocardial strength
8. Increased probability of cardiac failure
9. Increased internal body temperature
10. Increased gastrointestinal motility
11. Increased secretion of digestive juices
12. Increased intestinal absorption
13. Increased rate of cerebration
14. Fine muscle tremors
15. Anxiety, paranoia, insomnia

As we have mentioned, the noticeable symptoms of the thyroxine axis appear about ten days after the triggering event. Suppose some serious stressor, like the unexpected death of a close friend, hits you. In just under two weeks, you may get diarrhea or feel jittery and have trouble sleeping. Often we experience stomach problems or the manifestations of increased cerebration, or we have unexplainable anxious days and sleepless nights, but we do not associate these problems with stress because the stressor happened so long ago. When you experience such difficulties, look back about ten days and see if a major stressor might explain the problem. If so, realize that the noticeable effects will soon wane.

The Vasopressin Axis

This pathway begins as a hypothalamus-pituitary interaction, but it does not involve the hypohypophyseal portal system. It uses a direct neural connection between the hypothalamus and the pituitary, which allows its somatic influence to be manifested more quickly than is true for the portal system axes of ACTH and thyroxine. The effects of vasopressin can be observed following those of the medullary catecholamines and prior to the corticoids.

The **vasopressin axis** operates in the following manner. The neuronal axons of the **supraoptic nucleus**, in the anterior hypothalamus, extend all the way down the infundibulum to the cells of the **posterior pituitary gland**. This facilitates a more immediate link with the pituitary than that used by the two pathways we have discussed. Figure 5.13 illustrates this link.

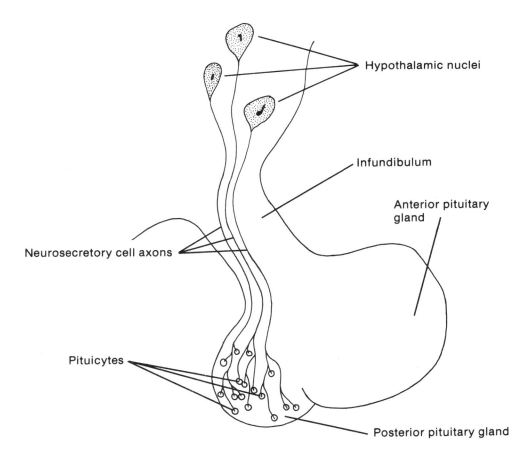

Figure 5.13. Hypothalamus-posterior pituitary connection.

The neurosecretory cells of the supraoptic nucleus secrete a hormone called **vaso-pressin** into the cells of the posterior pituitary. Vasopressin is manufactured at the nerve endings of the neurosecretory cells. It is released into the posterior pituitary cells, which are called **pituicytes**. A pituicyte is a cell of little maturity and simple function. Pituicytes do not have the capability to manufacture hormones; they merely serve as small storage vessels for the chemicals created and released by the neurosecretory cells. Vasopressin is stored until sudden discharges of supraoptic activity cause the pituicytes to release the vasopressin into systemic circulation.

Unlike the hormones of the anterior pituitary, vasopressin is not a trophic hormone. It operates directly on the organs, without the necessity of an intermediary gland, which is one reason why the effects of this pathway are manifested prior to those of cortisol or thyroxine.

The vasopressin axis is illustrated in Figure 5.14.

The role of vasopressin is to elevate blood pressure. Although this pathway is technically not part of Cannon's original description of the fight or flight response, it plays a role in the biological concept. In a physically dangerous situation, there is a good possibility of blood loss. If the body loses too much blood, pressure will fall and there may no longer be sufficient hydrostatic pressure to deliver oxygen from the blood into the tissues of the brain. This is called shock, an undesirable state to fall into while trying to survive a wild animal attack. Vasopressin enters to raise blood pressure and lower the probability that maladaptive shock will occur.

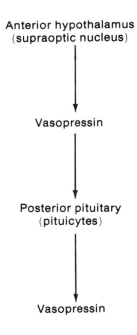

Anterior hypothalamus
(supraoptic nucleus)

Vasopressin

Posterior pituitary
(pituicytes)

Vasopressin

Figure 5.14. Vasopressin axis.

Vasopressin uses two independent mechanisms to elevate arterial blood pressure. The first is just what its name implies: vasoconstriction. Vasopressin is a powerful vaso-constrictor. The smooth muscle walls of most systemic arteries will constrict in the presence of this hormone. Vasopressin can significantly raise blood pressure through this mechanism alone.

Vasopressin is also called **antidiuretic hormone**, or ADH. Vasopressin and ADH are different names for the same thing. Antidiuretic hormone works against the process of diuresis, or the liberation of water from the body, principally through urination and perspiration. ADH works on the kidneys in a fashion similar to that of aldosterone. It first causes increased permeability of renal tubules to water; water reabsorption then follows, and blood volume subsequently rises, resulting in an increase in blood pressure. ADH also inhibits the excretion of fluid via the sweat glands. Vasoconstriction and water retention operate synergistically to effectively and quickly raise blood pressure.

The following list summarizes the effects of the vasopressin axis:

1. Increased smooth muscle contraction
2. Vasoconstriction
3. Increased renal permeability to water
4. Water reabsorption
5. Decreased perspiration
6. Increased blood volume
7. Increased arterial blood pressure

The anterior hypothalamus and the pituicytes also release oxytocin, a powerful smooth muscle contractor, but there is no current evidence to suggest that stress plays a direct role in the release of oxytocin.

Figure 5.15 illustrates the complete neuroendocrine stress response presented in this chapter.

SUMMARY

As a stimulus enters the brain via perception, it goes first to the thalamus to be directed to the appropriate cortical sensory area. The information is forwarded to the cortex for interpretation and appraisal. If it is appraised as a stressor or threat, a neural message travels down to the limbic system, an area associated with emotional arousal. The resultant emotional arousal stimulates the nuclei of the hypothalamus, which in turn alter somatic activity via direct innervation of the organs and through the endocrine system by way of the pituitary gland.

There are five principal pathways to the somatic neuroendocrine stress response. The first to manifest its effects is direct organ innervation from the sympathetic nervous system. Sympathetically innervated autonomic arousal prepares the body for physical action. The next pathway to manifest itself is the release of catecholamines from the adrenal medulla. Medullary release perpetuates the autonomic arousal originally triggered by the sympathetic nervous system. Next, vasopressin (or ADH) from the posterior pituitary operates on the kidneys and vascular system to elevate blood pressure in anticipation of a probable blood loss. The ACTH axis next shows itself, primarily through the effects of cortisol from the adrenal cortex. Cortisol provides the fuel for physical activity by breaking down the body's fat and protein. Finally, the thyroxine axis reveals

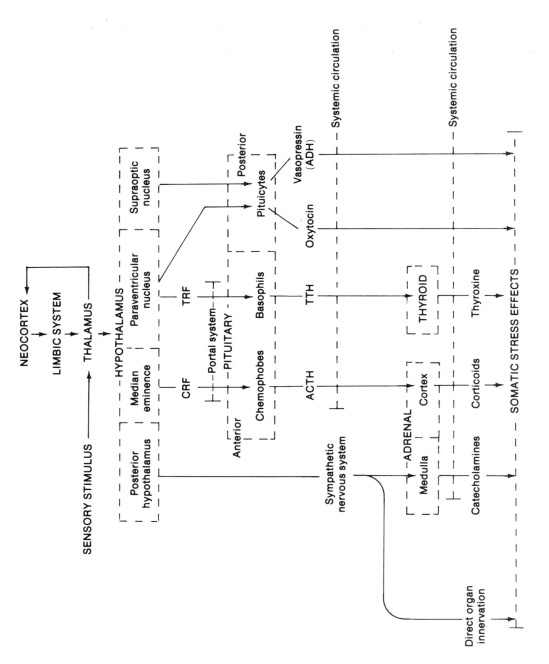

Figure 5.15. Comprehensive neuroendocrine stress response.

its effects. Thyroxine elevates metabolism, stimulates gastrointestinal activity, and increases rates of cerebration.

The effects of stress can be observed as quickly as 2.5 seconds and can persist for up to eight weeks following exposure to a single stressful event.

All of the stress pathways begin at the same moment (with hypothalamic arousal), yet they are timed to manifest themselves at different moments following perception of the stressor. This is accomplished through the varied communication mechanisms used in the different pathways.

REFERENCES

Allen R. J. "Development and Application of Psychophysiological Testing Protocol for Evaluating the Efficacy of Diverse Stress Control Strategies," University of Oregon Microforms, Eugene, 1980.

Bridges, P. K. "Recent Physiological Studies of Stress and Anxiety in Man," *Biological Psychiatry*, v. 8(1), 95-112, 1974.

Cannon, W. B. *Bodily Changes in Pain, Hunger, Fear, and Rage*, C. T. Branford, Boston, 1953.

———. "The James-Lange Theory of Emotions: A Critical Examination and an Alternative Theory," *American Journal of Psychology*, v. 39, 106-124, 1927.

Daniel, J., et al. "Mental and Endocrine Factors in Repeated Stress in Man," *Studia Psychologica*, v. 15(3), 273-281, 1973.

Engel, B. T. "Stimulus-Response and Individual-Response Specificity," *Archives of General Psychiatry*, v. 2, 305-313, 1960.

Everly, G. S., and Rosenfeld, R. *The Nature and Treatment of the Stress Response*, Plenum Press, New York, 1981.

Furst, C. *Origins of the Mind*, Prentice-Hall, Englewood Cliffs, N.J., 1979.

Greenfeld, N. S., and Sternback, R. A. *Handbook of Psychophysiology*, Holt, Rinehart and Winston, New York, 1972.

Guyton, A. C. *Textbook of Medical Physiology*, 5th ed., W. B. Saunders, Philadelphia, 1976.

Hafner, R. J. "Relationship Between Personality and Autonomic Nervous Reactions to Stress," *Journal of Psychosomatic Research*, v. 18(3), 181-185, 1974.

Hollinshead, W. H. *Textbook of Anatomy*, Harper and Row, Hagerstown, Md., 1974.

Junge, D. *Nerve and Muscle Excitation*, Sinaner, Sunderland, Mass., 1976.

Kurstin, I. T. *Theoretical Principles of Psychosomatic Medicine*, John Wiley and Sons, New York, 1976.

Lacey, J. I. "Somatic Response Patterning and Stress: Some Revisions of Activating Theory," reprinted in Appley, M. H., and Trumbell, R., *Psychological Stress: Issues in Research*, Appleton-Century-Crofts, East Norwalk, Conn., 1976.

Lacey, J. I., and Lehn, R. "Differential Emphasis in Somatic Response to Stress: An Experimental Study," *Psychosomatic Medicine*, v. 14, 71-81, 1952.

LeBlanc, J. "The Role of Catecholamines in Adaptation to Chronic and Acute Stress," *Proceedings of the International Symposium on Catecholamines and Stress*, Bratislava, Czechoslavakia, July 27-30, 1975.

Mason, J. W. "A Historical View of the Stress Field," *Journal of Human Stress*, v. 1(2), 22-36, 1975.

———. "Organization of Psychoendocrine Mechanisms: A Review and Reconsideration of Research," *Psychosomatic Medicine*, v. 30(5), 6-12, 1968.

Oatley, K. *Brain Mechanisms and Mind*, E. P. Dutton, New York, 1972.

Penfield, W. *The Mystery of the Mind*, Princeton University Press, Princeton, N.J., 1975.

Porges, S. W., and Coles, M. G. H. *Psychophysiology*, Benchmark Papers in Animal Behavior, v. 6, Dowden, Hutchinson, and Ross, Stroudsburg, Pa., 1976.

Sarason, I. G., and Spielberger, C. D. *Stress and Anxiety*, v. 3, John Wiley and Sons, New York, 1976.

Selye, H. "General Adaptation Syndrome and Disease of Adaptation," *Journal of Clinical Endocrinology*, v. 6, 117-230, 1946.

———. *Stress in Health and Disease*, Butterworth, Boston, 1976.

———. *The Stress of Life*, McGraw-Hill, New York, 1978.

Shepherd, G. M. *The Synaptic Organization of the Brain*, Oxford University Press, New York, 1975.

Usdin, E., et al. *Catecholamines and Stress*, Pergamon Press, Oxford, 1976.

Wenger, M. A. "The Measurement of Individual Differences in Autonomic Balance," *Psychosomatic Medicine*, v. 3(4), 427-434, 1941.

CHAPTER 6

The Role of Stress in Disease

There is a story of a yogi who met Cholera on the way to Calcutta. The yogi enquired where it was going. "To Calcutta," answered Cholera, "to slay ten-thousand" - and departed. The yogi, unafraid of the plague, continued and finally arrived at the city, where he heard that a hundred thousand had died. Later on, the two travelers met again, and the yogi asked Cholera why he had lied to him. "Oh no, I have not lied to you,' replied the Cholera, "I slew only ten-thousand, the rest died of fear!"

Wings of Power

Stress is the leading cause of death in this country. If you look at mortality statistics over the last several years, you will notice that cardiovascular disease kills between 52 and 54 percent of all people who die each year in the United States. Diseases of the heart or vascular system kill more people than all other causes of death combined in this country. More than half of the remainder die from some form of cancer. As we will see in this chapter, stress plays a major role in the development and progress of both cardiovascular disease and cancer. In fact, stress can be such an important precipitating factor in so many dangerous diseases that we can consider many physical disease states to be simply the long-term effects of stress.

PSYCHOSOMATIC DISEASE

Nearly all physical diseases that we experience are psychosomatic. As we discussed in Chapter 2, a psychosomatic illness is not an imaginary one; imaginary diseases are called hypochondria. A psychosomatic disease is one in which the mind influences the state of the body so that measurable, observable physical damage occurs.

Psychosomatic diseases can take on several characteristics. First, the mind may simply weaken the body so that it becomes easier for a pathogen to evade the body's defenses and precipitate disease conditions. Second, states of mind can further weaken the body's resistance to disease so that disease progress is accelerated. Third, in some instances, states of mind can actually cause a disease problem to begin. In the third instance, we say the disease is psychogenic. Some disease states are psychogenic, but nearly all physical disease problems are psychosomatic. In fact, it is difficult to conceive of any physical disease condition that could not in some way be influenced by states of mind.

In any physical disease condition there are many many causes and intervening factors. When we talk about psychosomatic or psychogenic disease conditions, we refer to the potential of stress or states of mind to cause or mediate the disease problem. In psychogenic disease states, it does not mean that stress was always the cause of the problem; it means that states of mind have the potential to initiate the problem. A psychosomatic disease is one in which a state of mind has the potential to exert influence on disease susceptibility or disease progress.

We will begin by exploring cancer and cardiovascular disease in detail. We will begin with these diseases because they represent the two leading killers in this country and because we tend to think they are purely physically based. We assume that only physical causes and environmental agents or nutritional factors can cause or mediate conditions like cancer or cardiovascular disorders. We will soon discover, however, that there is a huge stress component to both. In fact, it may be that stress is *the* most important factor in determining whether you are going to get cancer or encounter some kind of cardiovascular problem.

CANCER

Nearly one out of every four persons who will die in this country this year will die of some form of cancer. Everyone fears it, but the incidence of mortality from cancer is not necessarily what makes it the most frightening. We fear it because it is mysterious; it all seems to go on inside the body, with few outside signs. We associate cancer with long-term illness, severe chronic pain, and death. Most of us assume that if the physician tells us we have cancer, we are going to die. Much of the danger of cancer, then, may be due to the way we think about it. If we can understand cancer and cure our ignorance about it, we can temper its lethal nature by eliminating our own internal fears.

According to the American Cancer Society, cancer is "a large group of diseases all characterized by the uncontrolled growth and spread of abnormal cells." This is the most widely accepted definition we have. It has several important facets. First, cancer is not one disease, it is many. Cancer is a collective term. All the diseases that we collectively label cancer are characterized by an uncontrolled growth and spread of abnormal cells. These abnormal cells are from the victim's own body. Cancer is *not* an infectious disease; organisms do not come in and infect the system. Cancer is a disease in which the cells of the body turn against themselves. All cancers convert normal cells into what we call malignant cells, which are abnormal cells that grow, reproduce, and spread in an abnormal, unrestrained fashion. Malignant cells are derived from cells that used to be normal, healthy cells that performed vital functions in the body. Something changes the cells inside the body to produce a malignancy.

Characteristics of Cancer Cells

There are five ways in which malignant or cancerous cells differ from the normal cells of the body. These five characteristics are:

1. Relative inviability
2. High nutrient demands
3. Weak attachment to surrounding tissue
4. Abnormal growth and reproduction
5. Lack of contact inhibition

Relative Inviability

Viability refers to the ability of a cell or organism to live. When we say that cancer cells are relatively inviable, we mean that they have a high mortality rate. When a new cancer cell forms, its chances of surviving are much lower than those of a normal cell. In fact, most cancer cells die immediately following their formation; they lack the machinery necessary to sustain life. The reasons for this inviability will become clear as we explore the other characteristics of the malignant cell.

High Nutrient Demands

Cancer cells have higher nutrient demands than normal cells because they often lack the cellular machinery necessary to manufacture many of the enzymes, proteins, and other products that cells need for normal behavior and existence. They cannot make their own, so they rob the external environment and other adjacent cells of the nutrients and enzymes they need to survive. Cancer cells often deplete the surrounding area of vital nutrients. The reason for this efficiency on the part of cancer cells will be clearer when we explore how cancer cells form and reproduce.

Weak Attachment to Surrounding Tissue

Normal cells of the body cling to each other. Heart muscle cells, cells of the lung tissue, skin cells, bone marrow cells all stay together. Cancer cells, however, do not adhere to each other nor do they stick to tissues well. It is easy for a cancer cell to break off from the central colony and float around to some other area within the body. Cancer cells do adhere to each other in colonies to a certain extent, but it is easier for a cancer cell to break loose and go to some other spot in the system than it is for a normal cell. This characteristic will be important when we discuss the development and spread of cancer.

Abnormal Growth and Reproduction

Normal cells reproduce through a process called binary fission, which means that one cell divides into two pieces. Each of these two pieces is a complete cell capable of reproducing itself. You probably remember this process from high school biology. Several things happen during the process of normal cellular reproduction. Before cellular division takes place, the cell manufactures two of everything necessary for a cell to survive. Two sets of chromosomes are made, two sets of mitochondria, two sets of ribosomes, and so on. After replication is complete, the cell wall pinches off. Half of the contents of the cell go into one side and half go into the other. Two complete cells have been formed.

Cancer cells do not follow the normal rules for cellular growth and reproduction. They reproduce in a haphazard, almost random fashion. Two distinctions separate the reproductive habits of cancer cells from normal cells. The first is that cancer cells divide quickly, often while they are still immature. In fact, cancer cells sometimes are described as immature cells. The second distinction is that instead of dividing into two parts, they may divide into three or five or six in a totally unpredictable fashion. These two deviations from normal reproductive patterns create a lot of problems for the cancer cell. First, because they divide before complete replication of all cellular machinery and genetic information has been accomplished, there are not enough components to form two complete new cells. This is further complicated by the fact that cancer cells divide into many parts in a totally unpredictable manner. Think about the problems this is going to create. A cell divides before it has made enough parts to sustain life in even two cells, yet it divides into three or four or five. Clearly, most of the cells formed are going to have an incomplete complement of cellular machinery and incomplete genetic information. Many cells that form are simply empty cell walls; the cell wall closes off around nothing but fluid. This is the primary reason for the high inviability of cancer cells. Most cancer cells do not survive because they do not have enough material inside them to sustain life. Those cells that do survive often lack a lot of the cellular machinery necessary to make their own enzymes and essential proteins, which is why cancer cells have such high nutrient demands.

You may have the impression that cancer makes a systematic assault on the body because it seems to be such an effective killer. Cancer is not systematic; it is random. Cancer cells totally ignore the rules that govern a living system. That is why it is deadly. Cancer cells grow and reproduce without any concern for whether conditions for growth are right or whether the resulting cells are going to live. Although most cancer cells die, some develop and spread and create significant problems because division happens so quickly.

To envision the reproductive process in cancer cells, imagine that you are trying to make human beings. Normally you collect enough parts to make two people and then assemble them so you have two complete human beings. You make sure you have four arms, four legs, twenty fingers and twenty toes, two heads, two torsos, and so forth. In a malignant situation with cancer cells, however, the new organism does not wait until it has all the parts, and it tries to assemble more than just two from the parts it does have. Imagine the kind of people that turn out. A malignant craftsman may try to form four or five human beings from only three arms, one head, two torsos, and three feet. The organisms that result will have a low capacity for survival and, if they do survive, will be highly dependent on the resources of the surrounding area to sustain their survival. Cancer cells reproduce in just this fashion; they do it quickly and they do it in high numbers. The result is a lot of abnormal cells, a high mortality rate, and high nutrient demands from the surrounding environment.

Lack of Contact Inhibition

This may be the single most important characteristic distinguishing cancerous cells from the normal cells of the body. Contact inhibition is a type of cellular behavior that helps restrict the growth of cells. This phenomenon helps to maintain the normal size, structure, and function of healthy organisms. Imagine that you could watch normal cells growing in a jar. The cells have everything they need to survive: their only limitation is space. After the first day you would notice that the size of the population had grown a little. After the second it would have grown more. Growth would continue until it seemed rapid because of the sheer number of cells that would be dividing. When the cells reached the lid, however, you would notice that they had stopped growing. As soon as the space limitation for such a colony of cells had been reached, all reproductive effort would cease.

Further reproduction would occur only if a cell within the population died. The space left behind by that cell would be filled by the reproductive effort of another, but the population size and space would not increase. This phenomenon is called contact inhibition. Whenever cells reach their limit of growth as a group, they send out a message to each other saying that the population size is big enough, so growth can stop. The mechanisms of contact inhibition are not well understood, but it is clearly a facet of the behavior of normal cells.

For some reason, cancer cells do not inhibit their reproductive effort when they fill their alloted space. If you could watch cancer cells grow in a jar, they would grow through the cover, break the glass, and take over your house. The point is that as long as food is available, cancer cells will continue to grow, whether or not there is space for them. This is another instance in which malignant cells ignore the restrictions that living systems place upon themselves in order to thrive. The absence of contact inhibition is another reason why cancer can be so dangerous inside a healthy organism. Malignant cells have the potential to grow until they fill every space inside a healthy body, choking off normal cell growth completely.

How Cancer Develops and Spreads

We now have some understanding of the basic component of cancer—the malignant cell. The next phase is to look at how cancer develops and spreads within the body. Cancer has four stages:

1. Single cell initiation stage
2. Localized stage
3. Regional involvement stage
4. Advanced stage

Single Cell Initiation Stage

Cancer begins with just one cell. During single cell initiation, one normal, healthy, functioning cell inside the human body is altered so that it possesses those five characteristics of malignant cells. It takes just one cell to trigger an entire disease process.

Single cell initiation is accomplished through a process called mutation. A mutation is an alteration in the structure or sequence of cellular DNA. DNA is a chemical, a long chain of nucleic acid, that is made up of four nitrogenous bases. These four bases act as letters in an alphabet. The bases store the information on how a cell is to be structured and how it is to function. The DNA inside every cell is essentially the same. Each cell contains enough information, simply stored in this four-letter alphabet, to create an entire new functioning human. In fact, you have inside every cell in your body the complete complement of DNA necessary to make an entire human organism that will look like you and function exactly as you do.

A mutation occurs when this sequence of information is altered in some fashion. Mutations simply rearrange the letters or shift around the positions of some of the bases in DNA. Think of DNA as a series of written instructions on how to build a human being. A mutation is simply some kind of change in the instructions, as though pages have been rearranged or left out. The cell that is created after a mutation often dies. The change produced by altering the structure of DNA often will be lethal, leaving the cell with insufficient equipment to survive. Sometimes a mutation goes unnoticed and affects nothing. On rare occasions, a mutation is beneficial. About 1 out of every 1,000 times that human cells mutate, a cell is formed that possesses the five characteristics of malignancy.

Cancer is caused by a specific kind of alteration in the structure of cellular DNA. Agents that cause mutation are called mutagens. Mutagens that specifically result in malignant cells are called **carcinogens**. A carcinogen is any agent capable of causing cancer. General categories of carcinogens include chemicals, radiation, and chronic irritants. Chemical carcinogens include things like saccharin, red dye #2, and benzopyrene from cigarette smoke. Most forms of radiant energy—sunlight, X rays, and radiation from nuclear blasts, for example—can be carcinogenic. A prime example of a chronic irritant is asbestos fibers. Although malignancy is triggered by an external agent that causes a change in cellular DNA, remember that cancer cells are cells from within the body. Even though external agents trigger the process, cancer is not an infectious disease. Cancer starts when the structure of DNA within a single cell of the body is altered and produces a malignant cell.

Localized Stage

Imagine what that single cell is going to do. As quickly as possible, it is going to divide, not just into two parts, but into many. Most of those resulting cells will die, but one or two may survive. They, too, are going to divide as fast as they can, forming many new cells. Again, many of the new cells will die, but several may survive. That single cell triggers a frantic reproductive effort. Soon, rather than just one malignant cell, there will be an entire colony, a small mass of malignant cells continuing to grow and reproduce. When this mass of cells is detectable, either near the surface of the body or through equipment such as X rays, it is called a **tumor**. A tumor is simply an observable or detectable mass of abnormal cells. Not all tumors are malignant; many are benign. A benign tumor is a colony of cells that imposes restrictions on its own growth. Warts and moles are common examples. A malignant tumor possesses no growth restrictions at all.

The existence of a tumor within the body is the characteristic of the second stage of cancer. This localized stage is the phase of the disorder that defines the type of cancer a person has. Remember from our definition that cancer is a large group of diseases. Cancers are considered different diseases when they originate in different parts of the body. If cancer starts on the skin surface it is skin cancer, if it begins in the lung tissue it is lung cancer, and so on. There are two reasons why cancers that originate in different parts of the body are considered different diseases. First, because the cells of origin are different, their inherent reproductive capabilities and rates will be different. Cancer that begins on the skin grows and develops much faster than cancer that originates in bone tissue. Second, different kinds of cancer require different kinds of treatments. Cancer on the skin surface can be treated more simply than can cancer inside the delicate structures of internal organs.

Regional Involvement Stage

Remember the third characteristic of cancer cells: they form weak attachments to themselves and to surrounding tissues. This characteristic of malignant cells becomes important during the third stage of cancer. Imagine what is going to happen to the cells on the surface of a tumor. It is highly likely that a number of those cells are going to break loose from the central tumor mass and migrate to other areas of the body. The migration of cells from a central tumor to adjacent regions of the body is called **metastasis**. Metastasis is the characteristic of regional involvement, the third stage of the spread of cancer. During regional involvement, cells commonly migrate into the lymph glands, into nearby bone tissue, or into muscle masses. Now an entire region of the body is involved.

Advanced Stage

Each cell that has metastasized, or floated to another area of the body, is now capable of dividing. Each metastasized cell is going to start frantically reproducing just like the cell that started the original tumor. Instead of one tumor there will soon be many. This is the characteristic of the advanced stage of cancer. Each cell that is metastasized during the stage of regional involvement is capable of establishing a new tumor in another area of the body.

Generally, cancer is not difficult to treat in the early stages, such as the localized stage. By the time it reaches the advanced stage, however, cancer is extremely difficult and many times totally impossible to treat. In fact, treatment of cancer becomes more and more difficult the longer a person waits.

Why Is Cancer So Dangerous?

We now know that cancer is simply a condition characterized by the presence of abnormal cells. The more prolific the cells are, the more serious is the disease. That is all that cancer involves. There are no poisons and there are no invading organisms. Why then is cancer so dangerous? Why does it kill one in four?

There are two reasons why cancer is dangerous. The first reason is that cancer cells have high nutrient demands, as we have already mentioned. Cancer cells cannot manufacture many of the enzymes and essential nutrients they need to survive, so they rob surrounding healthy body tissues of essential proteins, enzymes, and vitamins. By taking away the resources that normal healthy tissues need, cancer impairs the functioning of vital organs of the body. The second reason is that the presence of masses of malignant cells can block off vital passageways. Cancer takes up space. If cancer is located in the lung tissue, or if tumor masses are wrapped around the trachea or vital vascular spaces, the flow of important products through the body can be restricted or blocked. Simply by taking up space, cancer restricts vital communication and flow of important elements throughout the body. The longer cancer is allowed to progress and spread, the more these two problems are amplified.

How Often Does Single Cell Initiation Occur?

An interesting question is how often during a human being's lifetime one cell changes in such a way as to become malignant and capable of starting the cancer process. Realizing that it takes only one cell to start this disease, we might assume that single cell initiation happens only a few times in a lifetime. In fact, we believe that in the average human, one cell becomes malignant every six to eight hours. In other words, three to four times every day, one of the cells in your body goes through a change that could potentially trigger the growth of cancer. How then does anyone live beyond the age of five? Why aren't we all doomed to die within the next five years? Five years is about as long as one can expect to live with cancer if something does not intervene. What prevents us from getting cancer?

The Role of White Blood Cells

Lymphocytes, or white blood cells, provide us with cellular immunity that fights off infectious disease and keeps malignancies in check. White blood cells check every cellular organism in the human body to make sure it belongs where it is, to make sure that every cell is normal, and to make sure there are no invading cells that might cause disease problems. The same mechanism that protects us from developing cancer protects us from infectious disease.

How white blood cells function is not well understood. We believe that they float through the circulatory system and enter the interstitial spaces, the fluid spaces between the cells, where they reach out with little arms called pseudopods. The pseudopods somehow scan each cell that they encounter. They either feel for certain trace chemicals on the membrane of the cell or they enter the cell and in some fashion read the sequence of DNA within it. Through some unknown process, the white blood cell determines whether the DNA contained within each cell matches its own. Remember that every cell in the body has the same DNA. If the cell is malignant, or if instead of a human cell it is invading bacteria or an invading organism of some other kind, the white blood cell will not recognize the DNA as similar to its own and will destroy the cell. The destruction of the cell is called lysis, which means to take apart or break down. The cell membrane is destroyed or degraded by chemicals released by the white blood cells and, because of the fluid pressure within the cell, an explosion results.

To prevent you from getting cancer, your lymphocytes have to check every cell in your body every six to eight hours, or three to four times a day. That is an awesome task, especially when you realize that you have more cells inside your body than there are stars in this galaxy. Each one has to be checked four times a day to make sure that its DNA is normal. There are enough biochemical letters and words contained in human DNA to direct the construction of another human being. If those instructions were printed in a book, surely it would be as thick as Webster's Unabridged. We could liken the task performed by white blood cells to checking thousands and thousands of unabridged dictionaries for a single typographical error. The magnitude of such a task is overwhelming, but this is exactly what the white blood cells have to do, and they have to do it constantly. A malignant cell forms every six or eight hours, and the white blood cells have to find it. If they miss it, it will start to reproduce and cancer will begin to develop rapidly.

What Determines Whether You Will Get Cancer?

Your chances of getting cancer depend on two factors. The first is how quickly malignancies occur in your body. The second is how well your body's immune system works, or, in other words, how your white blood cells are. Malignancy rate can be affected by many factors. We think that in the average human being in this country, a malignancy occurs every six to eight hours. If you frequently encounter a large number of carcinogens, however, your malignancy rate will increase. If you smoke cigarettes, if you get excessive amounts of sunlight and sunburns during the summer, or if you are exposed to asbestos fibers or to a lot of X rays, your malignancy rate will increase and so will your chances of developing cancer. Avoiding carcinogens is no guarantee that you will not get cancer however; it is only one factor.

Getting cancer is a matter of balance between your malignancy rate and your body's ability to keep those malignant cells in check. If your immune system is healthy and functioning well, you can tolerate a large degree of exposure to carcinogens. If, on the other hand, your immune system is weak, even the inherent malignancy rate (with no exposure to carcinogenic agents in the environment) might be enough to cause the disease. Cancer is not something that happens once or twice in a lifetime because you smoked too many cigarettes. Cancer is a chronic disease. All of us have it all the time because malignant cells are being produced in our bodies constantly. Your most important natural weapon against cancer is to make sure that your immune system is functioning well.

Some white blood cells live only long enough to destroy a given number of invading cells; others live for several weeks. To maintain a sufficient amount of white blood cells in your system, you need to manufacture new white blood cells all the time. If your body stopped producing white blood cells today, you would have none within two months.

The main ingredient in a white blood cell and in all cells is protein. If you are going to make white blood cells at a rate that will keep you safe from disease, you must have plenty of protein. This is the clue as to how stress can influence the development and spread of cancer.

The Link Between Stress and Cancer

As you may recall from Chapter 5, cortisol, one of the hormones released during the stress response, mobilizes protein in the body. Cortisol chews up fat and protein to make sure the body has plenty of energy to fight off physical threat situations. During chronic stress situations, or if the stress response is triggered on a daily basis throughout life, the presence of cortisol will ensure that protein availability is very low.

You may also recall that immunosuppression is another result of cortisol release. Immunosuppression means that because cortisol is converting the protein in the body into energy, there is no longer enough protein to manufacture new cells. During chronic stress, a person's white blood cell count drops significantly. The implication is clear: if cortisol burns up the protein that would have gone into making new white blood cells, the body is left with impaired cellular immunity. No longer will it have enough white blood cells to make sure the body is thoroughly checked for abnormalities every six or eight hours. The chances of a malignant cell getting through and establishing a tumor are greatly increased. Therefore, cortisol, released through the ACTH axis of the stress response, can mobilize protein, impair cellular immunity, and vastly increase the probability of getting cancer.

Stress does not cause cancer. The ACTH axis of the psychogenic stress response weakens the body's defense system so that cancer can develop more easily. We know of no mechanism by which the effects of stress can cause changes in the structure of cellular DNA. Therefore, cancer is not a psychogenic disease. Cancer is a psychosomatic disease, though, because changes in mental states can trigger a change in physiological conditions that can weaken the system, impair immunity, and allow cancer to develop. This means that the experience of stress increases our chances of getting cancer. It also means that if we can learn to control stress effectively, we can help prevent the development of the disease.

Take this one step further. Imagine that your physician has just told you you have cancer. That knowledge is going to be a profound stressor for you. When you hear your physician's words, your adrenal cortex is going to release a massive dose of cortisol. That cortisol is going to chew up protein and impair the effectiveness of your body's immunity.

Knowing that you have cancer—feeling the fears you may have about the disease—is going to weaken your body further and make it easier for cancer to develop. Several studies have shown that people who are not informed that they have cancer typically experience a slower malignancy growth rate than patients who are told immediately. We are not advocating that people be left ignorant. What people with cancer should realize is that their state of mind, their attitude about the disease, is an important factor in determining how quickly it develops. The same mechanisms that protect against cancer are involved in keeping it in check and slowing its development. Therefore, once a person gets cancer, it is essential that the person learn how to control stress, maintain a proper attitude, and use all the body's natural defense mechanisms to help fight the disease. The body can fight cancer, but excessive stress or excessive emotional and mental upset minimize its capability.

If we can learn to control stress, we can have some influence on the probability we have of getting cancer. We can also influence how quickly the disease develops should we encounter it. The danger of cancer is due in part to the disease itself, but it can be made infinitely more dangerous through our experience of stress. Understanding the nature of the disease and understanding how stress influences it can help us mentally fight off the disease process.

CARDIOVASCULAR DISEASE

As we have already noted, cardiovascular disease kills more Americans than all other causes of death combined. Stress produces profound changes in almost every aspect of cardiovascular functioning, so it is directly involved in the etiology of most cardiovascular disease states.

There are different forms of cardiovascular disease. The cardiovascular system is designed basically as a transportation system. It is a vehicle by which products that are needed by the cells and structures of the body can get from where they are ingested or formed to where they are going to be used. It also serves as a waste disposal system that helps carry waste products from where they are created by the cells to the systems and structures by which they leave the body. Because the cardiovascular system delivers so many immediately essential products to the cells of the body, it is essential that its activity never be interrupted. Cardiovascular diseases occur when part of the flow of blood within the system is interrupted through one mechanism or another. Cardiovascular diseases can be diseases of either the heart or the vascular system. Diseases of the heart stop or interrupt blood flow to the body by damaging the central pump. Vascular disorders involve some kind of localized interruption in blood flow through damage to or blocked tissue in the passageways that deliver blood to the tissues. Most cardiovascular diseases are vascular in origin; even most diseases of the heart originate as vascular problems. Most breakdowns of the heart muscles themselves are due to an interruption of the blood flow that feeds the myocardium. Occasionally there is a breakdown or a dysfunction of the electrical fibers that innervate the heart muscles (tell the heart when to beat and coordinate the pumping activity), but most of the time, cardiac and vascular disorders are breakdowns in the flow of blood through the passageways that carry blood throughout the body.

Blood flow can be interrupted through breakage or through occlusion. If an artery or a vein bursts, blood can no longer be delivered to tissue areas downstream. An occlusion, the most common kind of vascular disorder, is some kind of blockage of blood flow. It can be caused by external pressure on the vascular walls or by the buildup of material inside the vascular system that clogs the passageways (like lime inside the pipes of an old house). There are many different manifestations of cardiovascular diseases. We are going to discuss several different cardiovascular diseases, particularly those that are dangerous or extremely painful.

Hypertension

Hypertension, or chronically elevated blood pressure, may be the single most important factor in the etiology of most cardiovascular diseases. It is considered both a disease in itself and a significant risk factor for the development of other cardiovascular problems such as myocardial infarctions (heart attacks) and strokes. High pressure exerts tremendous mechanical stress on the vascular walls and can set up the body and the vascular system for serious problems. Sudden bursts of high blood pressure above an already elevated level can break delicate arteries and can cause significant instant cardiovascular problems and even death.

Hypertension is an important issue to discuss in a text on stress because the most profound and universal effect of the psychophysiological stress response is to raise arterial blood pressure. Just as high blood pressure seems to be the most important internal factor in the development of other cardiovascular disease states, stress seems to be one of the most important factors in the development of chronically high blood pressure. As we explore the relationship between blood pressure and stress, two facts will become clear: (1) every facet of blood pressure regulation accessible to the body is influenced during the stress response, and (2) every axis or pathway of the psychophysiological stress response operates to raise blood pressure. This means that during stress, every mechanism the body has for controlling arterial blood pressure is influenced, so no matter how individuals respond to stress physiologically, their blood pressure is going to rise. It is therefore not surprising that most Americans over the age of 35 have hypertension.

To understand the role that stress plays in hypertension, let us first look at the factors involved in normal blood pressure regulation. The human body regulates its internal arterial blood pressure through three basic mechanisms:

1. Cardiac output
2. Peripheral resistance
3. Blood volume

Cardiac output is the amount of blood pumped per unit of time by the heart. It is the result of two elements: heart rate and stroke volume. If heart rate or stroke volume or both increase, cardiac output goes up. Heart rate is simply the number of times the heart beats per minute. Stroke volume is the amount of blood pumped with each beat. If cardiac output is increased through an elevation in either one of these two factors, blood pressure can rise. If cardiac output decreases, blood pressure may go down.

Peripheral resistance refers to how much resistance there is to the flow of blood in the vascular system. Specifically, it refers to the cross-sectional area within the vascular system that the blood has to flow through. If anything decreases that amount of space, peripheral resistance increases and blood pressure rises. Peripheral resistance can result from vasoconstriction, internal occlusions, or mechanical obstruction. Imagine a balloon filled with air. If we could measure the pressure on its surface, we would soon see that all we have to do to increase the pressure is to squeeze the balloon. By squeezing we make the balloon smaller inside, allowing less space for the air. The same thing happens in the vascular system. As the vascular space gets smaller, through something like vasoconstriction or through obstructions inside the arteries, blood pressure rises. The circulatory system is basically a closed system. There is a certain amount of fluid flowing through a given amount of tubing. If the size of the tubing shrinks, blood pressure goes up; if the size of the tubing expands internally, blood pressure goes down.

The third mechanism in blood pressure regulation is **blood volume**. Several systems in the body regulate blood volume, principally through the activity of the kidneys. If blood volume rises, blood pressure goes up; if blood volume goes down, blood pressure goes down. Again, think of the balloon analogy. If you keep blowing air into a balloon, eventually it bursts. If you let air out, its probability of bursting decreases. The same thing happens in the circulatory system. If you increase the amount of blood inside the system through something like fluid retention in the kidneys, pressure goes up. If, however, you decrease the volume of blood inside the system, say through blood loss or hemorrhaging, blood pressure goes down.

The three mechanisms of blood pressure can all compensate for each other, allowing the body to maintain normal blood pressure even though one facet of the system may be changing. If your heart rate goes up, for example, your vascular resistance can go down, thereby ensuring that no changes in pressure occur. The body operates to maintain normal blood pressure most of the time. This is part of homeostasis, a concept we discussed back in Chapter 1. Again, under normal circumstances, if one of the factors of blood pressure regulation increases, at least one of the others will decrease, maintaining an overall healthy balance. Short-term regulation in blood pressure is accomplished through cardiac output and peripheral resistance. Long-term regulation is accomplished through peripheral resistance and blood volume changes.

Under normal conditions, then, blood pressure should stay constant throughout life. Stress, however, is a unique situation, because stress increases every facet of blood pressure control. Stress can increase cardiac output, peripheral resistance, and blood volume under both short- and long-term circumstances. When we experience stress, blood pressure always goes up; we have no choice in the matter. The counter regulatory mechanisms that the body normally would use to bring blood pressure down during stress cannot function because they are also influenced by stress.

Pathways Capable of Increasing Cardiac Output

Several physiological stress response pathways are capable of increasing cardiac output directly. The first of these is direct sympathetic innervation to the heart. The effects of the sympathetic nervous system can increase both heart rate and stroke volume, resulting in increased cardiac output. Remember that the effects of the adrenal medulla are characteristically the same as those of the sympathetic nervous system because both use the same chemicals to produce the response. The catecholamines of the sympathetic nervous system and the catecholamines of the adrenal medulla can both increase heart rate and stroke volume. Of the two catecholamines, epinephrine exerts the principal influence on cardiac activity. Medullary release of epinephrine increases heart rate and stroke volume in exactly the same manner as sympathetic stimulation does. The only difference is that the epinephrine released from the adrenal medulla lasts longer, sustaining cardiac changes for about half an hour to one hour following a stimulus. Another pathway that exerts direct influence on cardiac output is the thyroxine axis. Thyroxine increases cardiac output by as much as 50 percent, and it sustains this elevation for several weeks. The result is a chronic rise in blood pressure and sustained stress on the heart.

Two of the pathways in the stress response can indirectly increase cardiac output by operating on blood volume. Aldosterone and vasopressin both operate on the kidneys to increase blood volume. When there is more fluid in the circulatory system, the heart clearly has to work harder. There is a law called the *Frank Starling law of the heart* that states that whatever comes into the heart must go out. If any factor increases the volume of blood in the cardiovascular system, the heart picks up its pumping activity to ensure that all blood is moved through the system. Therefore, even though aldosterone and vasopressin do not operate directly on the heart, they can increase cardiac output by elevating blood volume.

In summary, all five axes of the stress response can increase cardiac output and hence play a role in increasing blood pressure. These five pathways are direct organ innervation, medullary release of catecholamines, the ACTH axis releasing aldosterone, the thyroxine axis releasing thyroxine, and the vasopressin axis releasing vasopressin. In terms of blood pressure regulation at the level of the heart, all the axes of the stress response increase blood pressure in both the short-term and long-term sense.

Pathways Capable of Increasing Peripheral Resistance

Four of the stress response pathways can increase peripheral resistance. Both direct sympathetic stimulation and release of norepinephrine from the adrenal medulla can cause vasoconstriction. Vasopressin released from the posterior pituitary acts as an intermediate and powerful vasoconstrictor. Finally, cortisol operates in two ways to increase resistance and blood flow through the arteries. The first mechanism, discussed in Chapter 5, is called stress polycythemia. As you will recall, cortisol provides energy for long-term physical adaptation by converting body parts into readily available fuel. To ensure that this fuel can be used by the cells, cortisol expands or increases the numbers of red blood cells that carry oxygen to the tissues. The blood becomes thicker and more resistant to flow as its cellular density increases. As blood attempts to flow through the tiny capillary spaces, cells begin to clog the flow of fluid. The result is a significant amount of back pressure, which increases peripheral resistance and hence increases blood pressure.

Cortisol also contributes to peripheral resistance by way of its unique contribution to atherosclerosis. Atherosclerosis is a chronic disease process through which material slowly builds up inside the arteries, eventually blocking off the flow of blood. Atherosclerosis is such a central process involved in the chronic elevation of blood pressure that we will discuss it in detail later in this chapter.

Pathways Capable of Increasing Blood Volume

Blood volume is a long-term mechanism for regulating blood pressure. Therefore, only the long-term pathways of the stress response are capable of changing arterial pressure by operating on blood volume. Two stress response pathways can elevate blood volume: the ACTH axis, through the release of aldosterone, and the vasopressin axis, through the release of the antidiuretic hormone (vasopressin). As discussed in Chapter 5, these two hormones both cause the kidneys to retain salt, resulting in an increase in water retention. This water enters the bloodstream and raises the volume of fluid in the blood. The circulatory system is a closed container, so elevating the amount of fluid within it increases pressure.

Normally, if a factor increases the activity of one facet of blood pressure in the regulatory system, at least one other facet decreases in order to maintain homeostasis and normal blood pressure. For example, if blood volume increases, peripheral resistance usually goes down to accommodate the increase in fluid volume. The net result will be no change in blood pressure. As we have noted, every component of the blood pressure regulatory system increases under stress. Further, in one way or another, each of the five axes of the stress response increases blood pressure, and several of the axes operate in several ways to increase pressure. Each individual reacts differently to stress. In some people the ACTH axis may be dominant; in others it may be the vasopressin axis. No matter how individuals respond to stress, however, their blood pressure is going to rise, because every pathway of the stress response increases it. Hypertension is almost a universal disease in this country. One reason may be that stress plays such a dominant role in overriding the body's ability to regulate blood pressure.

For the average American, blood pressure rises with each year of life. Increasing blood pressure is so common that physicians often assume it is a natural part of the aging process. Medical science even assigns different values for hypertension in the old and in the young; physicians assume that if you are over 40, your blood pressure is going to be higher. Consequently, it takes a much higher pressure reading to consider an individual over 40 hypertensive than it does for someone who is under 40. This distinction has little medical utility. The vascular system of an older adult is no stronger than that of a younger person. It makes no sense to assume that a higher level of blood pressure is required to produce damage in an older adult. It is normal for a person's blood pressure to rise with age. All this means, however, is that it happens to most people. It may well be that this "normal" rise in blood pressure throughout life is not a natural part of the aging process but is something induced by stress.

The Role of Baroreceptors

During chronic stress, blood pressure remains at a high level. The important question is whether blood pressure returns to normal after the stress experience. Bringing blood pressure down to normal is a function of structures called **baroreceptors**. Baroreceptors are pressure sensors located in many different parts of the body. The principal baroreceptors for regulating blood pressure are the carotid arteries, which are located in the neck. These arteries supply blood flow to the brain. Pressure is usually controlled at the carotids because the brain is a delicate organ that requires fine control of blood pressure. Baroreceptors sense the pressure within the system and feed that message to the hypothalamus, which sends out regulatory messages to the body. Chronic high blood pressure stretches the baroreceptors. If high pressure is sustained long enough, this stretching alters the sensory capabilities of the baroreceptors. They begin to think that this elevated pressure is normal. When the stress response is over and the body returns to a normal level of functioning, the baroreceptors return to an elevated level of functioning. This is called resetting the baroreceptors. We can liken the process to turning the thermostat in a house a little higher each day until the heat gets out of hand. Chronic elevated pressure damages the baroreceptors, causing them to set themselves at a higher and higher level. The body never gets an opportunity to come back down to what was once a normal level of functioning. Frequent stress-induced elevations in blood pressure contribute to the stretching and resetting of the baroreceptor mechanism. The end result is that chronic stress alters the body's pressure regulatory mechanism so that blood pressure slowly rises throughout life.

The Role of Atherosclerosis

The disease process called atherosclerosis is considered independent of hypertension, but it is an important factor in the development of chronic high blood pressure. Stress plays a major role in the progress of this disease.

As you read over the next few paragraphs, realize that the disease process being described is probably going on inside your body. Atherosclerosis is common to Americans. It is so common, in fact, that it probably will contribute to your premature death.

Atherosclerosis is a gradual process whereby fatty material slowly builds up within the walls of the arteries. This buildup of fatty deposits increases peripheral resistance to blood flow because it helps shrink the interior diameter of the arteries, allowing less space for the blood to flow. In the advanced stages of the disease, arteries can become completely occluded or blocked off, so that no blood flow is possible. The common result of complete occlusion is the death of all tissue that should receive the blood supply from those arteries that have been blocked off. The disease process has three stages:

1. Atherogenesis
2. Atherosclerosis
3. Arteriosclerosis

Atherogenesis. Two things occur during atherogenesis. The first is that the linings of the arterial walls become irritated. Sometimes mechanical irritation causes damage to the walls of the arteries; other times chemicals cause the irritation. A number of chemicals in the foods that we consume, such as the nitrites used to preserve meat, can irritate the delicate internal lining of the arterial walls. The second thing that happens is that the body tries to soothe the irritation. When you get a severe sunburn, you may soothe the irritation by smearing a thick layer of cream over it. The vascular system does this, too. Whenever the internal linings of the arteries get irritated, a creamy substance is deposited on top of the irritation. The deposit helps to smooth over the irritation so blood flow is not disrupted. The substance that is deposited on the irritation is called cholesterol. Cholesterol is a lipid—a fatlike substance. It has about the same consistency and appearance as Crisco. Atherogenesis, then, is characterized by the irritation of the arterial walls and the subsequent depositing of cholesterol on the walls to soothe the irritation.

Atherosclerosis. The second stage of the disease, atherosclerosis, is characterized by the existence of chronic deposits of cholesterol—called plaque—throughout the interior linings of the arteries. As Americans enter their twenties, it is a pretty good bet that they have a layer of cholesterol plaque in most of the arteries in their bodies. As life continues, further layers of cholesterol can be deposited. As the layers of plaque begin to thicken, the space available for blood to flow through the arteries gets smaller and smaller. This increases peripheral resistance to blood flow, thereby increasing blood pressure in a chronic sense. This is one of the most important basic mechanisms through which blood pressure gradually increases throughout life.

Arteriosclerosis. What happens in this stage is that, as life goes on, cholesterol plaque begins to harden. Think back to the analogy of putting cream on sunburn. Imagine that you smeared a nice thick layer of cream all over your sunburned skin and then fell asleep. Imagine what that cream is going to look like when you wake up. It will have lost its smooth appearance and texture. It may have dried out and begun to set up like plaster. It may be hard on the surface and may crack as you move. The soft substance that you used to soothe the irritation of your sunburn will have hardened. This is exactly what happens inside your vascular system. As life goes on, cholesterol deposits gradually begin to set up like concrete. When it is initially laid down (and for many years thereafter) cholesterol retains its soft, pliable consistency. It easily flexes and expands as pressure changes within the system. As time goes on and the plaque begins to harden, the arteries do not give as much anymore. They become brittle and cracks begin to appear. During this stage, a sudden shift in blood pressure can break a delicate, now brittle, arterial wall. By this time, the arteries have taken on the character of an old plastic garden hose. When it was new, it was flexible; you could tie it in a knot and water would still run through. But after 20 years of laying in the sun beside the garage, it has dried out and become brittle and cracked. If you tried to bend it even a little it might break into pieces. This is exactly what happens to the arteries. Arteriosclerosis, the third and final stage of this disease process, is often called **hardening of the arteries**. Not only has blood pressure been elevated because of peripheral resistance from this hard occlusion, but the arteries are brittle and susceptible to damage through breakage.

What About Cholesterol? Cholesterol is not simply an evil thing. It is an essential substance that makes our bodies watertight. It is cholesterol that keeps water from seeping out through your stomach when you take a drink. The surface of your body stays impermeable to water because of the presence of cholesterol. In fact, even the depositing of cholesterol within the linings of the arteries is a good idea. Without it, the irritation and mechanical damage done inside the artery walls would create a lot of turbulence and blood could not flow efficiently through the system. Cholesterol is important stuff. The problems from atherosclerosis do not arise because of the presence of cholesterol, or even from the initial plaquing. They arise when too much cholesterol is deposited. Only a thin layer is required to reduce the irritation inside the artery linings. When too much is deposited, occlusions begin to build up and blood pressure begins to rise.

The Importance of Lipolytic Enzymes. The body is equipped with a natural mechanism to keep the amount of cholesterol present in the artery linings at the right level. The mechanism operates through chemicals called lipolytic enzymes. The term lipolytic is derived from lipid, meaning fat (referring to cholesterol), and lysis, or the process of taking something apart. A lipolytic enzyme is a piece of protein that takes apart cholesterol. As a lipolytic enzyme encounters cholesterol in the walls of the artery, it simply chews it up, making that wall of cholesterol thin. A person's risk of developing a problematic level of atherosclerosis depends on two factors: (1) the amount of cholesterol present in the bloodstream and (2) the efficiency of lipolytic enzymes in keeping cholesterol plaque in check.

Now think back to the physiological stress response. Remember that the cortisol released during this response converts proteins into fuel that the body can burn. Cortisol chews up antibodies and burns up the protein needed for new white blood cells. Cortisol also takes apart lipolytic enzymes. When cortisol is released during stress, it converts lipolytic enzymes into fuel. The number of lipolytic enzymes drops, and the mechanism that keeps plaque in check is gone. Without the lipolytic enzymes, the layer of plaque gets thicker and thicker, rapidly occluding the arteries and raising blood pressure.

The American diet does contribute to the problem of atherosclerosis, hypertension, and premature death, but the experience of stress helps to accelerate that entire process. There is an interesting empirical observation that lends some support to this contention. During the war in Vietnam, a lot of young men died—men who were 18, 19, and 20 years old. Autopsies showed that many of these young men had advanced arteriosclerosis. Not atherosclerosis, but arteriosclerosis. Arteriosclerosis, or hardening of the arteries, usually occurs in people who are 70, 80, or 90 years old. After the stress of this wartime situation, it was observed in men who had not yet reached 20. At first dietary factors were blamed, but it turned out that the diet of Americans in Vietnam was not that different from the normal domestic diet and that any differences probably could not account for the rapid development of this disease. It is now thought that the atherosclerotic process was tremendously accelerated due to the high levels of stress these men experienced.

Atherosclerosis may be the most common disease state affecting people in this culture. It is influenced to a high degree by the experience of stress.

Is hypertension a *normal* result of the aging process in Americans? Yes, it is. A more important question, however, is whether hypertension is a *natural* part of the aging process in human beings. The answer is no. The chronic, life-threatening elevation of blood pressure as we go through life is not a natural phenomenon inherent to the process of aging. It is something that is induced through our diet and through our experience of stress. It is an unnecessary, ubiquitous, and severe threat to human life. Hypertension can be thought of as a psychogenic disease because five of the pathways of the stress response cause increases in blood pressure. The noted exception is atherosclerosis. Atherosclerosis is not psychogenic. Stress does not initiate the problem, but stress definitely mediates its progress and determines whether it becomes life threatening. Most elevations in blood pressure are caused by a change in state of mind and the experience of psychogenic stress. High blood pressure is one of the most significant factors contributing to cardiovascular disease. It is certainly not stretching the argument to conclude that the experience of stress is one of the most important factors in the premature (and often unnecessary) death of Americans.

Heart Attacks and Strokes

Besides playing a role in the development of hypertension, stress also is important in triggering sudden cardiovascular accidents. By chronically elevating blood pressure through life, stress sets up conditions in the body that can lead to heart attacks or strokes. Stress also can be the trigger for the event itself.

A heart attack occurs when the blood supply to part of the heart muscle is interrupted. The muscle fibers of the heart have to work all the time, so uninterrupted blood flow is essential. If blood flow is interrupted, either through arterial occlusion or breakage, the muscle fibers fed by that damaged artery die. This death, or necrosis, of heart muscle fibers is called a **myocardial infarction**. When heart muscle cells die, the pumping capacity of the heart is severely impaired. If enough of the cells die, cardiac failure results. **Cardiac failure** is a condition in which the heart fails to meet the body's demands for blood flow. If a great deal of heart muscle tissue is damaged, the heart can no longer pump, and the person dies. Hypertension and atherosclerosis can set up conditions whereby blood flow to the heart muscle cells can easily be interrupted.

Any sudden surge of blood pressure occurring in a weakened artery can cause an artery to break. We call this breakage a **stroke**. When arteries break, all tissues downstream suddenly lose their blood supply and hence receive no oxygen and nutrients. Tissues that are not nourished can die within several minutes. Strokes can occur anywhere within the body. They are particularly common in vascular areas where an aneurysm is present. An **aneurysm** is a thin spot in the wall of an artery that easily balloons out and can burst when pressure is high. Our most common reference to strokes is when arterial breakage occurs in the brain. When part of the blood supply to the brain is lost, brain cells die immediately. People frequently die from cerebral strokes. If an individual survives a cerebral stroke, recovery is often difficult and lengthy. The damage that results from a cerebral stroke depends on the area of the brain affected by the loss of blood supply. Stroke victims commonly lose capabilities such as memory, language, motor coordination, and a host of other basic cognitive and motor functions.

Stress can be the trigger in vascular accidents. If the vascular system is weakened through the presence of either aneurysms, arteriosclerosis, or occluded arteries, a sudden elevation in blood pressure can quickly terminate blood flow to a given area. The effects of epinephrine and norepinephrine, which you recall are the products of the immediate response to stress, can easily trigger an accident. Epinephrine acts on the heart to increase cardiac output quickly. Norepinephrine acts on the vascular system to increase vasoconstrictive activity suddenly. These two effects together can raise blood pressure quickly. Sudden surges of catecholamine activity, triggered by the experiences of psychogenic stress, are capable of raising blood pressure so sharply that a vascular accident can occur. In such a case, a person becomes so excited or so frightened that a heart attack or a stroke occurs. While visiting Las Vegas as a child, I heard the story of a patron who had won an instant $25,000 purse playing Keno. He got so excited that he had to run into the men's room to relieve himself. While he was telling another patron about his sudden good fortune, part of his vascular system ruptured. He suffered a myocardial infarction and died on the floor of the restroom.

Stress can play a role in potentially fatal cardiovascular disease states, either by contributing to the development of chronic diseases and problems within the cardiovascular system or by suddenly raising blood pressure and cardiac activity, thereby triggering a vascular accident. Cardiovascular diseases are therefore psychosomatic diseases. In some instances, cardiovascular problems can be considered psychogenic, because in many cases the experience of sudden psychogenic stress can be the principal agent that triggers the final breakdown of the system.

Peripheral Vascular Diseases

Stress contributes to other cardiovascular diseases that are not necessarily life threatening but that can be unpleasant, painful, and sometimes disabling. These diseases fall into the general category of peripheral vascular disease.

Raynaud's Disease. This peripheral vascular disease is characterized by a hypersensitivity of the peripheral blood vessels to norepinephrine. During times of sympathetic discharge, vasoconstrictive activity is sometimes so pronounced that peripheral body tissues do not get an adequate oxygen supply because they have been deprived of blood flow. Death of peripheral tissues is common. This process begins in the fingertips and sometimes in the toes. When the body tissue dies, the only medical treatment available is progressive amputation of the dead material. People who suffer from Raynaud's disease often do not experience the extreme tissue death that necessitates amputation of body parts, but they do suffer severe problems. One of the most notable is hypersensitivity to cold. Because of the intense vasoconstriction, exposure to even moderately cold temperatures produces severe pain in the hands and feet.

Buerger's Disease. A similar condition, called Buerger's disease (thromboangitis obliterans), is common in cigarette smokers. Buerger's disease is characterized by a hypersensitivity to nicotine. Nicotine artificially stimulates the sympathetic nervous system, and intense vasoconstriction of the peripheral blood vessels results. There are numerous cases in which Buerger's disease, exacerbated by excessive cigarette smoking, has resulted in the amputation of an individual's arms and legs. (I met a man who had lost both legs, one arm, and half of the other arm who requested that a clip arrangement be fastened to the stub of his remaining arm so he could continue smoking!) Vascular disease problems like Raynaud's disease and Buerger's disease are severely exacerbated and sometimes principally caused by the excessive presence of norepinephrine, so it is easy to understand how stress plays a role in their development.

Currently, medical treatments for these peripheral vascular disorders are limited to amputation and sympathectomy or removal of the sympathetic nerves. A sympathectomy leaves the individual with no vasomotor control, a highly unsatisfactory treatment. Recently, the greatest success in treating problems of this nature has come through thermal biofeedback training, which we will discuss in Chapter 17.

Migraine Headaches. A migraine headache is not a muscle tension phenomenon, although muscle tension headaches can be caused by excessive stress. The most common form of migraine is experienced as an intense throbbing pain. Often dizziness, disorientation, and nausea accompany the headache. The throbbing is simply from the beating of the heart, indicating that this is a vascular problem. Most migraines begin with vasoconstriction in the peripheral blood vessels. A frequent sign of a migraine coming on is sudden coldness of the hands and feet. Often the result of peripheral vasoconstriction, or restricted blood flow to the arms and legs, is an increase in blood flow to the cranium or head. This increase in cranial blood flow often causes intense fluid pressure within the skull, which results in the sensation of pain. Each time the heart beats the pressure rises and falls, accounting for the throbbing pain of a migraine headache. The release of norepinephrine from the sympathetic nerve endings and from the adrenal medulla, which causes intense vasoconstriction at the periphery, is often the cause of a migraine. In many cases, migraine headaches are clearly related to stress. Current medical treatments for migraine are limited and largely unsatisfactory. Here again, biofeedback training (discussed in Chapter 17) has contributed to the effective treatment of the problem.

RESPIRATORY DISEASE

Besides affecting the body's immune mechanisms and the cardiovascular system, stress has been found to play a role in respiratory diseases.

Asthma

One disease that has long been thought to be psychosomatic is asthma. Remember that psychosomatic does not mean imaginary. A psychosomatic disease is one in which state of mind plays a role in physical change. An asthma attack is characterized by bronchiole constriction; the air passageways in the lungs constrict, inhibiting an adequate flow of air into the lungs. An asthma attack is characterized by shortness of breath, sometimes a panicky gasping effort to try to get air into the body, and occasionally coughing or sneezing. It is not uncommon for sudden emotional stress to trigger an attack.

The mechanism by which stress can play a role in asthma is somewhat of a paradox. You may recall that one of the immediate effects of stress is bronchodilation. This makes sense as part of the fight or flight response because it allows more air to get into the air sacs, or alveoli, which facilitate the transfer of oxygen into the bloodstream. In some people, however, the experience of sudden emotional stress triggers the opposite reaction, or bronchoconstriction. The reason is that about 1 person in 25 responds to stress in the parasympathetic rather than in the sympathetic system. A **parasympathetic respond-er** has an immediate reaction to stress that is exactly opposite to what we would expect. The overall physical effects of this kind of activation include decreases in blood pressure, constriction of the bronchioles, and increases in gastrointestinal activity. During normal fight or flight reactions the sphincters in the body constrict. In some parasympathetic responders, the sphincters relax during stress. We think this helps explain the unusual phenomenon of people soiling themselves when they are frightened suddenly. Parasympathetic stress responders are susceptible to bronchoconstriction and increased gastrointestinal activity during times of stress. Some of them have difficulty breathing when they are emotionally aroused and others experience serious gastrointestinal problems. Although it is not as common a psychosomatic disorder as hypertension, in many individuals asthma is most certainly a psychosomatic disease.

There are two kinds of asthma: extrinsic and intrinsic. Extrinsic asthma, which we have just discussed, is caused by external agents like chemicals or stress. Intrinsic asthma is induced by a biological agent like bee stings or microorganisms. This intrinsic category introduces another issue relating stress to respiratory disease. Stress seems to play a role in hyperimmune responses. Hyperimmune responses are things like allergies, which are characterized by an overactive response on the part of the body's immune system. The overt reactions include such things as constriction, swelling, and itching. Hay fever is an example of a hyperimmune response in which the immune system overreacts in the presence of antigens like pollen. Hyperimmune reactions seem to increase in frequency and intensity during times when a person feels helpless and overwhelmed by events in life. Psychogenic stress seems to set the stage within the body for allergies to manifest themselves. In many instances, allergies appear only when a person is experiencing stress. You may be allergic to bee stings, for example, but if life is going smoothly for you, you can be stung by a bee with no severe reaction. During times of stress, the same bee sting could cause a severe hyperimmune response. A lot of evidence suggests that stress makes one more susceptible to allergic reactions, but no one knows what mechanism is involved. In fact, the hyperimmune response is exactly opposite to what stress normally produces in the body. Stress usually impairs the functioning of the immune system, but in many individuals stress makes the immune system hypersensitive and can help precipitate severe allergic reactions. It is a mysterious case.

Tuberculosis

Tuberculosis is another respiratory disease that seems to be related to stress, yet no one understands why. Evidence suggests that patients who become chronically ill from tuberculosis have high life change scores and seem to score low on measures of coping ability. In other words, they are people who experience a lot of stress in life and lack the skill to cope with it. Possible mechanisms have not been suggested.

Emphysema

Emphysema is a serious disorder in which airflow within the lung tissue is drastically impaired. Emphysema is most commonly characterized by the destruction of tissue within the lungs and sometimes the filling of lung tissue with fluids. Basically, the lungs lose the surface area necessary to facilitate proper gas exchange and oxygenation of the blood. This disease is common in cigarette smokers. During emphysema, a person experiences a chronic shortness of breath; physical activity must be severely restricted. People who have severe emphysema must stop and rest often, even when just walking down the street. To develop an appreciation for what emphysema feels like, find a clothespin and a small straw. Clamp your nostrils shut with the clothespin and stick the straw in your mouth. Now try to perform your daily activities for about an hour, allowing yourself to breathe only through the straw. You will notice that you have to slow down. You may even experience moments of panic after you move too quickly and find yourself gasping for breath through the limited air space. The breathing of an emphysema victim is restricted to at least this degree all the time. Emphysema is considered an irreversible condition. There is no mechanism known, or evidence to suggest, that psychogenic stress plays a role in the development or etiology of emphysema. Stress can, however, exacerbate the problem. During times of stress, the body's tissues demand more oxygen; the heart beats faster; the muscle tissues crave oxygen. During the hypermetabolic stress response, the breathing difficulty that a person with emphysema normally experiences is amplified. The difficulty that such a person has in performing even simple physical tasks will be exaggerated.

GASTROINTESTINAL DYSFUNCTIONS

Ulcers

Ulcers are the classic example of a psychogenic disorder. Many factors can cause an ulcer, but psychogenic stress can trigger the mechanism all by itself.

The stomach is made up of muscle tissue. We eat meat, the muscle tissue of animals, as a regular part of our diet. If the stomach is made of the same material as the meat we digest, what prevents the stomach from eating itself? The answer lies in a physiological balancing act. The stomach protects itself from its own digestive enzymes and acids by coating its lining with a thick layer of mucus. This mucous layer prevents the digestive enzymes from getting through to the wall and muscular tissue of the stomach itself. The food inside the stomach can be broken down, but the stomach itself stays safe, protected by this mucous coating. The safety of the stomach depends on two factors: (1) the thickness of the mucous layer and (2) the amount of digestive enzymes present. If the mucous layer gets too thin, the digestive enzymes can penetrate it and begin to digest the stomach. If the amount of digestive enzymes secreted begins to increase, even though the mucous layer remains thick, again the stomach will begin to digest itself. An ulcer is often described as a hole in the stomach or intestinal lining. This hole is created by the digestive enzymes produced by the gastrointestinal system itself. If you have an ulcer, your body is eating itself from the inside out.

What role does stress play in ulcers? Stress can alter the balance between the presence of digestive enzymes and acids and the thickness of the mucous lining of the stomach. Stress operates on acidity through several pathways. The first is through catecholamines, which, as part of the fight or flight response, shut down gastrointestinal motility. This means that the stomach and intestines stop moving. The sphincters also contract. The digestive system is nonessential during times of physical danger, so it shuts down. Since the sphincters constrict and all motility stops, the food just sits there. One mechanism that triggers the release of digestive enzymes is the presence of food in the stomach. It is just like standing on the mat that controls an electric door at the supermarket. If you stand on the mat, the door opens. When food enters the stomach, it opens the door and digestive enzymes float in. During stress, the food continues to sit on top of the button because it is no longer being moved through the system. That is like continuing to stand on the mat. The door stays open and all the flies in the area rush in. While that food is sitting there in the stomach, it stimulates the release of more digestive enzymes. There will be a much higher than necessary concentration of digestive enzymes within the stomach, so the balance between digestive enzyme activity in the stomach and the protective mucous layer is shifted. Those digestive enzymes begin to break down the food inside the stomach; they also start to digest the stomach itself. This may be the mechanism that accounts for the sudden intense pain that some ulcer victims feel when they encounter sudden stress.

Other pathways of the stress response can play a role in gastrointestinal problems. Cortisol release, for example, increases the rate of basal nocturnal hydrochloric acid and pepsin secretion. This means that if high levels of cortisol are present, a person will release acid and digestive enzymes during sleep. As a further long-term mechanism, thyroxine tends to step up the activity of all gastrointestinal processes, increasing both motility and enzymatic secretion.

Diarrhea and Constipation

Diarrhea and constipation are also related to stress. The release of thyroxine can trigger diarrhea. By causing a decrease in gastrointestinal motility and contraction of the sphincters, epinephrine and norepinephrine can block excretory processes causing short-term constipation.

ORGANIC SEXUAL DYSFUNCTION

Think back again to the logic of the fight or flight response. During fight or flight, most of the organ systems decrease their activity level. The gastrointestinal system is one example. The organ systems that decrease their activity during fight or flight are those that are not essential in providing escape from a dangerous situation. The reproductive system also shuts down during the experience of stress. Studies with animals have suggested that there are changes in the structure of the reproductive system after exposure to chronic stress. Selye (1976) has hypothesized a mechanism—the **pituitary shift theory**—for this observation. During chronic stress, the resources of the anterior pituitary gland are devoted to the production of corticotrophins, specifically ACTH. Like every organ or system in the body, the anterior pituitary has limited resources. If it must produce high levels of ACTH for the stress response, it may have to cut back on its production of other trophic hormones. The pituitary shift theory states that during times of stress, the activity of the pituitary shifts from making gonadotrophins to making corticotrophins. Gonadotrophic hormones are responsible for the maintenance and functioning of the structures in the reproductive system. This kind of endocrine activity alteration may have an undesirable result. Its effect is called gonadal atrophy, or shrinking of the sexual organs. This phenomenon has been clearly observed in experimental animals. Accompanying behavioral results have included loss of sex drive and impotence. It is highly probable that during an extended period of stress, you may lose your sex drive and your ability to perform sexually.

EATING DISORDERS

Stress has been found to play a role in several undesirable physical conditions that are triggered, not so much by internal physiological changes, but through a stress-induced change in behavior. Two of these conditions are obesity and anorexia nervosa.

Obesity

One of the earliest findings regarding the physiological effects of stress was that chronic stress can result in decreases in body weight. The reason is that the ACTH axis releases cortisol, which breaks down the fat and protein in the body to increase levels of available fuel. If caloric intake remains constant, stress reduces body weight by breaking down fats and proteins. This is what happens in laboratory animals, but human beings are different. Many people get fat when they are under too much stress. How can this be when the physiological effects of stress operate to reduce body weight?

Most of us know the answer. Human beings use eating as a coping mechanism; we feed our faces in response to life's adversities. This overeating behavior more than compensates for the loss in body weight due to the fat and protein mobilization of cortisol. Why is overeating a common coping mechanism? There are two explanations. First, eating diverts our attention. If our hands and minds and mouths are occupied with feeding, we cannot spend as much time thinking or worrying about our problems. Second, eating has a tranquilizing effect on the mind and on the hypothalamus. One use for the fight or flight response is to mobilize the physical resources of the body to be able to hunt for food. Your body needs to be aroused when you are hungry, but there is no longer any need for this hypermetabolic activity after you have eaten. Therefore, eating can turn off the fight or flight response.

Eating affects the hypothalamus in two ways. First, it helps elevate blood sugar levels. Sensors that feed into the hypothalamus monitor levels of blood sugar. When blood sugar rises, the hypothalamus shuts down. Second, chewing and taking food into the mouth can produce an inhibitory effect on the hypothalamus. These are called head factors, or an awareness of the fact that you are eating something. This awareness results in an actual physiological tranquilizing effect. The head factors and the rise in blood sugar that inhibit the hypothalamus produce the phenomenon called postprandial lethargy. Postprandial lethargy is that sleepy sensation you get after finishing a large meal. Remember how people act after Thanksgiving dinner. At my house, those who do not make it to one of the couches simply roll around on the floor and groan. (This is the same reason why sometimes it is difficult to stay awake around the middle of the morning. You are experiencing postprandial lethargy from breakfast.) Eating definitely produces a physiological tranquilizing effect. Many of us overeat to divert our minds from our problems and to help our bodies calm down so we do not feel as upset over our stressors.

Obesity is not only an effect of a maladaptive coping mechanism. Being overweight can itself serve as a further stressor. Since excess weight is considered physically undesirable in this culture, being too fat can be a source of stress and can trigger more overeating behavior.

Anorexia Nervosa

Some people react differently. There is a disease condition, usually seen in girls and young women, characterized by almost complete abstinence from eating. It is called **anorexia nervosa**. Women who are anorexic purposely refrain from eating. They eat small meals if any at all. They refuse food when it is offered and if forced to eat a large quantity of food, will regurgitate it soon afterward. It is not the case that women who suffer from this disease are not hungry or that they think their bodies do not need food; they simply refuse to eat. This condition has damaging effects on the human body and, of course, results in severe weight loss. Often, women who suffer from anorexia are perpetually dissatisfied with their body size. They see themselves as too fat no matter how emaciated they become. In many cases, the condition is fatal. We do not understand why anorexia occurs. Some researchers believe it is related to severe life stress that is rooted in profound self-dissatisfaction.

The Relationship Between Stress and Nutrition

There is a great deal of interest in but little actual knowledge about how nutritional factors relate to stress. There are three ways in which eating habits relate to stress. First, as discussed in Chapter 3, substances called sympathomimetics—substances like caffeine, nicotine, and other related stimulants—can artificially trigger a stress response within the body and help make the nervous system more reactive in its response to stressors. The second and third ways in which nutritional habits relate to stress are through vitamin depletion and through the synergistic effects of poor nutritional habits and psychosomatic organ damage.

The release of cortisol through the ACTH axis of the psychophysiological stress response mobilizes protein. This mobilization creates a host of problems that we have already discussed. It chews up the antibodies, thereby impairing immunity. It breaks down lipolytic enzymes, thereby accelerating atherosclerosis. It burns up the raw protein needed for the creation of new cells, thereby further impairing the body's immune systems. Vitamins are a source of protein that fall easy prey to the mobilization effort of cortisol. For some reason, the vitamins that disappear during stress are largely the B complex vitamins. The B vitamins help us in the breakdown, absorption, and utilization of most of what we eat. In the absence of sufficient levels of B complex vitamins, digestion and food absorption are severely hindered. During chronic stress, vitamin depletion can help perpetuate the damaging effects of stress on the body. For this reason, vitamin supplements often are recommended for people experiencing chronic stress.

Nutritional habits can damage some of the same organ systems attacked during the long-term stress response. This is referred to as the synergistic effect, which means that the effects of stress and the effects of improper nutrition both contribute to the ultimate damage and degradation of an organ system, but through different mechanisms. A prime example of this is atherosclerosis, which we have already discussed. Several factors are required in the development of atherosclerosis. One is the presence of irritants in the vascular lining. This factor is related to the consumption of food additives such as the nitrites used to preserve meat. In order for cholesterol plaquing to occur in the arterial linings, relatively high levels of cholesterol must be present in the blood. Nutritional factors thus provide the basic products for atherogenesis. Then stress comes along to degrade and impair the efficiency of the lipolytic enzymes, thereby accelerating the process. In this fashion, poor dietary habits and the experience of chronic stress contribute in different ways to the development of atherosclerosis. The same situation occurs with cancer. Many of the foods we consume are carcinogenic. Our dietary habits can contribute to the appearance of malignant cells in the body, and then the experience of stress impairs the immune system so that those malignancies can further develop into a serious disease.

What Constitutes a Healthy Diet?

Recommending a healthy or "stress-free" diet is impossible. There is considerably more ignorance than knowledge regarding proper nutrition. Remember that any significant deficiency or imbalance in your pattern of food intake can serve as a profound physical stressor. Nutritional science will never be able to understand everything that the human body needs to survive. We can always hypothesize that undiscovered trace elements may be essential for the normal, healthy functioning of the body. There are only two recommendations that can be made regarding proper eating habits. The first is to eat from as wide a variety of sources as possible. Most fad diets and nutritional fanatics advocate some kind of restrictions such as not eating meat, or eating only red peanuts, or consuming only potatoes harvested under a full moon. We will never identify all the nutrients and trace elements necessary to keep a human being alive, so it seems obvious that the degree to which people restrict their diet may represent the degree to which they increase their probability of encountering a deficiency in some vital and as yet unknown nutrient. Diversify your diet as much as possible; do not restrict yourself. The second recommendation is that you should eat food in as close to its natural state as possible. In other words, avoid overly processed food products. Food processing usually strips food of important elements. As food is processed, it gets farther and farther away from the nutrients our bodies were designed to receive.

STRESS AND THE YOUNG, WOMEN, AND THE ELDERLY

Some specific effects of stress affect only certain segments of the human population. Let us take a brief look at the influences that stress can have on children, women, and the elderly.

Stress and the Young

Stress-related diseases are usually chronic problems that need time to develop, so we tend to think that only adults suffer from them. Several recent studies, however, have determined that maternal stress can be a significant factor affecting the birth weight of babies. There is also some evidence to suggest that excessive maternal stress impairs fetal growth and development. Physical damage from stress may thus begin even before birth. Some researchers have also suggested that the trauma of birth itself is such a significant stressor that it may affect the entire course of an individual's life.

As the levels of stress continue to increase over time in this culture, the age of onset of psychosomatic disorders seems to decrease. Stress-related disorders are beginning to affect people at earlier and earlier ages. A 1969 study investigated 83 families that had some history of hypertension. In these families, the investigators observed evidence of blood pressure abnormalities in children between the ages of 2 and 14.

Further evidence suggests that the age of onset of psychosomatic disorders is creeping into younger and younger age groups. Levine (1965) investigated families in which both fathers and sons developed cardiovascular diseases. By comparing the age of onset of symptoms and the severity of symptoms, he reported that the age of onset of the disease occurred 13.1 years earlier in sons than it had in their fathers. For the fathers, the average age of onset of cardiovascular disease symptoms was 61.2 years. Their sons began showing symptoms of cardiovascular disease when they were only 48.1 years old on the average. An even more frightening result was reported. We assume that medical treatment improves over the years, so, even though the sons had an earlier age of disease onset, we would assume that their chances for survival would be better than for their fathers. On the average, however, the fathers died 9.2 years after symptoms first appeared. Their sons, on the average, died only 7.5 years following the first appearance of symptoms. Stress not only seems to be hitting younger age groups, it seems to be killing people more quickly.

Benson et al. (1974) summarized this problem with the following clinical observation:

> Five to ten years ago it would have been a relatively rare event to witness a stroke or heart attack in a person in his thirties and it would have been astonishing if the patient were in his twenties. Now interns and house staff just starting in medicine consider heart attacks in men in their thirties to be commonplace.

We do not know much about the effects of stress in children. One reason is that until recently researchers have assumed that stress is not a problem for children. We assume that stress only affects people when they get older, but this is clearly not the case. Stress is a disease problem that people must learn to deal with at an early age or suffer the sudden and fatal consequences. We hope that within the next few years, a considerable amount of research will be done on the effects of stress on young people.

Stress and Women

Stress affects women in unique ways, some of which we discussed in Chapter 3. In many ways, particularly with reference to the endocrine system, women are more complex physiologically than men. Women therefore can experience some stress-related physical problems that men never have to face. One such problem that has been investigated has to do with stress-induced irregularities in the menstrual cycle, a potential result of the pituitary shift theory. When the pituitary gland begins to devote its resources to the production of ACTH, it shifts away from producing the hormones (luteinizing hormone and follicle stimulating hormone) that effect the changes a woman's body undergoes during the menstrual cycle. The precise influence of stress on menstruation is impossible to pinpoint, but significant irregularities can be induced by stress. Sometimes emotional stress triggers ovulation. At other times, chronic emotional stress prevents menstruation. Due to the nonspecific nature of the stress response and the widely varying pattern of endocrine activity in women, the effects of stress on menstruation are totally unpredictable. This represents another area that merits further intensive research.

Stress and the Elderly

There are many different theories to explain why we age. Regardless of what mechanism triggers the aging process, it is characterized by a slowdown in protein production, which reduces the body's ability to create new cells and repair wear or damage that occurred. The stress-mediated release of cortisol mobilizes existing protein with the body and severely inhibits the formation of new proteins. Therefore, it is theoretically possible that the stress-induced release of cortisol accelerates the aging process. So far, there is no physiological evidence to support this theory. We do know, however, that aging is characterized by a decrease in protein production and that stress can reduce the production of proteins in the body. Consider the example of holding a highly stressful job. Look at photographs of American presidents immediately following their election and then as they leave office. Clearly, the tremendous stress of that job rapidly accelerates the aging process.

We know that people of different ages experience qualitatively different kinds of stressors. The question here is whether the body of an elderly person reacts differently to stress than the body of someone who is younger. As humans age, many of their internal organs and glands begin to atrophy. As the adrenal glands atrophy, they have a decreased capacity to release catecholamines and corticoid hormones in response to psychophysiological stress. The body of an older person is therefore somewhat less reactive during the physiological stress response. This may sound desirable, but what it means is that the body is less capable of adapting to change. Although the release of the actual products of stress may be minimized, the organ systems of an older person may be open to greater damage because of their loss of physiological adaptability.

SUMMARY

Psychosomatic diseases are all physical disease problems in which state of mind can influence the disease. Psychogenic conditions are those in which state of mind can cause physical changes within the body that can result in disease. Most physical disease conditions that we consider to be stress-related are psychosomatic diseases; many can also be considered psychogenic. In other words, stress may be the principal cause of many physical disease problems.

A number of serious physical disorders are related to stress. The human stress response is a comprehensive physiological response, so stress can play a role in the development of serious physical problems in nearly any organ system of the body. It is difficult to conceive of a somatic disease that cannot be influenced in some way by the experience of stress. The most serious and life-threatening diseases that Americans face are closely related to the experience of stress. Stress can cause the problem or it can set up conditions in the body that allow serious or life-threatening diseases to manifest themselves easily.

Human stress is a disease condition in and of itself. Many medical problems that we consider to be distinct disease states may actually be just the long-term severe symptoms of chronic stress It is possible that the number one killer in this country is not cardiovascular disease but stress.

REFERENCES

Abrahamson, E., and Wunderlich, R. "Anxiety, Fear, and Eating," *Journal of Abnormal Psychology*, v. 79(3), 317-321, 1972.

Amkraut, A., and Solomon, G. F. "From the Symbolic Stimulus to the Pathophysiologic Response: Immune Mechanisms," *International Journal of Psychiatry in Medicine*, v. 5, 541-563, 1974.

Behnke, J. A., et al. *The Biology of Aging*, Plenum Press, New York, 1978.

Benson, H., et al. "The Relaxation Response," *Psychiatry*, v. 37, 37-46, 1974.

Bruch, H. "Death in Anorexia Nervosa," *Psychosomatic Medicine*, v. 33(2), 135-144, 1972.

————. *Eating Disorders: Obesity, Anorexia Nervosa, and the Person Within*, Basic Books, Inc., New York, 1973.

Burdon, A., and Paul, L. "Obesity: A Review of the Literature Stressing the Psychosomatic Approach," *Psychiatric Quarterly*, v. 25, 568-580, 1951.

Canter, A., et al. "The Frequency of Physical Illness as a Function of Prior Psychological Vulnerability and Contemporary Stress," *Psychosomatic Medicine*, v. 28, 344-350, 1966.

Christensen, N. "Catecholamines and Diabetes Mellitus," *Diabetologia*, v. 16, 211-224, 1979.

Cocchi, R. "Exogenous (or Essential) Obesity as Hypercompensation of a Humeostatic Bio-physiological Mechanism," *Acta Neurologica*, v. 31(6), 753-758, 1976.

Dally, P., and Gomez, J. *Anorexia Nervosa*, Faber and Faber, Boston, 1980.

Danowski, T. S. "Emotional Stress as a Cause of Diabetes Mellitus," *Diabetes*, v. 12, 183-184, 1963.

DeAraujo, G., et al. "Life Change, Coping Ability and Chronic Intrinsic Asthma," *Journal of Psychosomatic Research*, v. 17, 359-363, 1973.

Dillman, V. M. "Age-Associated Elevation of Hypothalamic Threshold to Feedback Control and Its Role in Development, Aging, and Disease," *Lancet*, June 12, 1211-1219, 1971.

Dreyfus, G. "Paradoxical Obesity: A Psychosomatic Syndrome," *Presse Medical*, v. 56, 409-431, 1948.

Dudley, D. L., et al. "Long Term Adjustment, Prognosis, and Death in Irreversible Diffuse Obstructive Pulmonary Syndromes," *Psychosomatic Medicine*, v. 31, 310-325, 1969.

Eigler, N. L., et al. "Synergistic Interactions of Physiologic Increments of Gluckgon, Epinephrine, and Cortisol in the Dog," *Journal of Clinical Investigation*, v. 63, 114-119, 1979.

Gendel, B. R., and Benjamin, J. E. "Psychogenic Factors in the Etiology of Diabetes," *The New England Journal of Medicine*, v. 234, 556-560, 1946.

Grace, W. J., and Graham, D. T. "Relationship of Specific Attitudes and Emotions to Certain Bodily Diseases," *Psychosomatic Medicine*, v. 14, 243-251, 1952.

Grissom, J., et al. "Psychological Correlates of Cancer," *Journal of Consulting and Clinical Psychology*, v. 43(1), 113, 1975.

Gutstein, W. H., et al. "Neural Factors Contribute to Atherosclerosis," *Science*, v. 199, 449-451, Jan. 1978.

Guyton, A. C. *Textbook of Medical Physiology*, W. B. Saunders Co., Philadelphia, 1976.

Holmes, T. H., et al. "Experimental Study of Prognosis," *Psychosomatic Research*, v. 5, 235-252, 1961.

———. "Life Situations, Emotions and Nasal Disease: Evidence on Summative Effects Exhibited in Patients With 'Hay Fever,' " *Psychosomatic Medicine*, v. 13, 71-82, 1951.

———. "The Nose: An Experimental Study of Reaction Within the Nose in Human Subjects During Varying Life Experiences," Charles C Thomas, Springfield, Ill., 1950.

Ilfeld, F. "Age, Stressors, and Psychosomatic Disorders," *Psychosomatic Research*, v. 21(1), 56-64, Jan. 1980.

Jacobs, M. A., et al. "Incidence of Psychosomatic Predisposing Factors in Allergic Disorders," *Psychosomatic Medicine*, v. 28, 679-694, 1966.

Kass, E. H., and Zinner, S. H. "How Early Can the Tendency Toward Hypertension Be Detected?" *The Millbank Memorial Fund Quarterly*, v. XLVII, No. 3, Pt. 2, July 1969.

Katz, L. N., and Pick, R. "The Role of Endocrine Stress and Heredity on Atherosclerosis," *Handbook of Physiology*, Section 2, 1197-1209, 1963.

Kimball, C. P. "Emotional and Psychosocial Aspects of Diabetes Mellitus," *Medical Clinics of North America*, v. 55, 1007-1018, 1971.

Kinal, S. "Emotions as a Cause of Cancer," *Psychoanalyst Review*, v. 42, 217, 1955.

King, B., et al. "Pituitary-Adrenocortical Response to Shock-Induced Stress in Normal and Hypothalmic-Hyperphagic Rate," *Psychology and Behavior*, v. 22(4), 753-756, 1979.

Kirk, J. "Steroid Hormones and Aging," *Journal of Gerontology*, v. 6, 253-261, 1951.

Kissen, D. "Personality Characteristics in Males Conducive to Lung Cancer," *British Journal of Medical Psychology*, v. 36, 27-36, 1963.

LeShan, L. Psychological States as Factors in the Development of Malignant Diseases, A Critical Review," *Journal of the National Institute of Cancer*, v. 22, 1-18, 1959.

LeShan, L., and Worthington, R. E. "Some Recurrent Life History Patterns in Patients With Malignant Disease," *Journal of Nervous and Mental Disease*, v. 124, 460, 1956.

Levine, S. A. "Angina Pectoris in Father and Son," *American Heart Journal*, v. 66(1), July 1965.

Lipowski, Z. J. "Physical Illness, the Individual and the Coping Processes," *International Journal of Psychiatry in Medicine*, v. 1, 91-102, 1970.

Menniger, W. C. "Psychological Factors in the Etiology of Diabetes," *The Journal of Nervous and Mental Disease*, v. 81, 1-13, 1935.

Parson, P. "The Genetics of Aging in Optimal and Stressful Environments," *Experimental Gerontology*, v. 13, 357-363, 1973.

Pepys, J. *Immunological Mechanisms in Asthma*, Churchill Livingstone, London, 1971.

Perrin, G., and Pierce, I. "Psychosomatic Aspects of Cancer," *Psychosomatic Medicine*, v. 21(5), 327-421, 1959.

Pincus, C. "Measure of Stress Responsivity in Young and Old Men," *Psychosomatic Medicine*, v. 12, 225-228, 1950.

Reznick, H. M., and Balch, P. "The Effects of Anxiety and Response Cost on the Eating Behavior of Obese and Normal Weight Subjects," *Addictive Behaviors*, v. 2, 219-225, 1977.

Riegle, G. "Chronic Stress Effects on Adrenocortical Responsiveness in Young and Aged Rats," *Neuroendocrinology*, v. 11, 1-10, 1973.

Ripley, V. "Psychoneuroendocrine Influences on Immunocompetence and Neoplasia," *Science*, v. 212, 1273-1278, June 1981.

Rosch, A. "Stress and Illness," *Journal of the American Medical Association*, v. 242(5), 427-428, 1979.

Rosenman, R. H., and Friedman, M. "Behavior Patterns, Blood Lipids, and Coronary Heart Disease," *Journal of the American Medical Association*, v. 184, 112-116, June 1963.

―――. "Neurogenic Factors in Pathogenesis of Coronary Heart Disease," *Journal of the American Medical Association*, v. 184, 269-277, June 1963.

Rowland, N., and Antelman, S. "Stress-Induced Hyperphagia and Obesity in Rats: A Possible Model for Understanding Human Obesity," *Science*, v. 191, 310-311, 1976.

Saul, K. "Improving the Body's Anticancer System," *Geriatrics*, v. 34, 122-129, 1980.

Schacter, S., and Rodin, J. *Obese Humans and Rats*, Earbaus Publishing Company, Potomac, Md., 1974.

Selye, H. *Stress in Health and Disease*, Butterworth, Boston, 1976.

Shafrir, E., and Steinburg, D. "Role of the Pituitary and Adrenal in the Mobilization of the Free Fatty Acids and Lipoproteins," *Journal of Lipid Research*, v. 1, 459, 1960.

Solomon, G. F., et al. "Immunity, Emotions and Stress With Special Reference to the Mechanism of Stress Effects on the Immune System," *Annals of Clinical Research*, v. 6, 313-322, 1974.

Stunkard, A. "From Explanation to Action in Psychosomatic Medicine," *Psychosomatic Medicine*, v. 37(3), 195-236, 1975.

Timmreck, T., et al. "Stress and Aging," *Geriatrics*, v. 35(6), 113-120, June 1980.

Treuting, T. F., and Ripley, H. S. "Life Situations, Emotions and Bronchial Asthma," *Journal of Nervous Mental Disorders*, v. 108, 380-398, 1948.

Uhley, H. N., and Friedman, M. "Blood Lipids, Clotting, and Coronary Atherosclerosis in Rats Exposed to a Particular Form of Stress," *American Journal of Physiology,* v. 197, 136, 1959.

VanItallis, T., et al. "Control of Food Intake in the Regulation of Depot Fat," *Diabetes, Obesity, and Vascular Disease*, Hemisphere Publishing Corporation, Washington, D.C., 1978.

Verzar, F. "Research on Aging of the Endocrine Organs," *Lectures on Experimental Gerontology*, Charles C Thomas, Springfield, Ill., 1963.

Walton, K. W. "Pathogenetic Mechanisms in Atherosclerosis," *The American Journal of Cardiology*, v. 35, 542, Apr. 1975.

Watson, C., and Shuld, D. "Psychosomatic Factors in the Etiology of Neoplasms," *Journal of Consulting and Clinical Psychology*, v. 45(3), 455-461, 1977.

Wittenberger, J. L. "The Nature of the Response to Stress With Aging," *Bulletin of the New York Academy of Medicine*, v. 32(5), 330-336, May 1956.

PART III

Stress Control

"It's very hard to live in a studio apartment in San Jose with a man who's learning to play the violin." That's what she told the police when she handed them the empty revolver.

Richard Brautigan

We all have our own ways of coping with stress. Unfortunately, most of them do not help the situation adequately and they usually mess up something else along the way. Many Americans, in fact, rely heavily on maladaptive coping methods like Valium or other depressant drugs, alcohol, or suicide. Even medical science does not treat stress effectively. It waits until disease, or the stage of exhaustion, has already set in before taking action. Then the treatment focuses only on a singular disorder, actually just one of the more severe symptoms of stress. Medicine treats only the symptoms and not the causes of stress.

We need effective ways to deal with stress. In the remaining chapters of this book we will explore in detail a diverse range of stress management strategies and skills.

To be useful and effective, a stress control strategy must satisfy three essential aims. First, the technique must be theoretically, experimentally, and practically capable of reducing psychophysiological arousal. It must decrease the probability of encountering psychosomatic disease by diminishing stress-related cognitive or physical responses or reactivity. This is

115

our basic evaluation criterion. Second, the technique must not require the sacrifice of such things as life goals, productivity, or level of achievement. Stress management does not involve cutting back on your standards of quality, quantity, and achievement or on the ends that you wish to realize in life. Appropriate stress control measures should actually enhance level of accomplishment by tuning out the maladaptive interference that stress creates, thereby permitting a more satisfying and productive existence. Stress control does not mean taking it easy; it means ridding oneself of one of life's constant sources of interference. Finally, an effective stress control technique should fit individual personality and life-style. For stress control to be effective on a pragmatic, daily level, it must be a frictionless fit with a person's personality. Adjustments or sacrifices in personal style should not be required.

We will rely on the psychosomatic model as our basic conceptual framework for understanding stress management. As discussed in Chapter 2, all we need to do to minimize stress-related disease is interrupt the chain of events at one of the eight stages of the model. We can therefore conceive of many different schemes for stress control, each intervening at a different stage.

We can derive four basic types of stress control techniques from the psychosomatic model. These include techniques that operate on the environment (stressors), the mind (cognition), or the body (physiological response and reactivity), and hybrid techniques that can affect many levels (such as systematic relaxation). The aim of all the techniques is to intervene in the psychosomatic disease process.

Stress control can be approached quantitatively or qualitatively. Quantitative stress management involves stress reduction, or a decrease in the amount of stress experienced. This is our usual connotation for stress control. It assumes that we are in distress conditions because we are experiencing more stress than we can handle. Qualitative stress management is also a valid approach. This concept involves shifting the character of stress so that distress situations can be converted to eustress opportunities. This means learning to use stress to your benefit rather than your detriment. Although most of the stress control techniques discussed in the following chapters emphasize stress reduction, many afford the possibility of converting distress to eustress.

There are two reasons for presenting such a wide variety of methods for handling stress. First, since everyone is different, no single technique will be right for every individual. Individuals need to explore and find the particular techniques that fit them best. Second, if you are serious about managing stress in your life, you will not employ one skill exclusively. Various situations require various approaches. Presenting a range of ideas will help you develop a colorful and complete personal program of stress control.

After reading the following chapters, you will know how to treat the disease of stress. You can expect many results if you practice what you learn. Your chances of encountering psychosomatic disease will go down. You should not experience harmful side effects, as you might with most traditional medical treatments. You will begin to control your own health.

You will be less tense and less anxious. Your performance and levels of accomplishment may improve. You will be on your way to a state of optimal health. Your life will be a whole lot more pleasant. Remember, however, that no one can control stress for you. You must take charge and practice the techniques that work for you. All of the answers you need to control stress within your life lie within yourself. The techniques that follow may help you to see yourself more clearly and to discover your own solutions.

CHAPTER 7

Social Engineering

Know when to let go of things which no longer serve you, but force you to serve them.

Suraci Nosof Suladed

The logical place to begin stress control is with the stressor. The sensory stimulus, or stressor, is the first step in the sequence of events leading to stress-related disease. We should not try to eliminate stressors from our lives, but if we can identify and weed out unnecessary stressors, we can effectively reduce our experience of stress.

Many stressors are unavoidable. We assume that there is little we can do to alter our circumstances, so we focus our energy on controlling our internal selves. To a certain extent, however, we can manage or reengineer our social environment and the stressors it provides. In this chapter, we will discuss two ways in which you can exert some control over your exposure to stressors. The two techniques are **social engineering** and **time management**. First let us consider another possibility.

AVOIDANCE: THE PERFECT SOLUTION?

There is but one completely effective scheme for stress management. It does not work for everyone, and it is not easy even for those who can pull it off, but it is completely effective. The technique has four basic steps.

1. *Compose a list of personal stressors.* On 3″ x 5″ index cards, write down every stressor you can think of that affects you. Use one card per stressor. Probe your mind, dig around, and record everything in life that bothers you. (You should buy lots of cards.)
2. *Field test and complete your list.* When you can think of no more, alphabetize your cards and carry them around with you for a few weeks. (You may need a small red wagon or grocery cart.) Each time you encounter something that bothers or upsets you, check you cards to see if you have included it yet. If you already have a card

for that situation, proceed with life. If not, make one. Do this for every problem you encounter for several weeks. In fact, keep it up until you are no longer encountering situations requiring new cards and you are well satisfied that your list of stressors is more or less complete.
3. *Memorize the list.* When your list is complete, sit down and memorize it. Be sure you have a complete mental listing of all your stressors.
4. *Never do any of those things again*! Avoid all stressors in your life. Never again expose yourself to any of the situations you have recorded and memorized. With no stressors, your problems will be over. You can go sit on the beach and drool.

The strategy just described is called **avoidance**. It is not a form of social engineering. We tend to think that if we could just avoid our stressors, our problems would be solved. Not so. There are several fundamental problems with avoidance that render it unacceptable as a legitimate form of stress management. First, it is not possible to avoid all stressors. If you successfully escape some, you will find that they will be replaced by other, perhaps more severe, stressors. Second, in attempting to avoid stress, you will avoid eustress as well as distress. Your life will be about as interesting as a bowl of lukewarm tapioca pudding. Finally, if you totally eliminate your stressors, you must also be prepared to forget about your aspirations, dreams, and goals. Stressors are necessary to get what we strive for in life. What can you do, then?

SOCIAL ENGINEERING

Social engineering involves minor reorganization of daily behavior to reduce the frequency of encounters with stressors without sacrificing life goals. The assumption behind this technique is that we do not always achieve our goals in the most stress-efficient manner. Social engineering assumes that there are many pathways that will accomplish a given goal and that each one has a different degree of stress associated with it. In other words, there are lots of ways to get something and some ways simply involve more obstacles (stressors) than others. If you can identify your goal, you should be able to outline a sequence of action for reaching it that entails a minimum of stress.

THE ROLE OF SOCIAL ENGINEERING IN STRESS MANAGEMENT

Social engineering operates on the psychosomatic model at the sensory stimulus level. It is designed to eliminate unnecessary stressors from life. This technique can be applied to any predictable, regularly occurring stressor. It works only when you know in advance that the stressor is coming, however; it will not help you calm down after a stressful event has taken place. You must do your engineering before the stressor actually appears. When you start using social engineering, apply it to frequently occurring stressors so you get plenty of practice in evaluating its efficacy.

HOW SOCIAL ENGINEERING WORKS

There are ten steps in the process of social engineering. The first eight come from *Investigations in Stress Control* (Allen and Hyde 1980). The recipe goes as follows:

1. *Identify a stressor.* Select a stressful event that occurs often in your life. It should be something you can predict, such as a certain traffic light, an unpleasant household task, or visiting an obnoxious individual. This process is not applicable to unexpected stressors like being fired from work or burning the toast.

2. *Define the stressor.* Determine what it is about the event that upsets you. A traffic light that causes you to be late for work may be a stressor but what really bothers you may be the embarrassment of walking in late or the prospect of losing your job. Analyze your thoughts and discover what it is about this stressor that causes it to trigger an emotional response. (Answering this question may be valuable in itself.)

3. *Ask yourself whether the stressor can be totally avoided.* Respond with a simple yes or no. On occasion, you may discover a stressor that you can avoid without sacrifice. All of us carry some useless stressors around. If you can honestly and without compromise answer yes, stop here and simply do not place yourself in a situation of encounter with that stressor again. If your answer is no, proceed to step 4.

4. *If it cannot be avoided, why not?* Ask yourself what goals are associated with this stressor or what it helps you attain. What would you lose if you totally avoided this particular stressor? Identify here the goal(s) that this event helps you acquire.

5. *Generate alternatives.* Think of as many alternatives as you can. Come up with alternate ways to acquire all the things you described in step 4, without experiencing the stressor you identified and defined in steps 1 and 2. In the traffic light example, for instance, you could find another route to work. Do not evaluate or judge the feasibility of individual alternatives; just think of as many as you can.

6. *Evaluate alternatives.* First, evaluate each alternative in terms of how well it meets your goals. Are sacrifices or compromises required? If so, the alternative may be undesirable. Next, determine which alternatives may increase the number of stressors you encounter, which ones involve a trade-off of one set of stressors for another, and which ones may reduce stress. Eliminate any alternative that does not meet all your goals or that increases the magnitude of stressors you may encounter.

7. *Select the best alternative.* After evaluating alternatives, select the one that will best meet your specified goals and will decrease the number or severity of stressors you must encounter to attain them.

8. *Try it!* When you run into this stressor, implement your behavioral alternative instead of following your old plan of action.

9. *Reevaluate the alternative.* Reexamine the alternative behavior. After testing it, ask yourself if it completely meets your desired goals and effectively reduces stress. If not, ask yourself if you have sacrificed other needs or goals that you were not aware of before. Then ask yourself whether the alternative reduces the stress of attaining your goals or simply replaces old stressors with new ones.

10. *Polish your behavioral alternative.* If necessary, revise your new style of action to meet any drawbacks you uncovered in step 9. You may wish to repeat the reevaluation each time you adjust the new strategy. Eventually, you should be able to arrive at a behavioral scheme that will get you everything that you are after in a more stress-efficient manner.

After applying the social engineering process to several of your common stressors, you will become aware that you are chasing after most of your goals in an overstressed style. Soon you will develop a subtle awareness of getting things done in a stress-efficient manner. With practice, the process of social engineering will occur simply and automatically in your mind; it will become second nature for you to seek out the most stressor-free pathways in your daily activities. Life will remain as rewarding, you will accomplish as much as ever, and life will be a whole lot simpler and more pleasant. Try this technique. You will find it to be an essential tool in an overall personal stress management program.

TIME MANAGEMENT

Time represents a common source of stress for most Americans. We never seem to think there is enough time to do all that we need to do, particularly in work settings. Time is a finite resource; the study of time management has evolved to help us use our limited allotments more effectively. Time management involves little more than a collection of easily implemented, simple-minded ideas and suggestions. As in the case of social engineering, however, putting these simple ideas into practice can help make our lives a little easier. The key is to practice the ideas presented and acquire a greater degree of self-discipline with regard to allocating time and energy. Self-management and self-discipline are at the heart of time management.

HOW TIME MANAGEMENT WORKS

Time management is a scheme to help you organize and effectively accomplish your daily tasks in a time- and stress-efficient manner. There are three fundamental steps to effective time management: **planning**, **setting priorities**, and **implementing**.

Planning is based on the notion that most time wasters are internally generated and are derived from unclear objectives, lack of priorities, and an inability to anticipate clearly the time and energy demands of the day The first activity in planning is to analyze the nature of your regular tasks and break them down into general categories such as returning phone calls and correspondence, studying, writing, attending meetings or classes, exercising, eating, and taking naps. Next, determine what percentage of your time is taken up by each activity. After you have a rough idea of how you spend your time, the next step is to list your anticipated activities for each day. Do this either first thing each morning or, preferably, the night before. When you have listed all your activities, estimate the time required to perform each task. Total the required times and then add 15 percent for interruptions and unexpected delays. Use this total figure as a reasonable estimate of your required time investment for the day.

Next, arrange your activities in order of importance. At the top of your list place those activities that have the most direct or central bearing on your objectives. This list of priorities will be your guide to the ordering of your work throughout the day. When setting your prioiities, it is a good idea to put the most difficult or distasteful tasks first. This leaves you with the easiest tasks to perform at the end of the day, when your energy is lowest. This way, instead of dreading the end of the day, you can enjoy it.

Once you have planned your activities and set your priorities, you can start doing something. This is often the most difficult part of time management. We usually know what we should do, but we lack the self-discipline to do it. Use your list of priorities to identify those tasks that are most closely associated with your goals first, regardless of how difficult they may be or how long they may take. Do not be tempted to clear away the easy stuff first, for you may never get to what is really important. Do not put off activities simply because they are complex, laborious, or unpleasant. If you get them done early, you will not waste energy dreading them all day. When you worry about doing something you end up doing it many times in your mind; why not do it just once?

The most important facet of implementation is to perform one task at a time and stick with it to completion. This may take some discipline, but remember that self-management is the key to time management. Also remember that if you do not have time now to do something right you probably are not going to have time to do it over.

ELIMINATING GOAL DISPLACEMENT

By implementing these strategies, you can abandon some trivial tasks and behaviors that hinder your attempts to attain your goals. According to Mackenzie (1977), "Refusing to do the unimportant is a requisite for success."

Many of us fall into a trap called goal displacement. We lose track of our objectives and become involved in secondary tasks that are merely tools to help us attain our goal. This happens to teachers when they get so busy marking tests, making seat assignments, and checking attendance that they forget to teach. We are often so busy being busy that we forget our overall goals and produce nothing.

Social engineering and time management techniques can help reduce your exposure to stressors, thus allowing you to get more accomplished in life and do so with a more stress-free body. Do not go through life trying to look busy. Weed out those banal stressors, abandon the unimportant, relax, enjoy life, and be genuinely productive.

SUMMARY

A logical place to begin the management of stress is by reducing exposure to stressors. Simply avoiding all unpleasant or stressful situations results in unacceptable sacrifices. If we could avoid all stressors, we would be forced to abandon most of our life goals and our ability to make meaningful contributions to the world. We cannot eliminate all stressors from our lives, but we can learn to trim away the unnecessary ones and reduce the quantity of damaging stress we must face.

Social engineering and time management are two strategies that can be used to identify and eliminate unnecessary stressors without sacrificing productivity, accomplishment, or life goals. They involve identifying goals and objectives and then engineering behavior (or time) in a way that accomplishes goals in the most stress-efficient manner.

REFERENCES

Allen, R. J., and Hyde, D. H. *Investigations in Stress Control*, Burgess, Minneapolis, Minn., 1980.

Barrett, F. D. "The Management of Time," *The Business Quarterly*, Spring 1969.

Bird, C., and Yutzy, T. D. "The Tyranny of Time: Results Achieved Versus Hours Spent," *Management Review*, Aug. 1965.

Cooper, J. D. *How to Get More Done in Less Time*, Doubleday, Garden City, N.Y., 1962.

Engstrom, T. W., and Mackenzie, R. A. *Managing Your Time*, Zondervan, Grand Rapids, Mich., 1967.

"Executive Workloads—The Triumph of Trivia," *The Wall Street Journal*, August 13, 1968.

Girdano, D., and Everly, G. S. *Controlling Stress and Tension: A Holistic Approach*, Prentice-Hall, Englewood Cliffs, N.J., 1979.

Hummel, C. E. *The Tyranny of the Urgent*, Inter-Varsity, Chicago, 1967.

Laird, D. A., and Laird, E. C. *The Technique of Getting Things Done*, McGraw-Hill, New York, 1947.

Mackenzie, R. A. *The Time Trap*, McGraw-Hill, New York, 1972.

Peter, L. J., and Hull, R. *The Peter Principle*, Morrow, New York, 1969.

Updegraff, R. R. *All the Time You Need*, Prentice-Hall, Englewood Cliffs, N.J., 1958.

Walker, C. E. *Learn to Relax: 13 Ways to Reduce Tension*, Prentice-Hall, Englewood Cliffs, N.J., 1975.

Webber, R. A. *Time and Management*, Van Nostrand Reinhold, New York, 1972.

CHAPTER 8

Cognitive Reappraisal

Advice on what to do when you have fallen into a crack in the earth, trapped under a boulder the size of a small cathedral, with no hope of rescue:
A) Reflect on the fact that life has overall been generally good to you so far, or
B) Realize, considering your present circumstances, that life has probably not treated you favorably so be comforted by the fact that it won't be lasting much longer.

The Hitchhiker's Guide to the Galaxy

Dealing with stressors themselves is an effective way to control stress, but it is of no value in helping us handle events that have already happened or events that we cannot predict. Some of our most severe stressors are unexpected situations. The factor that determines whether a given event is going to be a stressor is usually not the nature of the event, but rather how we choose to interpret it. Another direct way to intervene in the psychosomatic stress process, then, is to learn how to control our interpretation of events.

Learning to reappraise potential stress situations relates back to Selye's concept of distress and eustress. If we consider the events of life to be threats, we are in a distress or pathogenic situation. If we can look at the same event as a challenge, it can promote growth and health. This is a powerful concept. The impact of life's adversities lies not in the events themselves or in the outside world but inside our minds.

Cognitive reappraisal is a strategy to help us rethink potential stressors. Most of our stressors are psychogenic. This means that our interpretation of the event or our mental state is the prime element that triggers further physiological arousal. We can control almost any stress situation if we can first simply learn to control our thoughts and how we interpret events that are potential stressors.

GOALS OF COGNITIVE REAPPRAISAL

The goal of any kind of cognitive reappraisal strategy is to learn to rethink potential psychogenic stressors, thereby interrupting the psychosomatic model at the cognitive appraisal level. The technique of cognitive reappraisal is one that will help you condition your mind to interpret events in an adaptive, health-promoting fashion as opposed to maladaptive and stress-fostering patterns of thought. Cognitive reappraisal is one of the most useful and effective techniques we will cover in this text. You can use it any time you are in a stress situation that is being mediated by the way in which you interpret events.

THE ESSENCE OF COGNITIVE REAPPRAISAL

The essential element in cognitive reappraisal is choice. William James, one of the first contributors to the science of psychology, spent a significant portion of his adult life in severe pathological depression. After years of suffering, he pulled himself out of this state through the simple realization that he always had the power to choose one thought over another. This may sound trivial, but the ability to select which thoughts we pay attention to may be the greatest single potential of the human mind. The simple ability to choose one thought over another may be our most powerful weapon against stress.

During World War II, Viktor Frankl was imprisoned in Auschwitz, the largest of the Nazi concentration camps. Frankl survived, but he witnessed the murder of his entire family in this grotesque and incomprehensible setting. Luck seemed to ordain his physical survival. His sanity and will to live survived due to his own efforts. Frankl survived with a strong drive to continue to live and grow. His book, *Man's Search for Meaning*, is a classic treatise on the ability of the human mind and spirit to use control over cognitive processes as a means of coping, even with life's most terrible and unthinkable adversities. Frankl's attitude was that no matter what the outside world stripped away from him or did to him, no external force could change his ability to think about the situation in whatever fashion he chose. According to Frankl, nothing can shake the sanctity of the human mind. No matter what the world does to us, no matter what the nature of external events may be, we always retain the power to think about them in whatever way we wish. This single element seems to be the key to survival. It is similar to a Buddhist concept. Tibetan Buddhists believe that we have no control over external events in life. They believe that we are predetermined beings. Yet they also believe that human beings have total control over how they interpret life's events. The idea is that you can never control the outside world, but you have the capacity for total control over your inner self. They believe that the person who can achieve control over his or her thoughts is the true master of the world.

Cognitive reappraisal was synthesized from these ideas. To reiterate: *you always have the capacity to choose what you are thinking about*. We all can be in control of our awareness. The fact that we often do not exercise this power is merely the reflection of another choice we make. We unconsciously choose to give up our power and let the world, the environment, or other people determine what we think about. The cognitive reappraisal strategy will reaquaint you with your own potential and give you a tool to help you decide what you will pay attention to and what the character of your thoughts will be.

There are many many cognitive strategies. We are not going to present a compendium of psychological theories and diverse intervention techniques related to changing cognitive processes. Rather, we will create a summary technique to help you control stress by gaining control over your interpretation of potential stressors.

The Immediate Reaction

Besides the central concept of choice, cognitive reappraisal is based on several other fundamental ideas. One idea is that events often become stressors for us because of the particular interpretation we attach to them at the moment they occur. There are, of course, numerous valid interpretations of any given event.

Imagine you are sitting at a red light all alone at an intersection. You hear loud music, glance into your rearview mirror, and see a large truck coming up behind you. You notice that the truck is packed high with furniture, that the cab is crowded, and that everyone in the truck, including the driver, is drinking beer and singing along with the radio. You also notice that the truck has one of those rusty steel I-beams for a front bumper. The last thing you notice is that the driver has not seen you or the red light and is not going to stop. That steel I-beam, the beer, several drunk people, and a lot of furniture come crashing into the back of your car. A potential stressor has just occurred. A lot of thoughts could enter a person's mind during such a situation. Find a piece of paper and jot down a dozen different thoughts that might enter your mind in a situation like this one the instant after it occurred.

Notice how easy it is to come up with many thoughts about one event. Anytime a situation like this occurs, you can choose how to interpret it.

The Role of Biology

Another idea important to cognitive reappraisal is that our attention often is automatically directed to a certain kind of interpretation. Rarely do we consciously choose how we are going to think about an event. We will discuss this part of our biological design in detail in Chapter 14. For now, remember that, because biological organisms are designed for survival, we tend to pay attention to the most threatening aspects of events. Many of us have conditioned ourselves to do this. We become tense and irritated every time we have to stop for a red light, for example. We do such a good job that we get tense even when we have plenty of time for stoplights. Although we may realize that there is no need to be upset we unconsciously focus in on these automatic negative or stressful interpretations of situations.

Choosing to Be Positive

There are positive and negative interpretations for every situation. Nothing is so horrible that it does not carry a positive element or possiblities for growth along with it. Even if a situation is as bad as anything can get, at least things cannot get any worse. Look back at your list of interpretations following the traffic accident. Most of them are probably negative or problematic interpretations of the situation. Try now to think about the good things that could come out of an accident like this. Push yourself a bit and write down six positive interpretations of such an accident.

The human mind has an interesting limitation. (Let us call it not a limitation but an interesting capability.) The awareness capacity of the human mind is limited, so we can pay attention only to a small fragment of ideas accessible to our consciousness at any moment. We cannot be constantly aware of every potential thought, memory, or idea at one moment. Also, we are not capable of being aware of all possible interpretations about a given event at any one moment. The scope of human awareness is limited; we can hold only a small number of sensations, thoughts, or ideas in our mind at one time. We can use this limitation to our advantage. We can choose to pay attention only to those interpretations that keep us calm and help resolve the situation, rather than to those that will upset us and make resolution of the condition difficult. Conditioning, biological design, and environmental determinates direct our awareness to one thought or another, but we determine for ourselves what we think about.

To summarize, then: (1) most stressors require interpretation to have any impact on us, (2) there are many possible interpretations of any given situation, (3) most of the time our attention automatically centers on threatening interpretations, and (4) we have the capacity to choose what we pay attention to.

HOW COGNITIVE REAPPRAISAL WORKS

Allen and Hyde (1980) have provided the following description of the steps in the process of cognitive reappraisal. As you read through these steps, recall a stressful situation from your recent past and apply the cognitive reappraisal technique to it.

1. *Identify a stressor.* It is best to begin with a frequently occurring event that you can predict with reasonable certainty. Choose an event that you currently interpret as threatening or emotion-evoking in some other significant fashion. This technique can be effective even with unexpected stressors because intervention takes place after rather than before the fact. To learn the skill, however, it is best to begin with a commonly occurring event so you have plenty of opportunities to practice rethinking the consequences.
2. *Analyze your original appraisal.* Describe how you currently appraise the event. What thoughts run through your mind during the event and immediately following it that cause you to get upset? What are you afraid of? What are you afraid might happen? Simply outline why you think of this event as a stressor.
3. *Generate alternative appraisals.* What are some of the other potential results of this event? In what other ways could you interpret the event as it occurs or immediately afterward? Come up with as many appraisals as you can that interpret this event as a benign occurrence, a challenge, or a stimulus for growth.
4. *Select a new cognitive set.* Review your list of alternative appraisals. Which ones sound plausible? Which ones sound like phony, sugar-coated avoidance or escapist thoughts? Select a sound, genuine, positive interpretation of what has occurred. Most important, make sure your selection leads to less mental anguish than your previous interpretation did. Choose one that will reduce your arousal and help you to deal more effectively with the event.
5. *Try it!* The next time you encounter this stressor, make a deliberate effort to focus your mind on your new, positive interpretation. Divert your attention from your previous stressful appraisal. Replace your old maladaptive thoughts with an appraisal that will reduce stress, promote growth, and help you perform better in the situation.
6. *Determine what is wrong with this technique.* From a practical perspective, this technique is not as simple or as effective as it sounds. If your new way of thinking seems comfortable right away, continue to use it and consider the stressor cured. If you have trouble accepting the new appraisal, consider two potential sources of interference. The first is conditioning. You probably are accustomed to thinking about this event in a negative way, so it will take time and practice for your mind to become reconditioned, adjust, and adopt a new style of thought in response to it. The more often you deliberately focus your attention on the reappraisal, the easier it will become to think positively the next time the stressor occurs. Practice, deliberate effort, and rehearsal are keys to success.

The second potential disrupting factor involves the notion of **secondary gains**. It is possible that there are some secondary factors or effects that actually reinforce or reward you for experiencing stress. Consider the example of the stereotypic American housewife. She works hard, performs all her duties well, and keeps the affairs of her family running smoothly. The better she performs her job, the more invisible she becomes. She receives few external rewards. Suppose, now, that she gets sick or starts to complain about physical symptoms. Suddenly people start paying attention to her. Her family and friends show concern and sympathy, her husband and children do more housework, people call her and send flowers. She gets lots of reinforcement for being sick. Often we derive many such secondary gains from experiencing stress. We may have to sacrifice something if we eliminate the impact of a significant stressor. The potential loss of secondary gains may hinder our desire to control a stressor and adopt a positive reappraisal. If you sense that something is holding you back, search your mind and try to identify the existence of secondary gains.

We may be tempted to say that people who appraise bad situations in positive ways are not facing reality. This is not the case at all. Cognitive reappraisal does not involve denial. Rather, in a highly rational fashion, we choose to focus our attention on the elements of a situation that help us stay calm and help us resolve the problem. When we worry, or get upset, or scream, or cry about negative situations, we often elicit a maladaptive response. The upset, the worry, the tears do not help us get the situation taken care of and they stimulate a stress reaction in our bodies. In contrast, if we adopt a positive interpretation in full realization of the negative elements of the event, we keep our bodies free of stress and at the same time establish a mental attitude suited to resolving the problem in a rational manner.

Another suggestion, outlined by Michenbaum (1975), is valuable in making cognitive reappraisal an ongoing process throughout life. It is called **stress inoculation**. The assumption behind stress inoculation is that the cognitive reappraisal process is not simply a single shot. Stress inoculation suggests that we deal with an event in an evolving fashion as it changes over time. As you reappraise an event its character is going to change, and as you work on a situation its structure will change. Be prepared to modify your interpretation continually so you can effectively adapt to the changes in your life.

Exercising your power of choice is difficult at first, but the more you practice the more it will become your dominant style of mental activity. Remember, *you always have a choice.* You can learn to take command of your own mind.

SUMMARY

Cognitive reappraisal represents a synthesis of several different strategies for managing stress through rational interpretation. The key element in cognitive reappraisal is choice. Whenever a potential stressor occurs, we choose how we are going to interpret the situation. All events carry positive and negative interpretations. We can focus our minds only on a limited number of interpretations at one time. Cognitive reappraisal suggests that we choose to pay attention to elements that are adaptive and help us resolve a problem and that eliminate the stress-fostering nature of a situation.

Cognitive reappraisal operates on the cognitive appraisal level of the psychosomatic model. It can be applied to almost any cognitive stress situation, making it one of the most universal and useful strategies for controlling stress.

There are cognitive factors that work against positive interpretation of events in life. One of the strongest involves secondary gains, which are peripheral rewards that tend to reinforce us for experiencing stress. The threat of losing secondary gains can make us hesitant to change our style of thinking. By taking a close look at the secondary gains or rewards that you experience for being afflicted by stress, you may begin to get some valuable insight into factors that may be holding you back from realizing your full human potential and becoming a healthy human being.

REFERENCES

Allen, R. J., and Hyde, D. H. *Investigations in Stress Control*, Ed. 2, Burgess, Minneapolis, Minn., 1981.

Beck, A. T. "Cognitive Therapy: Nature and Relationship to Behavior Therapy," *Behavior Therapy*, v. 1, 194-200, 1970.

Bernardo, P. "Cognitive Strategies as a Means of Controlling Stress With Some Recommendations for Athletics," Unpublished Monograph, University of Maryland, College Park, 1980.

D'Zurilla, T., et al. "A Preliminary Study of the Effectiveness of Graded Prolonged Exposure in the Treatment of Irrational Fear," *Behavior Therapy*, v. 4, 672-685, 1973.

Ellis, A. *Reason and Emotion in Psychotherapy*, Lyle-Stuart, New York, 1962.

Frankl, V. *Man's Search for Meaning*, Beacon Press, Boston, 1962.

Glowgower, F., et al. "A Component Analysis of Cognitive Restructuring," *Cognitive Therapy and Research*, v. 2, 209-223, 1978.

Goldfried, M. R., et al. "Systematic Rational Restructuring as a Self-Control Technique," *Behavior Therapy*, v. 5, 247-254, 1974.

————. "Reduction of Test Anxiety Through Cognitive Restructuring," *Journal of Consulting and Clinical Psychology*, v. 46, 32-39, 1978.

Jaremlco, M. "Cognitive Strategies in the Control of Pain Tolerance," *Journal of Behavior Therapy and Experimental Psychiatry*, v. 9, 239-244, 1978.

————. "A Component Analysis of Stress Inoculations: Review of Prospectus," *Cognitive Therapy and Research*, v. 3, 35-48, 1979.

Jenni, M., and Wollersheim, J. "Cognitive Therapy, Stress Management Training, and the Type A Behavior Pattern," *Cognitive Therapy and Research*, v. 3, 61-73, 1979.

Keyes, K., Jr. *Handbook to Higher Consciousness*, 5th Edition, Cornucopia Institute, St. Mary, Ky., 1975.

Lazarus, R. *Psychological Stress and the Coping Process*, McGraw-Hill, New York, 1966.

Ledwid, B. "Cognitive Behavior Modification: A Step in the Wrong Direction," *Psychological Bulletin*, v. 85, 353-375, 1978.

Mahoney, M. *Cognition and Behavior Modification*, Ballinger, Cambridge, 1974.

Maslow, A. *Toward a Psychology of Being*, D. Van Nostrand, New York, 1968.

Meichenbaum, D., and Turk, D. "The Cognitive-Behavioral Management of Anxiety, Anger, and Pain," in Davidson, P., *The Behavioral Management of Anxiety, Depression, and Pain*, Brunner/Mozel, New York, 1976.

Meichenbaum, D. *Cognitive-Behavior Modifications*, Plenum Press, New York, 1977.

————. "Cognitive Modification of Test Anxious College Students," *Journal of Consulting and Clinical Psychology*, v. 39, 370-380, 1972.

————. "A Self Instructional Approach to Stress Management: A Proposal for Stress Inoculation Training," in Spielberger, C., and Sarason, J., *Stress and Anxiety*, v. 1, Hemisphere Publishing Corporation, Washington, D.C., 1975.

Meichenbaum, D., et al. "Group Insight vs. Group Desensitization in Treating Speech Anxiety," *Journal of Consulting and Clinical Psychology*, v. 36, 410-421, 1971.

Roskies, E., and Lazarus, R. "Coping Theory and the Teaching of Coping Skills," in Davidson, P., *Behavioral Medicine*, v. 1, Brunner/Mazel, New York, 1980.

Schachter, S. "The Interaction of Cognitive and Physiological Determinants of Emotional State," in Spielberger, C., *Anxiety and Behavior*, Academic Press, New York, 1966.

Spielberger, C., and Sarason, I. *Stress and Anxiety*, v. 4, Hemisphere Publishing Corporation, Washington, D.C., 1977.

Watts, A. *Does It Matter*, Vintage Books, New York, 1968.

Yorde, B. "A Comparison of the Effects of Cognitive Restructuring, Relaxation Techniques, and Frontalis Electromyograph Biofeedback Training to Induce Low Arousal Responses to Stress," Unpublished Doctoral Dissertation, Ohio State University, Columbus, 1977.

CHAPTER 9

Physical Activity

I cannot, and should not, be cured of my stress but merely taught to enjoy it.

Hans Selye

Physical exercise is a stressor. Muscular effort triggers neuroendocrine arousal in the same way fight or flight situations do. Ironically, there is now evidence to indicate that physical activity can reduce anxiety, long-term stress reactivity, and the probability of encountering psychosomatic disease. We can say that physical activity is the body's natural mechanism for reducing psychogenic, physiological arousal.

In the design of the human body, physical activity was meant to release the initial arousal that leads to maladaptive stress. We have discussed techniques for dealing with the environment and the mind. Physical activity, which affects the body directly, represents a third technique. As we will discover, physical activity can alter several levels of the psychosomatic model via somatopsychic feedback and the nature of the various activities themselves. Physical activity produces such profound and essential benefits that it represents an irreplaceable component of overall human health.

Consider this example from the animal world. A few years ago a small change was made at the National Zoo in Washington, D.C. Zoo personnel noticed that many of the animals were lethargic, seemed depressed, and were displaying hostile physical behavior toward each other (fighting, hair pulling, spitting, etc.). They decided to change the way they fed the animals. Instead of just flopping food down in front of an animal twice a day, they started hiding it in the animal's living environment. The animals had to search actively for their food if they wanted to eat. The result? The animals perked up, they stopped doing nasty things to each other, and positive physical behavior (grooming, licking, etc.) reappeared. The animals seemed much happier.

Animals are naturally physically active when aroused, so physical activity did not emerge as a way to control stress. Rather, stress emerged as one result of the disappearance of regular muscular exertion from our life-style.

The comforts and machines of contemporary life have made muscular work largely unnecessary. We no longer hunt for food, we stroll through grocery aisles. We do not attack one another physically, we argue and reason. We can survive without exerting ourselves physically, so we choose not to bother. We ignore the fact that physical activity is essential for the long-term, healthy functioning of any animal. In primitive conditions, we were always active, so few physiological stress problems existed. Technical and social changes have enticed us into becoming more sedentary and hence more prone to stress. A general awareness of the vast health benefits of physical exercise has appeared only in the last decade.

GOALS OF PHYSICAL ACTIVITY

We can view the goals of physical exercise from the perspectives of physical training and stress management. From a physical training standpoint, cardiovascular fitness is the first goal of exercise. As a result of an appropriate physical conditioning program the regular increased demand for blood flow by the skeletal muscles will stimulate growth and strength development of the myocardium and collateralization of coronary and peripheral arteries. The result is greater efficiency of the entire cardiovascular system, along with increased strength and redundancy to act as buffers against cardiovascular disease. A second goal of training is increased skeletal muscle tone and flexibility. An increase in muscular tone (not necessarily volume) results in a more positive physical appearance, which in itself may relieve a little stress.

From the standpoint of stress management, there are three goals of regular physical activity. First, muscular exercise should detoxify the body. In other words, it should burn off the stress-related hormones that perpetuate the arousal response. Second, exercise should decrease physical stress reactivity either through direct somatopsychic feedback or by altering cognitive states in a manner that decreases anxiety and other forms of maladaptive mental arousal. Finally, an exercise program should strengthen the internal organ systems in a manner that will make them more resistant to psychosomatic disease.

THE ESSENCE OF PHYSICAL ACTIVITY

Our discussion of physical activity will center around **aerobic exercise** or sustained, vigorous movement. By definition aerobic exercise increases the metabolic demands of the body, increases oxygen consumption, and places the cardiovascular and respiratory systems in a eustress condition. Aerobic exercise is designed to condition cardiovascular fitness. Any activity that involves continuous, sustained muscular action that elevates metabolic activity and cardiorespiratory activity is considered aerobic exercise. This type of physical activity is particularly effective for detoxifying the body of stress-released hormones and for conditioning long-term reductions in stress reactivity.

To facilitate a reduction in psychophysiological arousal, you should practice vigorous, sustained muscular activity. Examples of aerobic activities include running, swimming, cycling, and playing tennis. Activities like weight lifting or bowling are not aerobic activities and will produce no significant arousal reduction benefit because they do not involve continuous movement and sustained metabolic demand. For regular practice, choose whatever aerobic activity you enjoy the most. Exercise should not be dreaded, it should be enjoyed. Go out and play!

To condition your cardiovascular system and trophotrophically tune your psycho-somatic self, you need to perform an aerobic exercise for about 20 minutes at a stretch at least three times a week. Some evidence suggests that the body begins to decondition after only three days so three days of practice each week is desirable. This means running about 4 kilometers, swimming about 1 kilometer, or pedaling about 10 kilometers three days each week.

   Do not jump right into a heavy exercise program from a cold start. Work up to a conditioning level gradually. Push yourself only to a comfortable limit and always compete only with your own reasonable and safe level of ability. It is also a good idea to consult with your physician prior to beginning in order to establish a safe and smooth start and to set maximal tolerance limits for your body.

   For a comprehensive guide to aerobic exercise, see *The New Aerobics*, by Ken Cooper.

THE ROLE OF PHYSICAL ACTIVITY IN STRESS MANAGEMENT

   Physical activity can be used in a comprehensive stress management program as a somatopsychic technique for regular conditioning of decreased physical arousal and stress reactivity. Physical exercise represents a paradoxically effective method for achieving a trophotrophically tuned psychophysiological condition. (The term trophotrophic response, which is discussed in detail in the following chapter, basically means a relaxed reaction.)

   Physical exercise is just one of many options you can use to condition a trophotrophic response to stressors. Meditation, exercise, autogenic training, or progressive relaxation can all be equally effective. It makes little difference which technique you use, so long as you find it effective and it suits your life-style and personality. For overall health, however, there is no substitute for physical activity. Within reasonable, individual limits, everyone should engage in regular, muscular effort in the interest of personal health. We must return the physical activity component to our daily existence or suffer the consequences of disease, premature death, lethargy, excess weight, and a generally out of tune physical being. Even the mind cannot perform at its best when you are a physical waste.

VARIETIES OF STRESS-ALLEVIATING PHYSICAL ACTIVITY

   Two other types of physical activity that can be beneficial for dealing with stress are sexual activity and participation in high-risk sports.

   Of all the things we will discuss, sexual activity is far and away the nicest for controlling stress. This fact has little to do with physiological change or sensory experience. It is true because sexual activity represents one of the closest ways in which you can share an experience with another human being.

   There are, however, some biological changes accompanying sexual activity that can be beneficial for controlling stress. Perhaps the most interesting benefit is part of a recent discovery that is still little understood. Intense emotional experience can help trigger the release of hormonelike substances call beta-endorphins from areas of the brain that are functionally related to the pituitary. Endorphins have a close chemical resemblance to morphine. The analgesic (pain blocking) properties of morphine are well known, and the endorphins seem to produce a similar effect naturally. The release of these chemicals provides a natural mechanism for blocking the sensation of physical pain. It is possible that sexual activity can cause the release of endorphins within the brain and therefore eliminate all kinds of pain sensation. For example, it has been reported that sexual activity can significantly reduce arthritic pain for more than 12 hours. The possible release of beta-endorphins via sexual activity may represent a neurochemical antithesis to the onset of psychogenic stress.

Even in the context of controlling somatic stress, however, the potential physiological changes associated with sexual activity are of minor importance compared to the interpersonal effects. Recall that one of the most profound psychosocial stressors is social isolation. Intimate physical contact is perhaps the most powerful weapon we have against the devastating effects of loneliness.

Many people find that participating in high-risk sports is a powerful means of keeping stress under control. Evidence suggests that a tremendous endorphin release occurs during high-risk activities. In wartime combat situations, it is common for soldiers to be seriously injured and not realize they are hurt for hours because of the emotional intensity of the situation. Minor injuries and lacerations commonly occur during such sports as rock climbing, whitewater rafting, and hang gliding, but the pain is rarely felt as severely as it would be at the office or during a relaxed evening at home. The emotional rush, or possibly endorphin release, during high-risk activity effectively blocks the sensation of pain.

Researchers have recently suggested that some individuals have a kind of epinephrine addiction. These people need to experience stress regularly or they go through cognitive and physical withdrawal. The implication is that their bodies crave high serum concentrations of catecholamines. Such persons may be workaholics, Type As, mercenaries, or thrill seekers in general. If this is a valid phenomenon, it makes more sense to get your epinephrine fix from physical activity than from psychogenic stressors and sedentary behavior. Why not choose eustress over distress?

High-risk behavior provides a tremendous sensation of emotional cleansing. Standing on top of a pinnacle in the Tetons after a difficult two-day vertical climb or landing your glider after a five-hour powerless flight fighting through the turbulent winds of a mountain pass leaves a person totally drained of emotion and crystal clear in thought and sensation. When you have faced your own mortality and struggled to survive through skill and force of will, it is unlikely that parking tickets, phone bills, and midterm examinations are going to upset you. By their nature, high-risk sports set the human spirit free. The ineffable feeling of transcendent peace and calm that follows such activity can last for weeks and sometimes changes a person's life forever. The magnitude of the reward is in direct proportion to the risk.

THEORETICAL MECHANISMS OF EFFECTIVENESS

Physical exercise is a paradox. It is a stressor. It triggers catecholamine and corticoid release. Yet evidence indicates that it can help condition a trophotrophic response pattern and decrease anxiety. The question is how exercise operates physiologically. During exercise the body experiences the biochemical correlates of the stress response; following exercise, the body is in a trophotrophic state. Exercise usually elicits a greater magnitude of endocrine release than does the typical psychogenic stressor. During vigorous physical activity, the stress-related hormones disappear from the body and arousal is effected much more quickly than in the absence of a physically exerting response. The comparison between an exercise response and a sedentary response to a psychogenic stressor is illustrated in Figure 9.1.

In this figure, the arrow represents the onset of the stressor or the exercise period. Exercise initially triggers high arousal (such as high serum concentrations of catecholamines), but note that arousal returns to a resting level very quickly, in contrast to the delayed return in the absence of exercise. Remember that to produce a pathogenic condition, maladaptive arousal must be sustained. Notice also that before returning to the

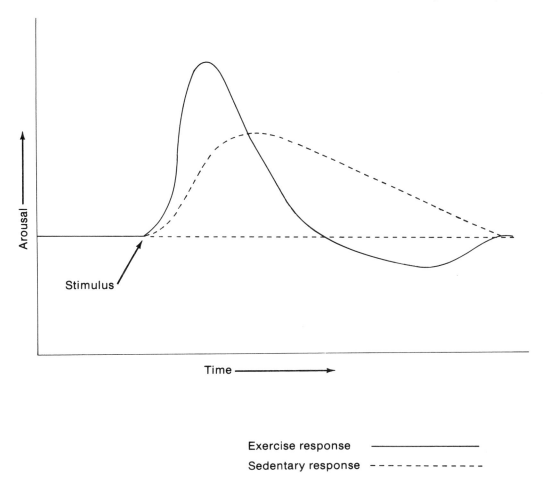

Exercise response ——————————

Sedentary response – – – – – – – – – – –

Figure 9.1. Somatic arousal response to exercise.

baseline, arousal goes lower than the resting state for a time after physical exertion. This is called a **parasympathetic rebound**. It may represent the body's effort to balance homeostatically the previous arousal. Obviously, physical exercise represents a healthier response than does sedentary behavior.

No one yet knows how exercise operates physiologically to relieve stress. There are at least two theories. First, since physical activity is a stressor, it may deplete the adrenals of catecholamines and corticoids, or it may use up all the ACTH from the pituitary or all the CRF from the hypothalamus, and so on. This **depletion theory** sounds plausible, but there is as yet only weak evidence to support it. A more likely explanation is called the **detoxification theory**. According to this theory, exercise detoxifies the stress-related hormones quickly. This means it gets them out of the body fast. Detoxification could be the result of overall stepped-up metabolism during exercise, or exercise could release stress hormones and an as-yet theoretical detoxifying enzyme at the same time. There is some evidence to support this theory, but the details are unclear. Exercise does reduce serum concentrations of stress hormones quickly, but we do not know how.

ADDITIONAL STRESS-RELATED BENEFITS

Exercise also results in cognitive changes that are beneficial for stress control. Decreased anxiety is one of these effects. People who exercise regularly find it difficult to become upset over anything after a hard workout. Perhaps the parasympathetic rebound has a calming influence on the mind. A peripheral benefit is the wonderful enhancement of self-esteem that accompanies good physical fitness.

Finally, physical exercise strengthens some of the organ systems that are attacked by stress, thereby reducing the probability of encountering disease.

CONTRAINDICATIONS AND COMMON DIFFICULTIES

Although vigorous physical activity is highly beneficial for stress management and physical health, it is a profound immediate stressor. Aerobic activity places a significant demand on the visceral organs, particularly the heart. You need to be aware of your physical condition before undertaking a strenuous exercise routine. As mentioned previously, it is highly advisable to consult with your physician before you start no matter how physically fit you think you are. It is also advisable, particularly if you are over 30, to have a complete cardiovascular fitness assessment. It will be well worth the expense. You will get the information you need to establish an exercise plan and maximum tolerance limits for your personal fitness level and current cardiovascular condition.

Other physical activities carry their own contraindications and cautions. Sex is rarely contraindicated for anyone. High-risk sports are wonderful for the individual spirit, but you must consider whether you are risking the well-being of other people in your life when you indulge in them.

WHAT TO EXPECT FROM PHYSICAL ACTIVITY

You should notice signs of increased endurance and stronger cardiac performance after a few months of regular aerobic activity. You will notice that you are not so out of breath when you run up flights of stairs or have to dash after a bus. You may also observe that while you are just sitting your heart is beating slower and stronger than before. Exercise makes the heart a stronger, more efficient pump. The result is that it does not need to beat as often to meet the body's need for blood flow, which gives it more time between each beat to nourish itself. You can plot this progressive increase in efficiency by taking and recording your pulse as soon as you wake up (and before you move around) each morning. If you chart your resting pulse rate over time, you will notice that it will begin to decrease steadily after a few weeks.

Most sedentary people think exercise drains energy and leaves a person tired and unfit to perform the rest of the day's activities. This is not the case. If you exercise in the beginning or middle of the day, your mind will clear and you will have much more working energy than if you just sit. No one yet knows why, but regular exercise is an effective way to combat fatigue. You do not spend energy, you gain it. Your increase in mental clarity, work efficiency, and stamina may even make up for the time you spend exercising. Exercise will make you feel so good you will wonder how you ever got along without it.

Many people report an increased sense of calm and decreased general anxiety as a result of regular, vigorous exercise. Again, no one understands why this happens, but active people commonly report that for several hours after hard physical exertion, it is difficult to get upset over anything.

Finally, because exercise tones the musculature and helps burn off unnecessary fat, you will be better looking. Also, high-risk sports may give you some handsome battle scars to show off to your friends, and sex is good for your self-esteem.

SUMMARY

Physical exercise is a natural mechanism of the body for preventing the harmful effects of stress. It effectively detoxifies the products of fight or flight arousal and terminates the lingering physiological changes that can ultimately wear out the body. At the same time, it strengthens the internal organ systems.

Physical activity is effective for managing stress because it can intervene in the psychosomatic model at many points, thereby affecting physical arousal, cognitive appraisal, and emotional arousal levels. Most highly effective stress management techniques operate on multiple facets of the reaction to stress in this manner.

Besides helping to control the experience of psychogenic stress, physical exercise is essential for enhancing personal health. It is irreplaceable in promoting high-level mental and physical well-being.

REFERENCES

Bellet, S., et al. "Effect of Physical Exercise on Adrenocortical Excretion," *Metabolism*, v. 18, 484-487, 1969.

Birrell, P., and Roscoe, C. "Effects of Intensive Aerobic Exercise on Stress Reactivity and Myocardial Morphology in Rats," *Physiology and Behavior*, v. 20, 687-692, 1979.

Buuck, R., and Tharp, G. "Effect of Chronic Exercise on Adrenocortical Function and Structure in the Rat," *Journal of Applied Physiology*, v. 31, 880-883, 1971.

Collingwood, T. "The Effects of Physical Training Upon Behavior and Self Attitudes," *Journal of Clinical Psychology*, v. 28, 583-585, 1971.

Connell, A. M., et al. "The Contrasting Effects of Emotional Tension and Physical Exercise on the Excretion of 17-Ketogenic Steroids and 17-Ketosteroids," *ACTA Endocrinologica*, v. 27, 179-194, 1958.

Cooper, K. H. *The New Aerobics*, Bantam Books, New York, 1970.

Davies, C. T. M., and Few, J. D. "Effects of Exercise on Adrenocortical Function," *Journal of Applied Physiology*, v. 35, 887-891, 1973.

Davies, C. T. M., et al. "Plasma Catecholamine Concentration During Dynamic Exercise Involving Different Muscle Groups," *European Journal of Applied Physiology*, v. 32, 195-206, 1974.

de Vries, H. A. "Immediate and Long Term Effects of Exercise Upon Resting Muscle Action Potential," *Journal of Sports Medicine and Physical Fitness*, v. 1, 1-11, 1968.

de Vries, H. A., and Adams, G. M. "Electromyographic Comparison of Single Doses of Exercise and Meprobamate as to Effect on Muscular Relaxation," *American Journal of Physical Medicine*, v. 51, 130-149, 1972.

Few, J. D. "Effect of Exercise on the Secretion and Metabolism of Cortisol in Man," *Journal of Endocrinology*, v. 62, 341-353, 1974.

Folkins, C. H., and Amsterdam, E. A. "Control and Modification of Stress Emotions Through Chronic Exercise," in Amsterdam, E. A., et al., *Exercise in Cardiovascular Health and Disease*, Yorke Medical Books, New York, 1978.

Folkins, C. H., et al. "Psychological Fitness as a Function of Physical Fitness," *Archives of Physical Medicine and Rehabilitation*, v. 53, 503-508, 1972.

Galbo, H., et al. "Diminished Hormonal Responses to Exercise in Trained Rats," *Journal of Applied Physiology*, v. 43, 953-958, 1977.

————. "Hormonal Regulation During Prolonged Exercise," *Annals of the New York Academy of Sciences*, v. 301, 72-80, 1977.

Gilbert, M., et al. "Anxiety Reduction Following Acute Physical Activity," Unpublished Doctoral Dissertation, University of Wisconsin-LaCrosse, 1972.

Ismail, A. H., and Trachtman, L. E. "Jogging the Imagination," *Psychology Today*, v. 7, 79-82, Mar. 1973.

Lyon, L. S. "Psychological Effects of Jogging: A Preliminary Study," *Perceptual and Motor Skills*, v. 47, 1215-1218, 1978.

McPherson, B. D., et al. "Psychological Effects of an Exercise Program for Post-infarction and Normal Adult Men," *Journal of Sports Medicine*, v. 1, 95-102, 1967.

Michael, E. D. "Stress Adaptation Through Exercise," *Research Quarterly*, v. 28, 51-53, 1957.

Mitchum, M. L. "The Effects of Participation in a Physically Exerting Leisure Activity on State Anxiety Levels," Unpublished Master's Thesis, University of Florida, Gainesville, 1976.

Morgan, W. P., et al. "Use of Exercise as a Relaxation Technique," *Journal of South Carolina Medical Association*, v. 75(11), 596-601, 1979.

Morris, A. F., and Husman, F. B. "Life Quality Changes Following an Endurance Conditioning Program," *American Corrective Therapy Journal*, v. 32(1), 3-6, 1978.

Ostman, I., and Sjuständ, N. "Effect of Prolonged Physical Training on the Catecholamine Levels of the Heart and Adrenals of the Rat," *ACTA Physiology Scandinavia*, 82, 202-208, 1971.

————. "Reduced Urinary Noradrenaline Excretion During Rest, Exercise, and Cold Stress in Trained Rats: A Comparison Between Physically Trained Rats, Cold Acclimatized Rats and Warm Acclimatized Rats," *ACTA Physiology Scandinavia*, v. 95, 209-218, 1975.

Sarviharju, P. J. "Effect of Physical Exercise on the Urinary Excretion of Catecholamines and 17-Hydroxycorticosteroids in Young Healthy Men," *Journal of Sports Medicine and Physical Fitness*, v. 13, 171-176, 1973.

Tharp, G. D., and Buuck, J. R. "Adrenal Adaptation to Chronic Exercise," *Journal of Applied Physiology*, v. 37, 720-722, 1974.

Ulrich, C. "Stress and Sports," in Johnson, W. R., *Science and Medicine of Exercise and Sports*, Harper and Row, New York, 1960.

Viru, A., and Akke, H. "Effects of Muscular Work on Cortisol and Corticosterone Content in the Blood and Adrenals of Guinea Pigs," *ACTA Endocrinologica*, v. 62, 385-390, 1969.

Walsh, R., and Davidson, G. P. "Desensitization to Lactic Acid as a Possible Mechanism Mediating the Therapeutic Effect of Physical Exercise on Anxiety Neurosis," *Journal of Sports Medicine and Physical Fitness*, v. 20(2), 158-160, 1980.

Young, R. J. "The Effect of Regular Exercise on Cognitive Functioning and Personality," *British Journal of Sports Medicine*, v. 13, 110-117, 1979.

Young R. J., and Ismael, A. H. "Personality Differences of Adult Men Before and After a Physical Fitness Program," *Research Quarterly*, v. 47(3), 513-519, 1977.

CHAPTER 10

Theoretical Foundations of Systematic Relaxation

Relaxation is ease: giving in, letting go. Letting in; open flow; giving out. The natural state of the organism. A condition which nerves, muscles experience full sensation; set their within tone.

Bernard Gunther

We have presented techniques that facilitate stress control by operating on the environment (by minimizing stressors), the mind (by reappraising perceived events), or the body (by detoxifying the system or changing the pattern of somatic reactivity). Systematic relaxation techniques can be considered hybrids; they are capable of managing stress by intervening at many levels of the psychosomatic model. They can act on the mind, the body, and even the environment. Relaxation represents one of our most useful stress control tools because of the multifaceted nature of its effectiveness.

Systematic relaxation techniques are designed to reduce psychophysiological arousal. They produce a hypometabolic response pattern that is often the antithesis of stress. Relaxation methods can affect the disease of stress in its early stages; they represent a countermeasure for maladaptive arousal. Unlike medical treatments such as drug therapy, hormonal manipulation, or surgery, the secondary effects of systematic relaxation have beneficial effects on the body and on human performance capabilities.

This and the following two chapters explore the domains of systematic relaxation, altered states of consciousness, and sensory awareness. The material presented in these three chapters should give you a clear idea of the nature, effects, and appropriate implementation of relaxation before you learn specific techniques. If you first acquire an understanding of relaxation, the effectiveness of the individual techniques will be enhanced immeasurably.

MISCONCEPTIONS ABOUT RELAXATION

What do you think of when you hear the word relaxation? If someone tells you to go relax, what do you do? Stop reading and make a mental list of the things you do most often when you want to relax. If you are like most people, your list includes things like watching television, sleeping, soaking in a hot tub, sunbathing, listening to music, reading a novel, having a drink or a smoke, and going to a ballgame. We associate such activities with relaxation, but most of them are actually stressors because they either evoke emotional responses or require some cognitive or somatic adaptation.

There are four general misconceptions about relaxation. The first is that relaxation is associated with leisure activities. Most of the time, leisure activities are stressors. They either stimulate our emotional arousal, as in the case of television shows or exciting sporting events, or they require adaptation, as in the case of afternoon trips or vacations. As a general construct, we will not equate leisure with systematic relaxation.

The second misconception is that sleep is relaxation. Have you ever awakened from a full night's sleep and felt more tired than when you went to bed? Have you ever awakened in a sweat from the emotional response to an intense dream? One distinction between relaxation and sleep is that sleep has emotionally charged phases. The content of dreams represents a significant release of emotions unconsciously suppressed during waking life. Sleep can be a stressor.

The primary distinction between sleep and relaxation is that sleep is a psycho-physiologically dynamic state and relaxation is a stable state. During sleep, we go through many shifts in mental and physical arousal. Besides relatively random shifts in arousal throughout sleeping periods, regular 90-minute cycles of arousal exist. The result is that the body uses its resources to adapt to this ever-changing internal arousal. Although sleep involves periods of low arousal, it is fundamentally dynamic, which distinguishes it from true relaxation.

The arousal difference between sleep and relaxation is illustrated in Figure 10.1. The dashed line indicates base level arousal, the solid curve represents relaxation, and the dotted curve indicates sleep arousal levels. This figure illustrates that although sleep may elicit periods of arousal lower than those produced by systematic relaxation, relaxation is a stable plateau of somatic functioning, whereas sleep requires constant adaptation.

Whether high or low, dynamic arousal constantly calls the mechanisms of homeostasis into play. By definition, this adaptation effort is stress. Adjusting to increases and decreases in arousal requires the use of somatic resources. Real relaxation involves restoring products within the body (hormones, neurotransmitters, enzymes, etc.) that have been depleted during normal daily activity. Low arousal will help in this effort, but not if resources are being used for making adjustments. The stable arousal of relaxation allows the body to restore itself by temporarily eliminating the demands of adaptation.

Remember that one distinction between the sympathetic and parasympathetic nervous systems is that the sympathetics initiate change and adjustment whereas the parasympathetics stabilize functioning. The sympathetics are the adjusting, adapting, stress-related nerve tracts. The parasympathetics promote stability and somatic restoration. Stress begins as a sympathetic nervous system phenomenon; relaxation is a parasympathetic state.

The third misconception about relaxation is that it produces a state similar to that induced by tranquilizing drugs. Tranquilizers depress the nervous system, sensation, and awareness. Relaxation stimulates the nervous system, particularly the parasympathetic system. Drugs help a person "cope" by turning off sensation and awareness, whereas relaxation enhances sensation and increases awareness while relaxing the body. Again, the state produced by relaxation is not the same as that produced by depressants like tranquilizers and alcohol.

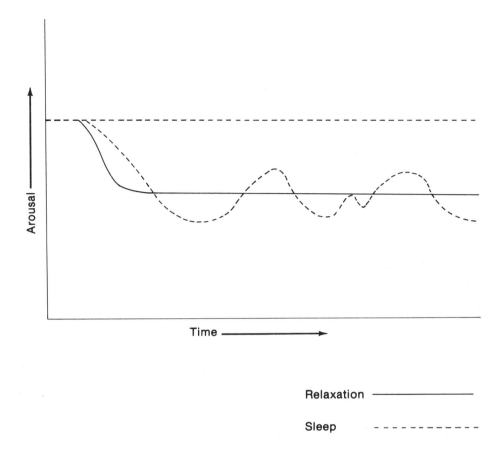

Figure 10.1. Arousal patterns of systematic relaxation versus sleep.

Finally, relaxation does not involve mental passivity. Think back to your list of relaxing activities. Most of them probably allow you to turn off your mind, sit back, and not be responsible for anything. Systematic relaxation, on the other hand, involves concentration and deliberate mental activity in order to achieve and maintain a steady plateau of low arousal. Relaxation requires some cognitive effort. When you begin practicing relaxation, it will probably "feel" different from what you expect.

To summarize, relaxation is *not* leisure, sleep, a state similar to that induced by tranquilizing drugs, or mental passivity. Rather, *relaxation involves activities that stabilize and maintain mental and physical arousal at a reduced level*. Relaxation involves a deliberate effort to stabilize and maintain low psychophysiological arousal.

VARIETIES OF RELAXATION TRAINING

There are two basic forms of relaxation training. **Centralized** forms initiate low arousal at the center of control—the mind. **Peripheral** techniques first relax the periphery—the body. The distinction is whether the effort to relax begins in the mind or in the body. More descriptive labels are **psychosomatic** relaxation, which begins with the mind, and **somatopsychic** relaxation, which begins with the body. Although they start in different places, both types of relaxation reduce arousal in both the mind and the body. Most forms of relaxation fit into one of these two categories.

Centralized, or psychosomatic, forms of relaxation begin with the mind and are effective in the early phases of the psychosomatic model. They have a generalized somatic effect on the body, altering activity in most organ systems. This type of relaxation is most effective for the general or random stress responder. A **general responder** reacts to stress with some activity in almost all systems. In such a person, the stress reaction is generalized throughout the body in response to almost any stressor. **Random responders** react to stress in different organ systems on different occasions; sometimes heart rate goes up, sometimes gastric movement ceases, sometimes excessive sweating occurs. Both of these responder types derive benefit from centralized techniques because they reduce activity in all organ systems. Examples of centralized, or psychosomatic, relaxation techniques include meditation, selective awareness techniques like hypnosis and guided imagery, and electroencephalographic (brainwave) biofeedback training.

Peripheral, or somatopsychic, techniques begin by reducing arousal at one of the end organs. These methods are effective at the physical effects level of the psychosomatic model. They mainly alter the target organ system, but they can have generalized effects by decreasing feedback in the psychosomatic model. Peripheral methods are useful for **rigid stress responders**—people who always respond to stress in a particular organ system, regardless of the situation. Peripheral techniques can focus the relaxation effort on the specific, problematic organ system. Such techniques are more physiologically specific than are centralized methods. Examples of peripheral, or somatopsychic, relaxation techniques include progressive neuromuscular relaxation, yoga, breath control, and most biofeedback training parameters.

EFFECTS OF RELAXATION

The specific effects of relaxation training will be discussed in detail as we discuss each technique in subsequent chapters. The principal effect of relaxation training is a physiological condition that is the antithesis of the stress response. According to Benson (1974), just as there is a human stress response, there is also a definable, physiological relaxation response that can be induced through systematic relaxation.

An important facet of the psychophysiological state produced by systematic relaxation training is that elements of it extend beyond the actual practice session. By virtue of regular relaxation practice, a person will have lowered reactivity to stressors throughout the day. This specific type of carryover effect is also called **trophotrophic tuning**.

The trophotrophic tuning concept is derived from the ideas of Gellhorn (1972), who indicated that there are two types of responses to a psychogenic stimulus: an **ergotrophic response** and a **trophotrophic response**. The ergotrophic response is a **hypermetabolic**, mobilization reaction. A trophotrophic response is a **hypometabolic**, relaxed reaction. By definition, we respond ergotrophically to stressors. In fact, most of us are ergotrophically tuned, or conditioned to respond in an uptight, hyperaroused fashion to many nonthreatening events. Think about how you have taught yourself to get upset when you have to stand and wait in long lines or when you have to stop for a traffic light. Even when you are not in any particular hurry, you may still get tense because you are ergotrophically tuned.

It is possible, however, to recondition yourself to respond to events in a trophotrophic, or relaxed, fashion. To do this, you must regularly experience trophotrophic states in order to make this a familiar pathway of psychosomatic reactivity. The more often you practice systematic relaxation and trophotrophic responses to potential stressors, the more likely it will be that you will naturally begin to react to life's sudden difficulties in a relaxed manner. As you recall from Chapter 1, our biological evolution is not capable of changing our bodies fast enough to help us adapt to a rapidly changing sociocultural environment. We must learn to take control ourselves.

Relaxation can intervene effectively in the etiology of psychosomatic disease, but its greatest potential lies in the prevention of disease. Generally, relaxation methods are of limited value in treating an existing disease. Use relaxation to gain control over your psychosomatic stress reactivity now; do not wait until you are sick.

Besides its psychophysiological effects, there is growing evidence to suggest that relaxation training has several positive side effects for cognition, perception, and human performance. Relaxation training may be capable of enhancing attention span, clarity of thought, and sensory acuity. In at least one investigation, grade point averages increased in students who practiced one form of systematic relaxation.

CONTRAINDICATIONS

Relaxation training lowers arterial blood pressure and blood sugar levels. If you have hypotension (chronically low blood pressure) or hypoglycemia (low blood sugar), relaxation training may exacerbate the condition. If you have either of these, consult your physician before you begin training.

Some medical conditions improve as the result of relaxation training. If you are taking regular medication for hypertension, diabetes, or epilepsy, your physician should periodically monitor the appropriateness of your dosage. This is necessary because you may get a little better, making overmedication a possibility. Relaxation training is not harmful to persons with these conditions. If you have one of them, just consult with your physician as you learn to relax.

SUMMARY

Systematic relaxation intervenes in the etiology of psychosomatic disease by altering many levels of the psychosomatic model of stress reactivity. Ideally, systematic relaxation reduces cognitive and somatic arousal and stress reactivity, while tuning out the maladaptive static in the mind and body that serves as a barrier to optimal human performance.

REFERENCES

Allen, R. J. *Relaxation Exercises for Controlling Stress and Tension*, Autumn Wind, College Park, Md., 1979.

Allen, R. J., and Hyde, D. H. *Investigations in Stress Control*, Ed. 2, Burgess, Minneapolis, Minn., 1981.

Benson, H., et al. "The Relaxation Response," *Psychiatry*, v. 37(1), 37-46, 1974.

Gellhorn, E., and Kiely, W. F. "Mystical States of Consciousness: Neurophysiological and Clinical Aspects," *Journal of Nervous and Mental Disease*, v. 154(6), 399-405, 1972.

Gunther, B. *Sense Relaxation*, Macmillan, New York, 1968.

Pagano, R. R., et al. "Sleep During Transcendental Meditation," *Science*, v. 191(4224), 308-310, 1976.

Walrath, L. C., and Hamilton, D. W. "Autonomic Correlates of Meditation and Hypnosis," *American Journal of Clinical Hypnosis*, v. 17(3), 190-197, 1975.

White, J., and Fadiman, J. *Relax*, Dell, Pine Brook, N.J., 1976.

Younger, J., et al. "Sleep During Transcendental Meditation," *Perceptual and Motor Skills*, v. 40(3), 953-954, 1975.

CHAPTER 11

Altered States
of Consciousness

These two ways of thinking, the way of time and history and the way of eternity and timelessness, are both parts of man's effort to comprehend the world in which he lives. Neither is comprehended in the other, nor reducible to it; each supplementing the other, neither telling the whole story.

Robert Oppenheimer

Two modes of thought. Two modes of knowing. Two modes of human understanding and consciousness. For thousands of years, human beings have understood that there are two distinct ways in which to know and experience existence. There is a rational mode—analytic, time-centered, verbal, and structured—and there is an intuitive mode—experiential, timeless, holistic, and receptive. Both of these modes are equally real. Both of them are equally valid ways to understand and to know about those things that are accessible to our consciousness. We can experience the sensory delights of a misty early morning sunrise, and we can try to describe how refraction patterns in the atmosphere created the rainbow of colors. We can experience the ineffable sensation of love, and we can strive to communicate it by attaching words to our feelings. Within human consciousness there is a mode of operation that feels, senses, and receives and there is one that analyzes, thinks, and evaluates.

Robert Ornstein (1972) has called this duality of operation within the human mind the **theory of bimodal consciousness**. This theory asserts that there are two qualitative patterns to human consciousness—one analytic and one intuitive. These have been called the **normal state of consciousness** and the **altered state of consciousness**. The term normal simply refers to the state that occurs most frequently. It does not imply that the normal state of consciousness is the only one that is valid. As we will see, both modes of consciousness are required for the healthy and creative functioning of the human mind. Altered states of consciousness are simply deviations from the type of thought we normally associate with waking life.

Many of the mechanisms we use to control stress were designed not to alter physiological functioning, but to facilitate a shift in state of consciousness. This is particularly true of activities like meditation, yoga, guided imagery, and hypnosis. Most of the relaxation techniques covered in subsequent chapters involve the induction of some mild altered states.

The experience of altered states of consciousness is a normal part of everyday life, but we do not often associate it with waking life. The changes in the way the mind works under an altered state are perfectly natural and normal, although they may seem strange at first.

One note before we begin: There is evidence to suggest that the ability to achieve altered states is associated with one's ability to learn to control autonomic functions and ultimately gain a high degree of control over the experience of stress or gain high levels of personal health and well-being.

WHAT ARE ALTERED STATES OF CONSCIOUSNESS?

Charles Tart (1969) has provided us with the most widely accepted definition for an altered state of consciousness. It is, he says, "a qualitative shift in the pattern of mental functioning." He emphasizes that an altered state is not necessarily a quantitative shift in consciousness. A person experiencing an altered state is not more or less conscious, more or less alert, or more or less awake. An altered state represents a qualitative change in the way the mind operates that differs from the state of consciousness we normally associate with waking life.

Perhaps the best way to understand an altered state is to use some examples. According to Andrew Weil (1972), we have an innate drive to experience altered states of consciousness. Think of how much time we spend sleeping and daydreaming. Think of all the antics children perform—like spinning around in circles until they get dizzy—to change consciousness for a moment. When people are not allowed to experience their normal altered states of consciousness, particularly sleep, nature induces such states for them. The thought patterns of someone who is deprived of sleep for an extended time become strange indeed, often resulting in hallucinations, changes in body image, and manic depressive states. The regular experience of altered states seems critical to the healthy functioning of the mind.

Sleep, the most common example of an altered state of consciousness, is characterized by a variety of different states of consciousness, including periods of near total unconsciousness and periods of visually creative dreams. In fact, few altered states that are induced through external means can compare to the imaginative fireworks that go on during dreaming.

Highway hypnosis is another interesting example of an altered state that occurs in normal life. This phenomenon often occurs when we drive for long periods of time or over familiar roads. You can be driving across familiar territory when suddenly you notice you have gone 10 or 15 miles and have no recollection of it. You cannot remember driving, you cannot remember passing familiar landmarks, and you have no recollection of the passage of time. You wonder why you are still alive and how you drove the car. (Some people, it turns out, actually drive more cautiously during this state.) Highway hypnosis contains many of the essential characteristics of an altered state of consciousness. It involves a loss of immediate memory, a sense of timelessness, and intensive, focused awareness.

Watching a movie is another good example of an altered state. While we watch, we feel the emotions of the characters and forget about our own lives. Next time you go to a movie, look around. Observe the other people in the theater. They are totally unaware of what is going on in the real world. Their minds, for a time, are in a different place. They are in an altered state of consciousness.

COMPARISONS BETWEEN NORMAL AND ALTERED STATES OF CONSCIOUSNESS

In a general sense, the normal state of consciousness is characterized by *structure* and the altered state of consciousness is characterized by *experience*. During a normal state of consciousness, our thinking is mainly in terms of patterns and structures. We label our sensations and experiences. The normal state of consciousness is characterized by a constant internal dialogue; we convert experiences into words. We take all our observations and fit them into some kind of cerebral model or categorize them and shove them into a pigeonhole. In the normal state, we are more concerned with the models and the pigeonholes than with the experience itself.

During altered states, the mind focuses on the sensory experience itself. Rather than think, we experience and feel. The altered state is sometimes described as destructured consciousness. Our models of reality and our pigeonholing systems come apart. We feel no need to describe things to ourselves, and we tend not to evaluate things in terms of preexisting models or ideas.

The following lists show the complementary characteristics and orientations of the two states:

Normal State	Altered State
Verbal	Spatial
Intellectual	Experiential
Analytic	Holistic
Time oriented	Spatially oriented
Active	Receptive
Ego involved	Self-transcendent
Judgmental	Accepting

Verbal Versus Spatial. Since it is a state concerned with ideas and structures, the normal state of consciousness is permeated with verbal descriptions. Every time we have a sensation, our mind puts it into words. In fact, we often define thought in terms of this constant internal verbal chatter. We believe that when we think about something, we are talking about it to ourselves. Some people have even raised the absurd question of whether thought can exist in the absence of language. The altered state, we say, is more spatial than verbal. During altered states of consciousness, verbal description is considered banal. The altered state centers around experience, not the translation of experience into words. It is concerned with observing the spatial relationships of experience and sensation, not with categorizing those observations. In his essay "The Doors of Perception," Aldous Huxley described this distinction in a brief criticism of individuals who are stuck in the normal mode of consciousness. He speaks of "those resolute dead enders who have made up their minds to be content with the ersatz of Suchness, with symbols rather than what they signify, with the elegant precomposed recipe in lieu of the actual dinner."

Intellectual Versus Experiential. This contrast is close in character to the verbal-spatial contrast. In the normal mode, we think about things. In the altered state we simply experience them. Our intellectual processes are often associated with language. Intellect is believed to take observation and compare it to existing models or ideas. The altered state does not involve intellect because we are not hanging on to those cerebral structures. Rather we simply draw in life experiences. We make no attempt, in an altered state, to see experience as a component to an idea, just as we do not try to attach a verbal label to it.

Analytic Versus Holistic. Analysis is characterized by taking things apart. In the normal state, we try to understand something by breaking it into pieces, labeling each part, and trying to understand the whole as a collection of small pieces with their own function and character. Holistic thought means trying to understand something as the summation of its parts. In holistic thinking, one sees the commonalities between elements rather than the distinctions. The normal state understands by seeing how things come apart; the altered state understands by seeing how they go together.

Time Oriented Versus Spatially Oriented. The time orientation of the normal state of consciousness is just another example of the cerebral structures involved in normal thinking. Time is a concept created by the mind. Time is a cerebral structure that we attach to our observation of change in the natural world. The altered state is unconcerned with the passage of time. If you have experienced the highway hypnosis phenomenon you know that during such an altered state, time becomes unimportant and irrelevant. Rather than being centered around concepts like time, the altered state centers around spatial relationships, trying to see all the interrelationships between perceived factors rather than trying to quantify observations.

Active Versus Receptive. By active, we mean that in the normal state the mind tries to operate on the environment to change it and to make it fit its ideas. A mind in an altered state simply receives information. The normal state of consciousness is one that likes to be in control of surroundings; the altered state simply likes to experience those surroundings. The normal state manipulates. The altered state simply receives and learns.

Ego Involved Versus Self-Transcendent. In the normal state of consciousness, we have a keen sense of self and personal boundaries. We see ourselves as separate from the rest of the world. This falls in line with seeing distinctions rather than similarities. In the normal state of consciousness, we create an artificial shell around ourselves that in essence says this is me and anything outside this is something else. During altered states, we transcend differences. We do not see separateness. We no longer distinguish between what we consider ourselves and what we consider others. We see the commonalities. We dip into something of a transpersonal reality, where all things seem unified and all people are part of a larger, more comprehensive consciousness.

Judgmental Versus Accepting. Because normal consciousness carries with it many cerebral structures (ideas, categories, pigeonholes, etc.), it tends to evaluate or screen all incoming information and sensations. When we perceive something during a normal state of consciousness, we immediately categorize and evaluate it in relation to our existing mental constructs. During altered states, mental structures fall away, so that new sensations are experienced, not evaluated. We simply accept and perceive the sensations accessible to us without judging or categorizing them. The normal state attaches labels such as good or bad, threatening or nonthreatening, red or blue. The altered state places no value judgment or verbal label on any perception.

We could discuss many more distinctions, such as logical versus intuitive or controlling versus flowing, but all you need to remember is the primary distinction. The normal state is a structured state in which experience is compared, explained, and communicated in relation to constructs within the mind. The altered state is a destructured way of thinking in which reality is experienced and felt rather than labeled and evaluated.

The notion that the human mind operates in these two ways is called the theory of bimodal consciousness. There is evidence to suggest that philosophers who predate written history were aware of this duality and discussed the complementary nature of human consciousness. Some of the earliest written records go back to Kapila and Zarathustra, from the 6th century B.C. Both these philosophers discussed the dichotomous nature of reality and of human knowing. Written history is liberally sprinkled with references to the dichotomy of consciousness. Even though these references come from many different sources and cultures, they all say the same thing. Roger Bacon, the 13th century English scientist, wrote:

> There are two modes of knowing, those of argument and experience. They are complementary to one another. Neither is reducible to the other and their simultaneous working may be incompatible. One mode is verbal and rational, sequential in operation, orderly. The other is intuitive, tactic, diffuse in operation, less logical and neat, a mode we often devalue culturally, personally, and even physiologically.

(Ornstein 1972)

PHYSIOLOGICAL BASIS TO
THE THEORY OF BIMODAL CONSCIOUSNESS

New evidence has revealed that there may be a physiological basis to the bimodal consciousness theory. This evidence began with research following an unusual treatment for severe epilepsy. The findings from this research suggest that functionally we have two brains, that each may be capable of independent function and thought, and that each may operate in a different mode of consciousness.

Seizure Activity Within the Brain

Let us first look at what happens during a serious or grand mal epileptic seizure. During seizure activity within the brain, one or more neurons (or nerve cells) begin to fire spontaneously. No one knows for sure what initiates this activity, but it is thought that many things—such as flashing lights or emotional stress—can trigger this initial spontaneous firing of neurons. Through a process called recruitment, the original neurons begin to involve adjacent nerve cells, causing them to fire spontaneously as well. The seizure activity therefore spreads throughout the cerebral mass. Figure 11.1 illustrates a point of origin of seizure activity (it could be anywhere in the brain) and shows initial recruitment of adjacent nerve cells.

In this simple sketch, we see the brain from the top (looking down) and the cortex is represented as two structures connected by a bridge. In fact, the human brain has two cortical hemispheres that are connected by a central bridging structure called the corpus callosum, which ensures that the two halves of the cortex can communicate adequately with each other. During a grand mal seizure, the recruitment activity of nerve cells spreads across the corpus callosum from the hemisphere in which the seizure originated into the hemisphere on the other side of the brain. Once the recruitment activity crosses to the other hemisphere, the random firing of neurons can spread into that hemisphere as well. In a short time, seizure activity can involve the entire cerebral mass. This is illustrated in Figure 11.2.

When seizure activity is going on inside both hemispheres of the brain, the individual experiences considerable difficulty. There probably will be a profound change of

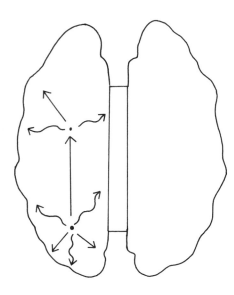

Figure 11.1. Onset of epileptic seizure activity.

consciousness, but a dangerous situation often results. Motor coordination is immediately lost, and all the muscles of the body begin to convulse violently. Such seizures occur spontaneously and periodically. No one understands what causes the seizure activity to begin, so this kind of epilepsy is difficult to treat.

The Split Brain Operation

In 1961, an unusual treatment for extremely severe epilepsy was tried out on a 48-year-old war veteran. A **split brain operation** was performed by P. J. Vogel and J. E. Bogen of the California College of Medicine. They reasoned that since the severity of epileptic seizure was related to the spread of spontaneous neuronal firing across the corpus callosum into the other side of the brain, that if the connection between the two halves of the brain were cut, the seizure would remain in one hemisphere, allowing the patient to retain control of the motor functions in half the body during a seizure. The structures severed surgically included the corpus callosum and the anterior and hippocampal commissures, two other sites of junction within the brain. This unusual and serious operation was performed initially with unknown results and consequences. It was done for people who had experienced severe epilepsy and for whom previous medical treatment had been inadequate. Fortunately, this surgical procedure did reduce the severity of seizure activity significantly. In fact, it was more effective than the experimenters thought it would be.

As early as 1952, Roger Sperry and Ronald Meyers of the University of Chicago had discovered that when you sever commissure structures within the brain, the two cerebral hemispheres function independently, as though they were two independent brains within

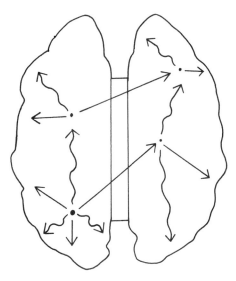

Figure 11.2. Contralateral recruitment of seizure activity.

the same animal. Sperry won the 1981 Nobel Prize in medicine for his pioneer work in studying how commissures integrate the activity of the two independent cerebral hemispheres.

By severing these structures, then, not only would the severity of a patient's epilepsy be minimized, but the two cerebral hemispheres of the brain might start operating as independent brains within the same skull. This phenomenon was not as immediately overtly striking as it may sound. Persons who had this surgery experienced no difficulty in talking or communicating and had no difficulty performing integrated motor tasks like walking. Soon, however, the independent functioning of the two hemispheres began to manifest itself in some interesting ways. Before we discuss them, let us take a look at the structure of the brain so we can better understand what these investigators discovered.

The Crossover Network

The two hemispheres of the brain receive information and control the activities of the left and right sides of the body. Through a crossover network, the right side of the brain controls the left side of the body, and the left side of the brain controls the right side of the body. Generally, information that enters your body from the left side goes to the right hemisphere, and information that enters from the right side goes to the left hemisphere. Consider the example of vision. Information that enters your eyes from the left side of a visual field enters the right hemisphere and vice versa. The eyes, however, do not send signals to opposite sides of the brain. The retina within each eye is divided so that when visual messages from the left field of vision enter both eyes, they pass through a structure called the optic chiasm and enter the right hemisphere. This means that both eyes are in communication with both sides of the brain. Half of each eye's visual input goes to the left and half to the right hemisphere. If the commissures and the corpus callosum are intact, the two hemispheres of the brain are in complete communication with each other and all physical and sensory activity is nicely integrated. Surprising things happen, however, when connections are severed and the two halves of the brain function independently.

What Was Learned

The split brain patients were given two types of psychological tests. In the first, pictures of words were flashed on a screen in front of them. The test was set up so that visual information could be presented to just one side of the brain at a time. It was flashed either to the left or to the right side of the visual field. The other type of test was tactile; the subject had to name objects by touching them. This test allowed the experimenters to instruct the subject to use one hand or the other, thereby sending information to either the right or left hemisphere.

When either visual or tactile information was presented to the subjects through the left hemisphere, they could easily describe it. They could write down a description and describe it orally. When words were presented to them through the left hemisphere, the patients could easily read them. They also had no difficulty solving problems that required calculation. When information was presented to subjects through the right hemisphere, however, they could not produce either oral or written responses. A patient shown a spoon through the right hemisphere could not say what it was. While holding a pencil in the left hand, so that the tactile information went to the right hemisphere, a patient might call it a can opener or a cigarette lighter. Some patients would not even attempt to describe it. The experimenters concluded that these incorrect guesses were coming from the left hemisphere and not the hemisphere that had received the information.

The right hemisphere could succeed at other tasks, however. For example, when subjects were shown a picture of a cigarette through the right hemisphere, they could easily feel around with their left hand and select an ashtray from among other objects that were unrelated to cigarette smoking. Yet, even after correct responses to tests of this nature, subjects were still incapable of either describing the object in the picture or the object they were holding in their hand.

Another interesting test that illustrated how the two hemispheres operate independently and in qualitatively different fashions involved flashing the word *heart* in the center of a visual screen. When this was done, the *he* section of the word was in the left visual field, so it entered the right side of the brain, and the *art* section of the word was in the right visual field, so it entered the left side of the brain. When patients were asked to tell the experimenters what they saw, they all said *art*. Then, when patients were asked to point, using their left hand, to which of the two cards they had seen, they all pointed to the *he* card.

It became clear from these investigations that the left side of the brain (which regulates and receives information from the right side of the body) possesses the language ability of the human mind. It was equally clear that the right of the brain has a minimal capacity for language. The initial assumption was that the left side of the brain was fairly well developed, whereas the right was operating at a reduced level of intellectual capacity. Later investigations proved, however, that although the right hemisphere is deficient in language ability, it possesses certain abilities that the left hemisphere does not.

Using their left hand, subjects could arrange blocks to match examples provided by the experimenter, and they could easily sketch a cube to indicate its three-dimensional nature.

With the right hand, however, they were totally incapable of performing either of these two functions.

Language ability, then, is located in the left hemisphere of the brain and spatial ability (recognition and reproduction of visual patterns) is located in the right. The observation that the mind has two modes of consciousness may well have a physiological basis. The two halves of the human brain may function in these qualitatively different modes, one in a structured, analytic fashion and the other in a more intuitive, spatial fashion. The left side of the brain may be responsible for such things as language, reason, logic, mathematical ability, and recognition of the passage of time, whereas the right side may be responsible for such skills as geometric pattern recognition, musical pitch recognition memory of melodies, and complex visual integration.

CHARACTERISTICS OF ALTERED STATES OF CONSCIOUSNESS

A number of varied changes in mental functioning occur during altered states of consciousness. Some of them are specific to states induced in a particular way. For example, the state of consciousness induced by sleep is not exactly the same as that induced by psychoactive drugs or by meditation. There are, however, several characteristics that most altered states of consciousness share.

Intense Focused Awareness. During an altered state, your mind is involved in one thought at a time. The scope of your awareness is severely limited. It tends to zero in on one thought, one idea, or one perception. In contrast, a normal state of consciousness is characterized by random thought activity. In a normal state, you think about many different things, and you are involved in the chattering of internal dialogue. During an altered state, you are not thinking about as many different things at one time, but what you are thinking about receives a greater amount of your cognitive energy and concentration. The Zen Buddhists use the example of the light from a lantern shining on a wall to explain this phenomenon. A normal state of consciousness, they say, is like the light on a wall when the distance between the lantern and the wall is great. The light spreads out and covers a wide area, and the intensity of the light at any one point on the wall is very dim. In contrast, they say, the altered state experience is like the light on a wall when the lamp is very close to it. As the lamp gets closer to the wall, the scope of illumination decreases, just as during the altered state of consciousness your attention limits its scope to fewer and fewer things. As the light begins to focus on one spot, the intensity of light on that spot becomes very great. During the experience of an altered state, you may not have the capacity to devote your attention to many different things at one time, but the things you do pay attention to receive your full capacity for concentration.

Presentcenteredness. A phenomenon related to this intense focused attention that occurs during altered states is presentcenteredness. Presentcenteredness means that your mind and your attention are occupied with the here and now, not with the past or the future. Your attention is directed to stimuli present at the moment. You are experiencing what is real and what is happening at the moment, not the leftover images of the past or the imaginings of the future.

Loss of Immediate Memory. Altered states are characterized by a focusing on the immediate, so a loss of immediate memory is quite common. People do not generally forget who they are or lose their ability to speak, but they may forget events that have just occurred. This happens because the mind is not hanging on to these things. It is devoting all its attention to what is happening at the present moment. You may even notice this phenomenon in yourself once in awhile. Remember back to the phenomenon of highway hypnosis. During this state, although you may have driven some distance, you have no recollection of it.

Distortions in Time Sense. Distorted time sense can take on one of three characteristics. In some instances, a few minutes seems like many hours. (You may have noticed this while trying to read the physiology chapter of this book.) In another instance several hours may seem like only a few minutes. Think about spending an evening with an attractive and interesting person. The hours seem to fly by. The most common distortion in time sense, however, is the complete absence of a sense of time. Altered states are sometimes described as timeless experiences. Time does not seem longer or shorter; it simply does not exist. Time is a creation of our minds. During an altered state of consciousness the whole idea of time simply fades away.

Ineffability. Ineffability means beyond verbal description. If you tried to describe a particular altered state of consciousness, you would have trouble putting it into words, and you would feel frustrated at how inadequately words convey the feeling and character of the state you were in. We can use words to describe the peripheral effects of sensations like love or hatred, yet we find adequately communicating the feeling itself to be nearly impossible. If you can describe the character of your state of consciousness, you probably are not in an altered state. When you no longer label perceptions that enter your mind but simply experience them, you are in an altered state.

Perceptual Alterations. The processing of sensory information changes somewhat during altered states. **Hallucinations** can occur during profound alterations of consciousness. Hallucinations are sensory perceptions with no external origin. You may see things or hear things or feel or even taste or smell things that have no external cause. More commonly, however, perceptual patterns are simply changed. The most common change is seeing familiar objects in a different way. You may notice shadows on the wall that you have not seen before. You may see patterns of reflection across metal objects or changes in color and contour across object surfaces that you never noticed before. While listening to music, you may hear interrelations between the instruments or even rhythmic or tonal patterns you have not heard before. Another common perceptual alteration is a **change in body image**. Sometimes you become acutely aware of sensations within your body. This is called an **increase in somatic awareness**. You can suddenly feel subtle changes going on inside your body that you never thought about or paid attention to before. Equally as often the opposite occurs. Your entire body, or parts of it, may feel numb. You may feel that a segment of your body has disappeared for a moment. A close friend of mine uses this phenomenon to gauge his progress with meditation. He knows he is meditating correctly when his elbows disappear. He gets a numbing sensation from his elbows so that he feels his forearms and hands are no longer connected to his body. It may sound a little weird, but this is a normal response during an altered state of consciousness. It is not something to worry about. Just realize that during the practice of altered states perceptual alterations and distortions can occur.

Self-Transcendence. A dissolving of personal boundaries is a common perceptual change during an altered state. The barriers that we put up around ourselves to define the self seem to break apart. People who have experienced profound drug-induced states of consciousness report sensations such as feeling that their bodies are melting into the chair they are sitting in. During this kind of sensation, a person begins to lose the sense of what is "me" and "not me." In a normal state, we can easily see where we stop and the chair begins. During an altered state, we can become confused over what is part of ourself and what is something separate from ourself. This confusion is related to a phenomenon called **expanded consciousness**, which means that our consciousness embraces a wider scope of experience than was possible during a normal state. (Expanded consciousness is not contradictory to focused awareness. Focused awareness refers to the number of thoughts going on in our head at one time. Expanded consciousness means that we realize that the scope and breadth of our consciousness extends far beyond the normal limitations that our minds impose on us.) Carl Jung (1958) has described this as the "transpersonal unconsciousness," a sea of consciousness in which each individual is merely the peak of one small wave. As we expand our consciousness we realize that seeing ourselves as distinct individuals is just as silly as looking at the peaks of each wave and saying they are not part of the ocean. In many ways, we are all interconnected. We share the same air, and the nutrients that compose our bodies have been transferred from one form to another for billions of years. Some people also believe that we share a collective consciousness. In Eastern literature, expanded consciousness is often described with the term **oneness**. The sense of oneness, or unity with all things, is based on the dissolution of personal boundaries that our normal mind has imposed on us. It can be a frightening phenomenon at first, but it can lead to valuable growth.

Hypersuggestibility. We no longer filter incoming information during an altered state, so we are more receptive to new ideas and we are more easily influenced by ideas that we may have rejected during normal consciousness. This phenomenon is valuable as part of the creative experience because it allows us to consider options we may have ignored before. It does, however, invite possibilities for abuse. Two notable examples of persons who have abused this phenomenon are Adolph Hitler and Charles Manson. Both these men understood how to manipulate states of consciousness. Although they used different techniques, the result was the same. They induced in their subjects an altered state of consciousness and then fed them ideas that would be accepted with little resistance. Although possibilities for the abuse of hypersuggestibility do exist, they are more than offset by its importance in the accessing of creative ideas.

In summary, then, an altered state of consciousness includes the following characteristics:

1. Intense focused awareness
2. Presentcenteredness
3. Loss of immediate memory
4. Distortions in time sense
5. Ineffability
6. Perceptual alterations
7. Self-transcendence
8. Hypersuggestibility

When you start noticing characteristics of altered states of consciousness while practicing different forms of relaxation, it usually means you are practicing the technique correctly or at least to the degree that it is capable of inducing a change in state of consciousness. Being able to recognize these characteristics while you are practicing is good feedback.

THE VALUE OF ALTERED STATES OF CONSCIOUSNESS

A human being cannot be truly creative or make any unique contribution without being able to balance both modes of consciousness, yet people often devalue the altered state. As Roger Bacon said, this is "a mode we often devalue culturally, personally and even physiologically." Imagine two extremes—a dreamer and an engineer. The dreamer is stuck in an altered state of consciousness, and the engineer is locked into the normal state. Neither has access to the complementary mode. The dreamer may have many creative possibilities in mind but is totally without the skills required to bring them out of the mind and into external reality. The engineer has all the skills necessary to bring an idea into existence and have it survive but has no ideas to work with. By themselves, these two persons are not capable of making an independent creative contribution. The truly creative individual possesses both these two modes of consciousness.

Imagination, intuition, and unique ideas come from the realm of the altered state. The normal state of consciousness operates on well-worn pathways. Unique thinking and novel solutions do not come to mind when you only think about what already exists. During an altered state, you pay no attention to structure, convention, or existing thoughts. This opening up to possibilities may be the source of imagination. Ideas generated during altered states can be communicated by applying to them the knowledge and skills that are the realm of the normal state of consciousness. The creative person can experience both states and use them to complement each other. One state is not normal and rational and real and the other weird and valueless. Both play a vital role in creativity and human endeavor of all types.

A good way to illustrate this point is to look at the history of science. Most of us think of science as a purely rational discipline involving logic, language, mathematics, and so on. We may doubt that scientists have any use for altered states of consciousness. Every major breakthrough or discovery in science, however, has involved a deviation from normal or accepted patterns of thought. If we think like everyone else, we do not think of anything new. Without intuition, science could not progress.

Copernicus, the first person to suggest that the earth was not the center of the universe, is a good person to start with. Prior to Copernicus everyone accepted the Ptolemaic model of the universe, which stated that the earth was at the center and the sun, moon, planets, and stars revolved around it. Certain celestial observations contradicted this theory, however, so Copernicus suggested an alternative model. He suggested that the sun might be the center of the universe and that its apparent movement around the earth was due to the earth revolving around its own axis. Copernicus's theory was insulting to the religious ideology of the day, but his model is far closer to the modern conceptualization of our solar system than was Ptolemy's. For Copernicus to formulate this theory, his thinking had to deviate from the conventions of his time.

Many scientists have made their greatest discoveries while in an altered state of consciousness. The French chemist Kekule is responsible for conceptualizing the ring structure of benzene. Chemists had long puzzled over the structure of benzene. The attributes of this molecule seemed to constitute an incomprehensible picture of what its structure might be. During this time (the 19th century), chemists thought molecules consisted of atoms arranged in linear chains. Kekule had pondered this question for a significant portion of his life. In frustration and despair, he ended up one night in a drunken stupor. As he was lying down after the evening's indulgence, the story goes, he had a vision of a circling snake. He saw the snake moving around and around in wheellike fashion until it bit its own tail. He suddenly realized that that must be the structure of benzene. People had never thought before that a molecule could turn around and connect to itself. They were totally used to thinking of molecules as linear chains. No one had entertained the idea that complete rings could exist in chemical structures. Kekule's discovery led to the birth of organic chemistry.

Nobel Prize winner Robert Millikan came up with his idea for the bubble chamber while in a similar state. The bubble chamber is a device that allows physicists to see subatomic particles and their movements. While staring into a glass of beer, Millikan observed that the bubbles form at the bottom and then rise to the top. He began to wonder why bubbles form in the bottom of the glass. He realized that a bubble begins as a tiny particle and that, similar to a raindrop, gas molecules collect around it until finally it is large enough to rise. His realization that the bubble is a lot bigger than the original particle led to the creation of the bubble chamber, in which subatomic particles pass through a supersaturated medium and leave trails as bubbles. This was a significant breakthrough for research in particle physics.

Another Nobel laureate, Niels Bohr, came up with the model of the atom while in a hypnogogic state—the state you pass through as you go from waking consciousness into deep sleep. Bohr had spent many years studying the structure of the atom in an analytic fashion. Then, while falling asleep one evening, all the information settled into place into a coherent model of the atom that we still use today.

Albert Einstein had one of the greatest scientific minds in human history, yet he did not learn to speak until he was three years old. His ability as a scientist, he said, was not due to his analytic or mathematical skills, but to his ability to turn off the thinking process. He used to say that "intuition is the thing." He believed that it was of great importance for a scientist to be able to access intuitive consciousness and thereby tap into the source of new ideas.

Science seems to be an analytic process, but discovery is often rooted in intuition. The ability to induce altered states of consciousness and use them in conjunction with normal states is essential to the creative process, whether it manifests itself as part of science or as healthy functioning.

HOW ALTERED STATES CAN ALLEVIATE STRESS

Altered states can help us cope with stress in two ways. During a normal state of consciousness, we judge and interpret events. As you will recall, many stress problems are triggered not by the event itself but by how we interpret it. Rehearsal in producing altered states of consciousness can liberate us from maladaptive judgmental kinds of thinking. The second way in which altered states can help us gain control over stress is through obtaining conscious control over internal physiological functions. Techniques that have evolved to induce changes in consciousness also induce psychophysiological changes. By learning how to induce altered states of consciousness, we may open up great possibilities for controlling the internal activity of our body and hence manage stress.

HOW ALTERED STATES CAN BE INDUCED

Altered states of consciousness can be induced externally through the use of chemical agents (like drugs) that alter the pattern of activity within the nervous system. Three behavioral methods can be used to facilitate a qualitative shift in consciousness. We can bombard the senses with information, we can deprive them of information, or we can present the senses with constant repetition. The chapters that follow present many different methods of systematic relaxation. Some of them involve decreasing sensory input and others involve the phenomenon of repetition.

SUMMARY

The human mind operates in two qualitatively different but complementary modes of consciousness. One is rational, verbal, and analytic; the other is intuitive, spatial, and holistic. The creative and healthy functioning of a human being depends on the ability to use both modes of consciousness. In this culture, we often consider the normal state to be the only valid way to experience reality. Altered states, however, are essential to creativity, and learning to induce them can liberate us from maladaptive thought patterns and give us control over the internal activity of our body.

REFERENCES

Assagioli, R. *Psychosynthesis*, The Viking Press, New York, 1971.

Barnett, L. *The Universe and Dr. Einstein*, Bantam, New York, 1968.

Bertini, M., et al. "Some Preliminary Observations With An Experimental Procedure for the Study of Hypnagogic and Related Phenomena," *Archivio di Psicologia Neurologia Psichiatria*, v. 6, 493-534, 1964.

Blackburn, T. R. "Sensuous-Intellectual Complementarity in Science," *Science*, v. 172, 1003-1007, 1971.

Bogen, J. E. "The Other Side of the Brain, I, II, III," *Bulletin of the Los Angeles Neurological Societies*, v. 34(3), 191-220, 1969.

Capra, F. *The Tao of Physics*, Shambala, Boulder, Colo., 1975.

Carroll, J. B., ed. *Language, Thought and Reality: Selected Writings of Benjamin Lee Whorf*, The M.I.T. Press, Cambridge, Mass., 1951.

Castaneda, C. *The Teachings of Don Juan: A Yaqui Way of Knowledge*, Ballantine, New York, 1968.

———. *A Separate Reality: Further Conversations With Don Juan*, Simon and Schuster, New York, 1971.

Deikman, A. J. "Bimodal Consciousness," *Archives of General Psychiatry*, v. 25, 481-489, 1971.

———. "Deautomatization and the Mystic Experience," *Psychiatry*, v. 29, 324-338, 1969.

DeRopp, R. *The Master Game*, Delacorte Press, New York, 1968.

Gazzaniga, S. "The Split Brain in Man," *Scientific American*, Offprint 508, 24-29, 1967.

Gurdjieff, G. *Views From the Real World*, Dutton, New York, 1973.

Harman, W. W., et al. "Psychedelic Agents in Creative Problem Solving: A Pilot Study," *Psychological Reports*, v. 19, 211-227, 1966.

Huxley, A. *The Doors of Perception*, Harper and Row, New York, 1954.

James, W. "The Stream of Consciousness," in James, W., *The Principles of Psychology*, Dover, New York, 1950.

———. *The Varieties of Religious Experience*, New American Library, New York, 1958.

Jouvet, M. "The States of Sleep," *Scientific American*, v. 216, 62-72, Feb. 1967.

Jung, C. G., "Aion," in de Laszlo, V. S., *Psyche and Symbol*, Doubleday, Garden City, N.Y., 1958.

Kleitman, N. "Patterns of Dreaming," *Scientific American*, v. 203, 82-88, Nov. 1960.

Kohler, I. "Experiments With Goggles," *Scientific American*, Offprint 465, 62-72, 1962.

Kuhn, T. *The Structure of Scientific Revolutions*, University of Chicago Press, Chicago, 1962.

Laing, R. D. *The Politics of Experience*, Ballantine, New York, 1967.

Lee, D. "Codifications of Reality: Lineal and Nonlineal," *Psychosomatic Medicine*, v. 12(2), 89-97, Mar.-Apr. 1950.

LeShan, L. "Physicists and Mysticism: Similarities in World View," *Journal of Transpersonal Psychology*, v. 1-2, 1-20, 1969.

Lilly, J. *Programming and Metaprogramming in the Human Biocomputer*, Communications Research Institute, Miami, Fla., 1967.

Ludwig, A. M. "Altered States of Consciousness," *Archives of General Psychiatry*, v. 15, 225-234, 1966.

Naranjo, C. "Present-Centeredness: Technique, Prescription, and Ideal," in Fagan, J., and Shepherd, I. L., eds., *Gestalt Therapy Now*, Harper and Row, New York, 1970.

Ornstein, R. E. *On the Experience of Time*, Penguin Books, Baltimore, 1969.

———. *The Nature of Human Consciousness*, W. H. Freeman and Company, San Francisco, 1973.

———. *The Psychology of Consciousness*, W. H. Freeman and Company, San Francisco, 1972.

Pearce, J. C. *The Crack in the Cosmic Egg*, Simon and Schuster, New York, 1973.

Sperry, R. W. "The Eye and the Brain," *Scientific American*, Offprint 465, 48-52, 1956.

Tart, C. T. *Altered States of Consciousness*, Doubleday, Garden City, N.Y., 1969.

——. "Science, States of Consciousness and Spiritual Experiences: The Need for State-Specific Sciences," in Tart, C. T. *Transpersonal Psychologies*, Harper and Row, New York, 1977.

——. *States of Consciousness*, Dutton, New York, 1975.

——. *Transpersonal Psychologies,* Harper and Row, New York, 1977.

Teyler, T. J. *Altered States of Awareness*, W. H. Freeman and Company, San Francisco, 1954.

Vogel, G., et al. "Ego Functions and Dreaming During Sleep Onset," *Archives of General Psychiatry*, v. 14, 238-248, 1966.

Weil, A. *The Natural Mind*, Houghton Mifflin Company, Boston, 1972.

CHAPTER 12

Sensory Awareness

The grass whispered under his body. He put his arm down, feeling the sheath of fuzz on it, and, far away, below, his toes creaking in his shoes. The wind sighed over his shelled ears. The world slipped bright over the glassy round of his eyeballs like images sparked in a crystal sphere. Flowers were suns and fiery spots of sky strewn through the woodland. Birds flickered like skipped stones across the vast inverted pond of heaven. His breath raked over his teeth, going in ice, coming out fire. Insects shocked the air with electric clearness. Ten thousand individual hairs grew a millionth of an inch on his head. He heard the twin hearts beating in each ear, the third heart beating in his throat, the two hearts throbbing his wrists, the real heart pounding in his chest. The million pores on his body opened. I'm really alive! he thought. I never knew it before, or if I did, I don't remember.

Ray Bradbury

As you sit here reading, take a moment out to notice all the things around you. Find a piece of paper and write down ten observations about your immediate surroundings.

Now go through your list and write beside each entry which of your five senses (sight, sound, scent, taste, or touch) you used to perceive each observation. Now add up how many times you used each sense. If you are like most people, more than half your observations were visual ones. You may have included a few auditory sensations, but you probably recorded few or no perceptions gained through scent, taste, or touch.

This exercise demonstrates that we are visual animals; we pay attention mainly to what we see. Consider some common expressions: seeing is believing, see for yourself, see you later, see what I mean. Most of a dog's information about the world comes from scent, a snake relies on thermal sense, a bat depends on auditory signals, a shark counts on its nose, but humans rely on what they see.

Aside from vision (and hearing, to some extent) our awareness of sensation is practically numb. We ignore scents, tastes, and touch so much that we are insensitive to most of the world. In fact, we are largely numb from a visual perspective as well. Most of us do not see color with high resolve, or notice variations in patterns of light and shadow, or even see the negative space in line drawings. Why do we ignore our senses?

Part of our insensitivity is due to our biological design. The limited awareness capacity of our nervous system originally helped facilitate survival by allowing us to pay attention only to things that were immediately threatening.

Cultural conditions also contribute to our sensory deficiencies. We are assaulted with stimulation from billboards, neon lights, crowds, traffic noise, television, stereos, automobile exhausts, deodorants, and so on. Our sensory attention is pulled in so many directions and assaulted with such great regularity that we adapt by tuning out. Our culture reinforces visual dominance by presenting most information to us visually. The prime villain is television. Notice how much television we watch. Watch someone who is watching television—eyes fixed on the glowing box, mouth hanging open, sense of self and the environment asleep. We should consider using television as a surgical anesthetic!

Notice how we are addicted to external sources of stimulation. We get home and immediately turn on the television or the stereo. The result is that our threshold for stimulation gets very high. We require loud, bright, obnoxious things to catch our attention. We lose our subtle, delicate senses.

As we lose our senses, we begin to ignore the sensations coming from our bodies. Somatic awareness is an essential component of effective stress management. To gain control over your health, you must know how your body works. Even more important than understanding how it functions is being able to feel it working and learning to sense its changes. You must train yourself to be receptive and aware of the ever-changing, dynamic state of your own body.

The activities on the following pages will help you develop your lost senses and refine and cleanse the ones you still use. Many of the ideas come from *Sense Relaxation*, a highly recommended book by Bernard Gunther. These activities may seem trivial or silly. Do them anyway. Only by doing them will your senses be able to reveal to you why the exercises are important.

SEEING

Although we are visual animals, we often see only gross shapes, movement, and lines. We unconsciously limit how much of what enters our eyes actually reaches our awareness. We are aware of very little that we can see. Take a look at Figure 12.1, the logo that is more powerful than a locomotive and faster than a speeding bullet. We immediately see a big letter *S*, as in Figure 12.2.

The *S* is easy to see and obvious to our awareness because it is a letter of the alphabet. Without looking back at Figure 12.1, close your eyes and try to visualize the shapes of the spaces that surround the *S*. Seeing them is difficult because they are not part of a familiar pattern. While trying to visualize them, you probably tried not to "see" them but to reconstruct them using the image of the S and the shape of the bordering shield.

Look at the logo again and notice the shapes of the negative spaces. They were there; you just ignored them. The negative spaces are illustrated in Figure 12.3.

As a child, that logo always confused me, because I never saw the *S*. All I saw were the negative spaces. Even though I did not understand the symbol, I liked it anyway. Those weird shapes seemed mystical to me. Had I known it was just an *S*, it would have lost all its appeal and wonder. One year I made myself a Superman costume for Halloween. I skillfully reproduced on my T-shirt my recollection of those odd, magical shapes. My logo

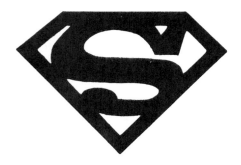

Figure 12.1. Our familiar logo.

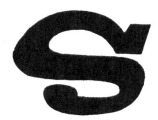

Figure 12.2. How we see the logo.

looked something like Figure 12.4. I had the negative space forms correct, but I never knew about that *S*, so it was not there.

Everyone laughed. I came to a tearful realization of my error. As I looked at the store-bought Superman costumes, however, I decided I liked my symbol better. I still do. We all see things differently. It would be valuable if we could learn to see things in many ways, so that we do not limit ourselves to the obvious and the mundane.

Go out and explore negative space. Look at the sky through tree branches. Do not just see the lines of the branches; notice the shapes of the little pieces of sky. Look at any wall in your home. Do not simply notice the objects on the wall; observe how they divide the background space. Learn to see not just what is there, but also the form of the surrounding void. Begin to see the dynamic relationships between the form and the space between the obvious and what is present but often ignored. See the light and see the shadow. See them at the same moment and watch them dance.

Color perception is another part of seeing. Do you think in color? Are your memories in color or in black and white? Do you dream in color? Spend some time noticing the subtle variations of shade intensity and hue of objects that seem to be simply colored. Look at

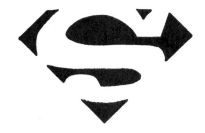

Figure 12.3. Negative space.

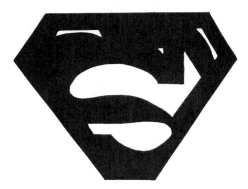

Figure 12.4. My interpretation of the logo.

trees again. Watch, from below, the leaves blowing in the wind, displaying their many faces and colors. Notice the dazzling flickers of many colors. It is not just green. See and be aware of all the colors and shades. Look down at the folds of your clothing. Notice the color shifts, the patterns, and the shapes of light and shadow. Begin to see as a painter must. During the next few days, look everywhere, notice detail, color, negative space, visual relationships, patterns of movement, depth, space, texture. Expand your visual awareness until you can almost taste what your eyes see. Restore your sight!

HEARING

There is a lot to be heard that we miss and many ways of hearing that we ignore. It is difficult to notice sounds with our eyes open because our visual dominance overrides auditory sensation. So close your eyes and listen. Take note of every sound in your immediate surroundings. Listen for the obvious sounds: doors closing, televisions and radios playing, people walking around or talking to each other, traffic outside. We notice those sounds that serve as the backdrop for all the others. It may be the distant drone of an air conditioning compressor, the humming of fluorescent lights, the quiet rushing of air entering the room through louvered vents, or the wind blowing past tree branches or across the tiny hairs of your ears. Hear these background sounds not just as noise; listen for their subtleties.

Become aware of the panasonic arrangement of sounds—their point of origin in the 360 degrees around your senses. Do not just notice a sound; note its location, depth, movement, and projection. Notice also the parasonic arrangement of sounds you hear. Parasonic refers to the vertical relationship of sounds, or whether they come from above you or below you. Imagine that you are seated in the center of everything and sound is happening all around you. Listen to the transient sounds. Listen for the steady, ever-present sounds. Then search for the tiniest, faintest sound you can hear. Focus on that tiny sound. Listen to what it is saying. Realize that an even tinier one exists. Listen for it. Keep listening, scanning for the smallest sound and listening closely to each one.

Finally, listen to the silence. In between the transient sounds are spaces of silence that we usually ignore. Listen for the silence. Experience the refreshing breathing spaces between sounds, like cool breezes on humid August afternoons. Listen as a composer must listen. The silent spaces communicate just as much as the sounds do. Learn to be aware of silence.

Learn to hear again, even with yours eyes open. Do not ignore sounds simply because they may not be immediately useful to you.

SMELLING

We do not just ignore scents, we go to great lengths to eliminate them. Think of how deodorant is sold in this country. A major industry of our country is dedicated to turning off our sense of smell.

Go into your kitchen and take out all the spice jars. Close your eyes and, one at a time, open each container and sniff, delicately, at the contents. Try to identify each spice by scent alone.

Now find a container of prepared food like instant stuffing or canned spaghetti and meatballs. Using your scent alone, try to identify the spices in the product. Search through the food with your nose and find every flavor.

Go to the zoo. Pretend you are blind. Close your eyes, wear dark glasses, and have a friend lead you around. Notice all the smells. Compare those of the animals with those of the people you pass and those from the concession stands. Do not look at an animal all day. Just smell.

TASTING

Our sense of taste is intricately associated with our sense of smell. They enhance one another, smell being particularly important to the full expression of taste.

Invite someone over for dinner. Prepare a meal of infinite variety in origin, spice, consistency, and texture. Place all the food on the table. Notice the location of all the food and any sharp objects. Then close your eyes. Eat the complete meal with your eyes closed. Use your hands instead of utensils. Experience every scent, every flavor. Notice the many dimensions of each thing you eat. Taste every spice, every ingredient of each bite. Become totally aware of taste. Finish the meal with a glass of cool water. As it passes through your mouth, feel and taste it washing all those sensations from your mouth down into your body.

Another excellent taste activity comes from Gunther. He calls it Orange A-peeling. It involves many senses, all of which stimulate, entice, and lead up to the sensation of taste.

Take an orange
in the palm of your hand.
See its shape,
its color, its top and bottom,
the markings on the skin.
Smell the orange.
Close your eyes
and move the orange
in the palms of your hands.
Listen to the sound that your
hands make contacting it.
Take the orange and roll it
all over your face.
With your eyes closed,
feel the temperature of the
orange on your face.
Experience how your face feels.
Open your eyes and see
the orange. Sensitively
break the skin and begin to
peel the orange. See
the juice come out of the skin.
Hear the sounds.
Feel the breaking of the skin.
Watch it come apart.
See if you can keep the skin
together so that it
comes off in a large piece.
Watch the peeling being
torn away from the flesh of
the orange. Take time—listen
to the sounds. Look
at the inside of the peeling.
Smell it. Look at the
flesh of the orange.
As slowly as you can, break
the orange in half and
watch it separate.
Slowly break off one section
and peel the skin off
in sections. Close your eyes
and eat that section
and the rest of the orange
one section
at a time.

TOUCHING

Americans rarely touch each other. Adults usually touch only during sexual activity, and then it is usually limited to small areas of the body. We miss a lot. Try the following activities to reawaken your tactile sensations.

First, wash your hands. While they are still wet, sprinkle lots of table salt on them. Now wash your hands with the salt. Feel them come alive. Wash and rinse them with cool water. Feel their tingling, their effervescence. Dry them gently and completely. Then rub some cream into them. Feel each pore drink it in. Wake up your hands.

When it gets dark outside, turn off all the lights in your bathroom. Go in and take a shower in complete darkness. Use lots of soap. Feel every sensation as you wash yourself clean. Do not turn on the lights until you are thoroughly clean, rinsed, and dry. Be aware of how much different your body feels now compared with how it felt before your shower.

SOMATIC AWARENESS

The most direct application of sensory awareness for stress control is in the development of somatic awareness—an awareness of all the various sensations of your body. Use your awakened senses to place yourself in closer touch with your physical self. Listen to your body.

As you sit here quietly, become aware and feel all the sensations from your toes. . . , then your feet. . . , your ankles. . . , your calves. . . , your knees. . . , thighs. . . , hips. . . , stomach. . . , chest. . . , arms. . . , hands. . . , fingers (each one). . . , neck. . . , head. Feel your breathing; hear it. Listen and feel your heart beating.

We usually feel our body only when it hurts. Learn to be aware of it all the time. Feel its function, its changes, its beauty.

Do not restrict your expanded sensory awareness to the brief activities presented in this chapter. Make sensation a part of each moment of your life. Seek out and experience the sensations around you. Open your senses. Ignore nothing.

SUMMARY

We have been conditioned to tune out or avoid the experience of subtle sensations. We use our eyes to the exclusion of our other senses. Through sensory awareness activities, we can reawaken our awareness to sensations from the body that we have been taught to ignore. By developing somatic awareness, we can enhance the effectiveness of relaxation exercises and reduce stress.

REFERENCES

Bradbury, R. *Dandelion Wine*, pp. 9-10, Bantam Books, New York, 1946.
Case, J. *Sensory Mechanisms*, Macmillan, London, 1966.
Gunther, B. *Sense Relaxation*, p. 95, Macmillan, New York, 1968.
Kohler, I. "Experiments With Goggles," reprinted in *Altered States of Awareness*, W. H. Freeman, San Francisco, 1972.
Prather, H. *I Touch the Earth, The Earth Touches Me*, Doubleday, Garden City, N.Y., 1972.

CHAPTER 13

Meditation

In an instant, rise from time and space. Set the world aside and become a world within yourself.

Shabistari

Meditation is the oldest form of systematic relaxation. It effectively alters human consciousness through the disciplined focus of attention. Although meditation originally evolved as a tool for reaching spiritually aware states of consciousness, recent research into its physiological effects has indicated that it has great potential for countering the somatic response patterns of stress.

We begin with meditation for three reasons. First, meditation is almost universally effective in reducing psychophysiological arousal; nearly everyone can derive some somatic benefits from it. Second, it can intervene at many points in the psychosomatic model, both in the cognitive and physical domains, making it one of the most effective stress control skills available. Finally, meditation is the most fundamental form of systematic relaxation; its simplicity embodies all the essential components of relaxation training. Once you have practiced meditation, grasped its fundamental concepts, and experienced its subtle effects, you will be well prepared to understand and implement any form of relaxation as an effective device for managing stress.

HISTORICAL EMERGENCE OF MEDITATION

Meditation has been an integral part of the religious, spiritual, and philosophical practices of nearly every culture. Presenting an accurate and comprehensive analysis of its development would be impossible. Each culture and each scholar has a different interpretation, and each is valid. We will look at the history of meditation from a broad viewpoint and draw some conclusions as to why it emerged at all.

The sixth century B.C. saw the birth of Pythagoras, Buddha, Lao Tsu, Zarathustra, Confucius, and Kapila, the enlightened creators of human spiritual history. The sixth century B.C. was as rich and concentrated in spiritual development and thought as the 20th century has been in scientific thought and technological development. The goals, directions, and purpose of meditation blossomed from the human mind during this time. The specific techniques were developed later.

According to Taoist legend, Lao Tsu, the founder of Taoism (pronounced dow'ism), was leaving China on foot to die, weary and sickened by the nature and ways of men. A gatekeeper recognized him and persuaded him to write down his wisdom to guide future generations. Although Lao Tsu asserted that "the Tao that can be told is not the eternal Tao," he quickly recorded his teachings in 81 verses, less than 5,000 words. This collection of vast illumination, stored in but a few words, was called the *Tao Te Ching*. It has served for more than 2,500 years as the source of inspiration and guidance for one of the world's dominant religions.

Kapila, the sage who founded the Sankhya school of philosophy, was one of several enlightened men who developed the idea that there are two fundamental reality systems. His teachings formed the basis for the development of Raja Yoga 400 years later.

Most notable to Westerners is the Hindu Siddhartha Gautama, whom history knows as Buddha, "the enlightened one." Guatama was struggling toward a goal of enlightenment, on paths formed by the Hindus, with great frustration. When he finally gave up Hindu methods, he experienced nirvana. This spontaneous, quantum leap in spiritual level was the first step in the development of his teachings. Buddha never wrote anything himself. What we know of Buddhism comes from the transcriptions of his followers.

Lao Tsu, Kapila, and Buddha never described or prescribed specific meditation techniques. They outlined the paths of spiritual enlightenment. Their followers developed the specific meditation exercises to be used as vehicles along those paths. The *I Ching* oracle and the moving meditation of "Tai Chi" of Taoism were developed long after the death of Lao Tsu. Kapila developed the philosophical system that was the basis for the development of Raja Yoga by Patanjali in 200 B.C. The 196 sutras composed by Patanjali represented specific directions for the eight-phased series of techniques leading to samadhi. Bodhidarma took Mahayana Buddhism to China in 527 A.D. to develop the discipline of Zen. In 1191 and 1227 A.D., Zen branched into the dominant schools of Rinzai and Soto, respectively. Zen involved the development of highly disciplined, specific exercises designed to facilitate a shift in consciousness from the rational to the intuitive mode. The aim of Zen meditation was to attain satori. Nirvana, samadhi, and satori all refer to the same thing: an ultimate, transcendent state of enlightened consciousness.

The methods and techniques developed by the followers of the original spiritual leaders all shared several fundamental elements. Nearly all of these activities are what we now collectively label meditation. Meditation was originally designed as a tool for accessing spiritually aware states of consciousness.

GOALS OF MEDITATION TRAINING

Meditation training is fundamentally designed to bring to the practitioner a mental state of calm, tranquility, and peace. From the standpoint of stress management, the primary goal of meditation practice is to reduce psychophysiological arousal. This aim has two facets. First, meditation should reduce immediate cognitive and physical arousal during the actual practice of the technique. Second, it should contribute to conditioning a trophotropic response pattern in reaction to most of life's activities and to stress.

Some secondary goals in relation to stress management include increases in somatic awareness, clarity of sensation and thought, and attentional abilities. Regular meditation practice should allow you to adopt appropriate cognitive responses to potential psychogenic stressors. You should experience an increased desire to avoid unnecessary stressors and a desire to avoid behavior that is unrewarding.

THE ESSENCE OF MEDITATION

Every man knows how useful it is to be useful. No one seems to know how useful it is to be useless.

Chuang-Tzu

Popular Western connotations about meditation are far removed from what it actually is. Let us begin by discussing what meditation is not. First, meditation is not a haircut. To practice meditation, you do not have to shave your head, or grow a beard, or sell incense in shopping malls, or wear long white robes and beads. Meditation does not require a significant change in life-style. You do not have to give away your worldly goods and move to an herb farm. Second, meditation is not a religion, even though it emerged from the religion and philosophies of the East. Meditation is actually a part of nearly every religious system, including—through prayer—the Christian religion, yet religion is not necessarily a part of meditation. This is just as wine is used in the sacrament of communion. Spending Saturday night getting buzzed on a fifth of Ripple does not mean you are taking communion. Clear your mind of the notion that meditation is a weird "pagan" ritual. Practicing it will not corrupt your mind, taint your soul, or quietly launch your Western reason into space.

Meditation is fundamentally an exercise for directing attention. We will define meditation in the words of Robert Ornstein (1971): "Meditation involves any activity which attempts to focus and maintain attention on a single, repetitive or unchanging stimulus."

Meditation involves exercises that focus attention on things that are either unchanging or repetitive. Sitting quietly and listening to a clock tick could be considered meditation. Other examples could range from contemplating a blank wall to watching ocean waves roll in and out, or focusing your attention on the beating of your heart. If you are exerting a deliberate effort to keep your attention on something that is either repeated or does not change, you are meditating. It does not matter what else you may or may not be doing. You may be sitting on a satin pillow with the Taj Mahal embroidered on it, or listening to sitar music, or burning lotus incense, but if you are not attending to a repetitive or unchanging stimulus you are not meditating.

Fundamentally, then, meditation is a simple activity. You simply make an effort to keep your attention on something that either repeats or does not change. That is all. We will discuss meditation simply as a collection of exercises that will help you perform this mental task, a context quite removed from its religious or spiritual applications. We will consider meditation to be simply a daily exercise that you perform in the interest of your personal health and quality of life, like jogging or taking a shower. The significance and applications of meditation training far exceed the scope of our discussion; we will merely apply this technique to psychophysiological stress management.

CHARACTERISTICS OF MEDITATION

Meditation is practiced in a variety of ways, some of which we will discuss later in this chapter. Regardless of how it is practiced, all forms of meditation techniques share five characteristics. The first four were outlined by Benson (1975). We have added a fifth characteristic that is important to the use of meditation for managing stress.

Quiet Environment

The first element of meditation training is a **quiet environment**. When attempting to keep your mind directed to an unchanging stimulus, it is helpful if you place yourself in an environment that is relatively free of sensory distractions. Meditate where you will not be distracted by the telephone, or sirens, or people interrupting you. As you will soon discover, meditation is difficult enough without any distractions. Benson's recommendation of a quiet environment is particularly useful for the initial sessions of learning meditation.

If your goal is to use meditation for stress control, however, a too-quiet practice environment may not be the most desirable setting. In studies done with people learning to meditate in quiet versus noisy environments, it was found that subjects in the quiet group lowered their psychophysiological reactivity to stressors much faster than did those in the noisy group. This evidence supported the notion that a quiet environment facilitates more rapid, effective learning of meditation than does an environment with auditory distractions. When tests were conducted on the same subjects three and six months later, however, it was discovered that people who learned to meditate in noisy settings were far better at lowering arousal to stressors in their real life settings than were those who meditated in silence. The implication is that if one continues to meditate solely in a distraction-free setting, there will be little transference of the state of calm produced by meditation into the busy activities of everyday life. If you can gradually learn to meditate amid distractions similar to your real life setting, meditation training will be all the more effective in helping you react calmly to stressors. Anyone can be calm and relaxed on an isolated mountain peak. The challenge is to learn to be calm and relaxed amid chaos.

We recommend that you begin meditating in as quiet an environment as possible and gradually wean yourself away from the silence, until you can comfortably meditate while surrounded by normal everyday distractions. You can, if you wish, use white noise—patternless sound—to mask auditory distractions. Examples include running water, radio static, and electric fans. If you are being disturbed by sounds while meditating, turn on a fan or play one of those nature sounds records. The latter idea is particularly useful, because the record can help you time your meditation session. For example, if you wish to meditate for 10 minutes, start the record at the halfway point. When you notice the sound has stopped, you will know that 10 minutes have elapsed.

If you use an external device to time your meditation session (a highly recommended practice initially; remember that distortions in time sense can occur), choose something that will turn a stimulus off at the end of a session. Do not use an oven timer or an alarm clock. Such an assault on the quiet environment will not allow you to emerge from your session properly. Rather, have a constant stimulus (like a nature sounds record) go off or fade away. This will allow you to reenter the external world softly as you notice that the sound is no longer there.

Specific Posture

Because of its somatopsychic effects, **posture** is important to effective meditation training. Theoretically, the position of the body during meditation influences states of mind. Meditative postures have evolved to facilitate the attainment of a desired state of consciousness. Think back to the old pop psychology concept of body language. This theory asserts that a person's mental orientation is unconsciously displayed by the way the person positions his or her body. The posture effect in meditation is just the opposite.

Instead of the mental state positioning the body, the position of the body affects state of mind.

The effects of body position on consciousness are subtle, but meditation is an activity in which subtle changes are highly significant. Sit down and place your hands over your stomach. Stop reading and notice how you feel in this pose. Now slowly open your arms and spread them out wide. Notice how you feel with your arms open. In which position do you feel the most secure? In which do you feel the most exposed or vulnerable? Repeat this activity, but this time close your eyes. Compare the mental sensation of security you have when your hands are folded over your stomach with the sensation of vulnerability you experience with your arms outstretched. The position of the body can quietly influence subjective states of mind.

Posture has long been associated with meditation practice. In fact, one form of Hindu meditation, called mudra, involves merely placing the hands in specified poses. Next time you see statues or illustrations of Eastern religious figures or deities in meditative poses, notice the hands. They will be in specific poses; this is mudra. Each position is designed to facilitate the attainment of a specific state of consciousness during meditation. Remember that meditation is a sensitive, quiet discipline; subtle changes produce significant results.

Each discipline has its own guidelines for correct posture. Christian prayer specifies a pose indicative of respect and humbleness, well in line with the character of the activity. Most Eastern forms of meditation specify variations on the padmasana, or lotus position. This is a seated position in which the legs are extensively folded. The point of this posture is not to see how much pain the meditator can endure. Rather, it aids in clearing the mind and sharpening awareness. The remarkable effectiveness of this posture may lie in the fact that it straightens the spinal column so it no longer bends and turns as it does during normal standing or sitting. In theory, spinal curves promote some sodium leakage in the spinal nerves, thereby sending false messages to the body and brain. Normally, we receive these false transmissions simply as background interference or static that we have become accustomed to. Supposedly, by straightening the spine, the lotus position clears the mind by removing the cause of neural static. Whatever the means, straightening the back results in a sharpening of attention and clarity of thought. The somatopsychic influences of posture are so effective that we will devote most of Chapter 15 to exploring them.

As you begin meditation, we recommend that you sit comfortably in a position that allows your back to be as straight as possible. Sit in a straight-backed chair or on the floor with your back against a flat wall. Maintain a pose that is comfortable, erect, alert, and well balanced. Do not lie down; you may become drowsy or fall asleep. Use postures that allow you to be relaxed yet alert. Meditation promotes and requires a clear, wakeful consciousness.

Meditation Object

This characteristic is the most important of the five for differentiating the various forms of meditation. The **meditation object** is the intended focus of all attention. It is the repetitive or unchanging stimulus referred to in our definition. The various types of meditation all involve a different, specific stimulus as the object of attention. This meditation object could be any stimulus that repeats or does not change. It could be a ticking clock, a vase of flowers, the sensations of your own breathing, repetitive physical movement, or even an imaginary chord being played over and over again by an orchestral string section in your mind. We will discuss many different meditation objects later in this chapter. The object in beginning meditation often is your own breathing. We will discuss the reasons for this later. As you learn to meditate using the brief directions provided in this text, we recommend that you use the repetitive stimulus of simply breathing as your attentional focus.

Passive Attitude

After you have practiced meditation for a few days, you will notice that keeping your mind focused on the meditation object is very difficult. The human mind was designed to focus on dynamic, not unchanging, stimuli. Therefore, the mind wanders easily. You will find it nearly impossible to keep your mind on one object for even two or three minutes. Your wandering mind will be a chronic source of frustration as you try to master the seemingly simple act of meditation. Just remember that this is a phenomenon that even the most experienced yogi or roshi cannot escape. Adopting a **passive attitude** simply means that when you notice your mind wandering, you do not worry about it. Meditation is not supposed to become a source of frustration (a stressor).

Recall that we defined meditation as any activity that *attempts* to focus and maintain attention. No one can actually maintain attention on a repetitive or unchanging thing, but merely can exert an honest effort. We expect your mind to wander. When you notice your attention drifting, gently steer it back on course. Realize that whatever has drawn your attention away can be thought about later. Adopt a passive attitude. The wandering mind is the single most common difficulty people have with meditation. When your mind wanders, accept it as natural and human. Do not worry about it. Quietly return your awareness to the appropriate object.

Regular Practice

Regular practice is of fundamental importance to the effective application of meditation to controlling stress. In order for meditation to help you recondition your psychophysiological response system, you must practice it regularly. This means daily. Think of it as you think of physical exercise. If you are going to use aerobic activity to condition your cardiovascular system, you must exercise at least three times a week. This is necessary to convince your body that it has a chronic need for increased cardiovascular performance. The same reasoning applies to meditation. Your aim is to retrain your mind and body to respond to stressors in a relaxed fashion. To override old patterns of behavior, you must rehearse this response pattern often, until it becomes your dominant mode of operation. Regular practice will ensure a carryover effect.

Instructions for Transcendental Meditation, the technique most widely used in the West, recommend that you practice for 20 minutes twice each day. This is excessive for beginners. If you think you have to spend 40 minutes of each day meditating, you probably will not bother with it. Or, because 20 minutes of focused attention on unchanging things will definitely tax the tolerance of most novices, you may end up meditating for 3 minutes and spend the remaining 17 anxious, bored, and impatient waiting for the time to pass.

When you start out, try to meditate for 5 to 10 minutes each day that you can. Five minutes of well focused attention beats 20 of boredom. Gradually, as you feel comfortable doing so, work your way up to about 15 minutes once each day. Set aside a regular, specific time each day for meditation. Some practitioners think that regularity of routine is beneficial by itself.

You should coordinate your meditation time with eating, sleeping, and physical exercise. Meditate before eating, not after. After a large meal, blood flow concentrates in and around the gastrointestinal system to facilitate food absorption. This helps you digest food, but it also makes you sleepy, a phenomenon called postprandial lethargy. You need to be awake and alert for meditation, so do it before eating.

Practice meditation during times of your waking day that are significantly removed from sleep periods. If you meditate first thing in the morning, you will go back to sleep. If you meditate before bed in the evening, you may either fall asleep while meditating or you may stay successfully alert and not be able to sleep afterward. Do not associate meditation with sleeping.

Finally, meditate after, not before, physical exercise. If you meditate before you exercise, it will relax your systems and temporarily diminish some of your physical ability. If you wait until after you have exercised, meditation will return your body to a resting state quickly. Also, the rebound from physical exertion combined with the cognitive effects of meditation will produce a profound change in your consciousness. Try it and enjoy it.

To summarize, meditation training for the management of stress has five basic components:

1. Quiet environment
2. Correct posture
3. Meditation object
4. Passive attitude
5. Regular practice

THE ROLE OF MEDITATION IN STRESS MANAGEMENT

Any personal comprehensive stress management program should include one technique that conditions the mind-body system to operate in a trophotrophic response pattern in the face of psychogenic stressors. Meditation serves that purpose for many people. Practiced daily, meditation can condition adaptive low arousal, enhance concentration ability, and increase attention span and mental acuity. Meditation is not an effective tool when used infrequently in the control of situational stressors. Techniques such as social engineering or cognitive reappraisal serve this purpose. Meditation is a preventive, trophotrophic conditioning activity that needs to be practiced regularly to be effective.

Meditation training produces a low-reactivity, psychophysiological carryover effect in most people. In fact, it is almost universally effective in this regard. Some people like meditation better than others do, and even though it is effective, some people do not like it at all. Recent research has indicated that people who relate best to meditation training are those who have a relatively well-developed awareness of internal states. Such people are generally sensitive to changes in internal activity, either cognitive or physical. They are comfortable with passive, internally focused activities like meditation. Strongly developed Type A individuals often become impatient while trying to sit still and meditate. People who are externally focused and time conscious and need to be constantly active may wish to look to other techniques, such as progressive neuromuscular relaxation, for conditioning trophotrophic responding. Another general group of people who have difficulty with meditation are those who have gone through life using some maladaptive habit as a coping device. These would be people who smoke, snack, or throw things to relieve stress. They are accustomed to physical action when under stress, so it is difficult for them to sit quietly. Meditating often makes them nervous.

Give meditation an honest try. Generally and for most people, this simple technique works well indeed. Try it for a couple weeks and see how it works for you.

HOW TO MEDITATE

First, read through these instructions completely. Now seek out a quiet space or create a quiet environment with some sort of white noise. Next, assume a comfortable, yet erect, seated posture. Try to sit in a position that seems balanced and requires little muscular effort to maintain. Your back should be reasonably straight. Your position should be one that keeps your mind alert, clear, and awake, not one that promotes drowsiness or sleep.

When you have achieved a comfortable, alert posture, slowly let your eyes close. Notice how your perception of the world changes as your eyes close. With your eyes open, most of your attention is devoted to what you see, so you tend to ignore your other senses. When your eyes close, your "secondary" senses suddenly become more vivid. With your eyes shut, you can easily focus attention on sensations that you usually ignore. Notice the new sounds you hear. Notice how easily you can feel tactile sensations from your body.

Direct your attention now to one of your subtle, somatic sensations. Focus your awareness on the sensations of a physical process that you ignore most of the time, a process that continually repeats itself inside your body each minute of each day of your life. Focus your attention on the quiet sensations of your own breathing.

Notice what it feels like to breathe in and breathe out. Just breathe in and out, naturally, at your own pace, and be aware of how it feels. Do not describe the sensations to yourself or try to put them into words; simply experience your breathing. Notice how it feels to draw air into your body, to fill your chest with renewed life and energy as you inhale. Notice how it feels to exhale, to release the spent air, to empty yourself again. Be aware of the sensations of air passing through your mouth or nostrils as you breathe in and out. Continue to breathe easily and naturally.

You will soon discover that no two breaths are exactly the same. Some are long, some are short. Some are deep and some are shallow. Breaths are like snowflakes—all are similar but no two are exactly alike. Focus all your awareness on your breathing; fully experience what it feels like to breathe.

As you continue to breathe quietly, in and out, passively aware of the sensations of every breath, say a silent word with each phase of each breath. Each time you inhale, say silently to yourself the word *one*. Each time you exhale, say to yourself the word *two*. Count one and two with every breath you take. This simple mental device will help you keep your attention on your breathing. For 5 or 10 minutes, breathe naturally, in and out. Be aware of the sensations of each breath, count one and two, and clear your mind of all things except the vital living process of breathing.

Remember, your mind is doomed to wander. When it does, just steer it gently back on course. Focus on your breathing.

After meditating on your breathing for 5 or 10 minutes, and before opening your eyes, bring your awareness back to the external world. Lift your attention from your breathing and remember where you are. Remember what clothes you are wearing. Bring your mind back to the outside world. With your eyes still closed, visualize the room you are sitting in. Remember what activities you have to do today after you finish meditating. Finally, remember and visualize what the physical space directly in front of you looks like. Just before opening your eyes, create in your mind a complete visual image of what you will see as your eyes open. Prepare yourself to arise from meditation.

Now, gently open your eyes. . . . Look around . . . breathe . . . feel. . . . Bring yourself back to the outside world feeling alert, alive, awake, relaxed, and refreshed. Stand up, . . . stretch. Proceed with life with a calmer, clearer mind and body.

That is it. Meditation is really very simple. Do this each day, at a regular time, for 5 to 10 minutes. Spend time at the end of each session slowly bringing your mind back to external reality. This will foster a smooth, effective transition from meditation to daily life, allowing you to feel alert and refreshed rather than drowsy.

VARIETIES OF MEDITATION TRAINING

The form of meditation just described is used as the introductory activity in most serious meditation disciplines. In yoga, it is called **pranayama**; in Zen, it is called **anapanasati**. Pranayama is often referred to as the science of breath. Its literal translation from Sanskrit is expansion, or manifestation of first energy (ayama: expansion or manifestation; pra: first unit, na: energy). Pranayama involves the process of drawing in the vital living energy—the process of breathing. Breathing and breath awareness meditation form the fundamental first steps of yoga.

Zen meditation begins with anapanasati, or breath counting. In anapanasati, consecutive breaths are counted from one to ten over and over. This meditation style is considered the essential introductory exercise to the more advanced exercises in meditation and cognitive development that constitute the rigorous training of Zen.

Breathing meditation is perhaps the most effective object, or style, for reducing psychophysiological arousal. It is not the only way to meditate, however. There are many different forms of meditation, each with its own object or specified focus of attention. The specific meditation object used separates one form of meditation from another.

There are three basic schemes by which we can categorize the various approaches to meditation. Some forms of meditation have external objects; others have internal objects. Some forms restrict awareness; others expand awareness. Finally, although most meditation practices are physically passive, a few are vigorously active.

Meditation With External Objects

Many forms of meditation rely on external stimuli to provide the focus of attention. Passively contemplating the image of a flower arrangement, or watching ocean waves roll in and out, or listening to the ticking of a clock, or feeling a steady autumn breeze blow through your hair could all be external focuses of meditation. A gentle branch of Zen, called Soto, often employs a form of meditation in which the practitioner sits on a hillside and visually drinks in the scene of the valley below. No thought is encouraged, just visual experience. The practitioner continues this activity daily, until he can close his eyes and visualize the entire landscape in every detail. This is an example of a type of meditation that emphasizes expanding awareness to take in all sensation, as opposed to restricting it to a single, minute thought or stimulus.

Another external object of meditation is the **mandala**, a geometric figure of circular motif with other concentric forms within it, usually other circles and squares. A mandala is usually highly complex, with deities and other elements positioned throughout it. The relative position of the elements is usually of spiritual or philosophical significance. An example of a Tibetan mandala is shown in Figure 13.1. The mandala is used as a visual focus for external meditation. The meditator looks at the mandala until he or she can close the eyes and visualize it in every detail. The mandala may then continue as an object of both external and internal focus, bridging the gap between external experience and the inner self.

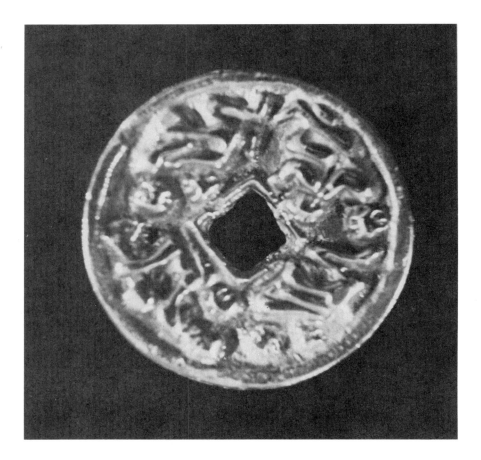

Figure 13.1. Mandala.

There is a story of a search for the Great Mandala by a sect of monks from the Soto school of Zen. They felt that as long as they were dedicating a significant portion of their lives to the contemplation of a mandala it might as well be **the** mandala. Some of the monks expressed the opinion that the earth itself was the Great Mandala. Others said no; the earth could not be viewed in its totality; the sun was the Great Mandala, they said. This seemed like a reasonable conclusion. The next day the monks assembled before dawn on a hillside facing the east. As the sun arose, they all fixed their eyes in wonder and contemplation on the Great Mandala, an orb of flame rising in the eastern sky. Their eyes traced its divine path until it disappeared behind their hillside in a grand display of color, light, and cloud. The monks were convinced they had indeed identified the Great Mandala. They were so inspired that they repeated their solar vigil for several days, from rising dawn to blazing dusk. After the third or fourth day, all were blind. It was a contented blindness, however, because the monks had the image of the sun, the Great Mandala, permanently burned into the retinas of their eyes.

Meditation Generated From Within

Generally, internal meditation restricts awareness to a specific stimulus. The most widely practiced form of meditation in the West, Transcendental Meditation, uses an internal focus called a **mantra**. Transcendental Meditation is actually derived from **mantrum yoga**. A mantra is a word or phrase repeated over and over, usually silently, that is used as an internal focus of attention for meditation. In our suggested exercise, the words *one* and *two* served as mantra. Other examples include the Kundalini mantra, *sat---nam*, meaning truth and light, or the universal mantra, *OM*. Some religious and philosophical disciplines assert that the particular mantra used by each individual is of critical importance. From a psychophysiological perspective, however, the various meditation objects used display no significant difference in their ability to reduce stress reactivity. Some complex mantra are recited aloud as chants and can produce profound changes in states of consciousness, particularly in group settings.

Ornstein has discussed a form of internal meditation that involves the use of internally generated sounds called **nadams**. These sounds are to be imagined and thus absorb all mental attention. A few examples include cin nadam, hum of the honey of intoxicated bees; ghanta nadam, sound of a ringing bell; tela nadam, sound of a small tight drum; and mega nadam, sound of rolling thunder.

Physiological processes are often used as internal objects. The body provides us with numerous repetitive sensations that are tangible and easily accessible stimuli for meditative attention. The best example is the process of breathing, as in pranayama and anapanasati, which we have already discussed. Breathing meditation is frequently employed as an introductory exercise to more advanced forms and also as the initial step of mastery for disciplines that teach control of visceral functions. Breathing meditation not only provides an effective attentional focus but also promotes an increased level of somatic awareness, the ability to sense subtle states and changes within the body. In terms of promoting decreased nervous reactivity to stressors and trophotrophic conditioning, breathing seems to be the most effective meditation object. We will discuss it in detail in Chapter 15.

The Rinzai school of Zen has evolved some interesting, and cognitively rigorous, meditation methods. In contrast to the Soto school, which operates on gentle, progressive development, Rinzai is an explosive, difficult discipline relying on sudden bursts of insight. Rinzai Zen uses a device called the **koan** as an absorbing meditation technique. A koan is an answerless riddle, or a question devoid of any possible logical solution. Examples include the classic "What is the sound of one hand clapping?" or "What did your face look like before you were conceived?" The koan can absorb and hold mental attention because no solution can be realized, no matter how hard one concentrates. Some practitioners think the real attentional focus of the koan is the answerless quality of the riddle (the concept of Mu). Others contend that the value of the koan is that by concentrating on its illogical nature, the rational mind is driven into submission by frustration, thereby allowing the intuitive consciousness to emerge and manifest itself. In either case, koan meditation is difficult mentally and requires master guidance to be of any value. It is not a modality recommended for general stress management but a step on the journey to high-level cognitive development.

Za-Zen is the most highly disciplined of all meditation variations. It is sometimes described as sitting meditation because it usually involves four hours per day of seated contemplation. Za-Zen is highly esoteric in practice and in focus. The sole object of meditation is merely the inner experience of meditative consciousness itself. Clearly, this is a technique for an advanced practitioner who has master guidance. It is suited to philosophical and cognitive development and is not recommended for the average person as part of a simple stress control program.

Physically Active Forms of Meditation

Our image of meditation is often one of physical passivity. Many meditation forms, including those we have just discussed, are physically passive. These forms are hypo-metabolic; they promote low levels of physical arousal. Meditation does not necessarily have to be physically inactive, however. Some of the most profound alterations in consciousness that can be induced by meditation are the result of its vigorous, physically active forms.

The best example of physically active meditation is a Sufi technique called the dance of the dervish. Sometimes referred to as the whirling dervish, this dancelike form of meditation bombards the sense with repetition. The activity usually involves circular, repetitive dancing in groups. Elaborate chants are combined with the dance steps. The result is that visual, auditory, and kinesthetic sensations are flooded with repetitive stimulation that is totally impossible to ignore. People frequently pass out during Sufi dancing. It is said that the Sufi dances with "feet on the ground and head in the clouds."

Kundalini yoga is another energetic discipline that involves hypermetabolic meditation. Kundalini meditation is designed to liberate energy from the lower chakras. This energy can be directed toward achieving phenomenal physical endurance or enhancing healing potential. Kundalini means coiled snake, a metaphor for the energy at the base of the spine that can be released through specific meditation and breath maneuvers, as a snake would strike, firing tremendous energy up through the vital systems. Little physiological research has been done with Kundalini, so nothing is known about its physiological effects, but clearly profound physical changes occur as a result of its practice. Unless directed by truly qualified masters, however, Kundalini can be extremely dangerous. Total celibacy is required of serious participants. Kundalini is an energetic discipline involving meditation. It is not specifically recommended for stress control.

Rhythmic exercise is one energetic meditation approach that does work well for managing stress effectively. Any form of physical exercise that contains a significant repetitive component can be used effectively as a form of meditation. Examples include running, swimming, and cycling. The key is that the practitioner focus attention on the repetitive facet of the task. Not only will the combined benefits of physical exercise and meditation be derived from this hybrid, but there will be a noticeable increase in endurance performance for the physical task. Marathon runners and long-distance cyclists commonly report that they use some form of repetitive attentional focus to help them conquer the agonizing physical endurance demands of their sport. Vigorous, repetitive physical activity and meditation together create a powerful psychophysiological weapon against stress.

The forms of meditation we have discussed represent only a few of the many forms practiced in different cultures around the world. By now you should understand what meditation is all about, and we can move on to a discussion of its benefits.

THEORETICAL MECHANISM OF EFFECTIVENESS

No one really knows how meditation works to reduce psychosomatic arousal. We will look at a few reasonable theories to get some idea how this simple mental activity can alter the long-term functioning of the mind-body system. The effectiveness of meditation is due to something more than just sitting quietly for a while. Most research into the physiological effects of meditation has compared it to simple, nonspecific relaxation and found it to be significantly more effective. Something about focusing attention on repetitive or unchanging things is capable of changing the operation of the mind-body system.

The most effective way to induce an altered state of consciousness behaviorally is through the use of repetitive stimulation. Meditation may even have been designed for this purpose. Through repetition, the dominant, analytic portion of the brain may be tied up with a menial task, thereby easing its suppression of the intuitive mind and allowing experiential consciousness to emerge. How, then, does changing states of consciousness help reduce stress responses?

Ornstein (1971) has indicated that the process of meditation "in psychological terms is an attempt to recycle the same subroutine over and over again in the nervous system." Remember that the essence of meditation is attention. When one fixes attention effectively over and over on the same stimulus, the conscious mind is tied up in a benign cycle of thought. Emotionally charged thoughts are barred from entering awareness. The cognitive result is the creation of an emotionless state. The physiologic result of this temporarily emotionless state is a stabilized, low level of arousal—a parasympathetic-dominant condition. By fixing all cognitive attention on a repetitive, emotion-free thought, the mind enters a state free of the normal, randomly pestering arousal from tiny flashes of worry, fear, joy, and anxiety. The mind stops sending mobilization messages to the body. The body can rest, truly undisturbed, for a time. We can liken this state to having the phone off the hook. With no more distracting messages calling you into action, you can relax and refresh yourself without disturbance.

Breathing meditation seems to be particularly effective for altering psychophysiological states. Again, no one understands how it works. The current theory is that since breathing regulation occurs in the brainstem along structures intertwined with the reticular activating system (a collection of cerebral structures that control the overall arousal level of the brain), regulation (or stabilization) of breathing helps stabilize adjacent areas as well. Since breathing control is located so close to the control center for cerebral arousal, careful regulation of breath may stabilize and lower the arousal level of the entire cerebral mass. The result is a neurogenic calming of the mind, reduced stimulation and output of the hypothalamus, and lowered physiological arousal. Keep in mind also that focused attention on bodily processes produces an enhanced sense of somatic awareness. This is highly beneficial for detecting the tiny early changes associated with stress-related disease so they can be dealt with before a real physical disorder results.

Meditation interrupts the psychosomatic model at the emotional arousal, physical arousal, and physical effects levels. Practitioners often observe that a significant early effect of meditation training is that they can keep events in perspective more appropriately. They do not get as upset at little things anymore. This indicates that meditation intervenes at the cognitive appraisal level as well. This same attitude shift often manifests itself as a desire to avoid unnecessary stressors. The mental tranquility produced by meditation can be highly addictive. People often lose their desire to hassle with life for insignificant rewards. The cognitive shift produced by meditation training can make you more keenly aware of the value of social engineering. Thus, meditation can even have impact at the sensory stimulus level. Some research indicates that perceptual changes, such as enhanced sensory acuity, accompany meditation training. Although the validity of this possibility is still somewhat open to question, it suggests that meditation may be found to affect perception as well. An obvious reason for the effectiveness of meditation, then, is that it can intervene in the psychosomatic disease process at many significant points, not only in the mind but in the body and the environment as well.

RESEARCH FINDINGS AND APPLICATIONS

Meditation is an old practice, yet its widespread use in the West for managing stress goes back only about 15 years. The Eastern mind easily accepted meditation long ago and practiced it because personal, empirical evidence indicated that it was a thing of value. Westerners seem to need analytic, objective, laboratory data to prove something is worthwhile before we will even consider trying it. According to our mind set, nothing is good until science says it is. The practice of meditation to control stress in the Western world blossomed only after laboratory tests indicated that meditation could measurably alter physiological states. This is a classic example of East meeting West. One of our fundamental tools for enhancing the quality of human health has gained acceptance and wide usage because Western scientific methods have been applied to study an ancient, intuitive discipline from the East.

The physiological investigation of meditation and related disciplines began in 1935 with an empirical study by Therese Brosse. She packed her portable electrocardiogram (ECG) for a trip from France to India. During her stay, she monitored the heart activity of a number of yogis who were said to be capable of performing unusual feats of visceral control. She reported observing that one of her subjects had stopped his heart (and presumably started it up again), based on her ECG recording. For two decades no one paid much attention to this significant observation or guessed at its tremendous implications.

In 1957, Bagchi and Wenger made an attempt to replicate Brosse's observation using superior instrumentation. According to their findings, none of the yogis measured could actually stop the heart. They did notice, however, that in striving to accomplish this task, the yogis were engaged in a "Valsalva maneuver." This action attempts to increase thoracic pressure through a specific breathing pattern and increased intercostal and pectoral (chest) muscle activity. Bagchi and Wenger thought that Brosse's subject had probably not stopped his heart, but that on her inferior equipment, the ECG signal had been masked by interference from skeletal muscle activity.

B. K. Anand had collaborated with Bagchi and Wenger. During the course of the study, he had noted that although the yogis did not actually stop their heart, they did produce significant reductions in heart and respiration rate. In 1961, he launched two studies that became the first indicators that meditation training could have a direct positive bearing on the experience of psychogenic stress.

One of Anand's studies involved Shri Ramanand Yogi, an experienced yoga practitioner. Reportedly, Ramanand Yogi could survive with little oxygen through the meditative techniques he had mastered. He was known for demonstrating his skill by having his assistants bury him in a small box underground and leave him there for several days. He always emerged, quiet and alive. Anand wanted to see whether Ramanand Yogi could survive at low oxygen concentrations under controlled laboratory conditions. He sealed him in an airtight box and left him to meditate while the oxygen concentrations in his enclosure were continuously monitored. He was given a panic button to press when he wanted out. By the time Ramanand Yogi signaled his desire to terminate the experiment, he had markedly reduced his oxygen consumption and carbon dioxide elimination. He had remained in the box during times when oxygen concentrations were at drastically low levels. Later, in 1964, Sugi and Akatsu reported that monks performing Za-Zen decreased their oxygen consumption by 20 percent and showed similar reductions in carbon dioxide production. These findings indicated that meditation could produce a hypometabolic physiological state.

Anand's second study involved exposing four experienced yogis to noxious stimuli. It had been determined that when the yogis were meditating, the occipital region of the brain produced a marked predominance of alpha waves. This wave form was thought to be indicative of a state of mental calm. In fact, during meditation, the yogis said they were inducing samadhi, a state of internal mental ecstasy in which one is oblivious to external events. The investigators wanted to see if they could disrupt this state. While they were meditating, two of the yogis were exposed to strong lights, loud banging noises, hot glass rods touched to the skin, and tuning fork vibrations. These stimuli would easily shatter the fragile alpha rhythms in any of us. The yogis maintained steady alpha waves throughout the experiment. The other two yogis were exposed to the cold pressor test, which involves immersing the hand in ice water (4° centigrade). This procedure, now used as a standard laboratory stressor, makes a human *very* uncomfortable after only 30 seconds and elicits a profound adrenergic stress reaction. The hands of two meditating yogis were placed in the ice water for 45-55 minutes, yet their alpha waves did not falter. All of the stimuli used in this investigation represented laboratory procedures that reliably induce a stress response in humans. Meditation placed the yogis in a psychophysiological state that was not reactive to strong stressors.

Anand's studies indicated that meditation can be of specific value for controlling human stress. They showed that meditation produces a hypometabolic physiological state, in direct opposition to the hypermetabolic condition of stress, and they established that during meditation practitioners do not display neurological or physiological reactions to profound sensory stressors.

The most influential research on meditation was published nearly a decade after Anand reported his findings. The original research project was carried out as a doctoral dissertation study by Robert Wallace and later expanded in conjunction with Herbert Benson. Basically, Wallace and Benson (1972) investigated the comprehensive physiological correlates of Transcendental Meditation. Their research represented the first attempt to identify the overall somatic effects of a basic form of meditation. At the time it was done, their research was significant for using subjects with relatively little meditation expertise. Earlier studies had used subjects with decades of devotion to meditation.

Wallace and Benson compared periods of actual meditation practice to simple rest periods. In this way, they felt that they could see what effects, if any, meditation had above and beyond simply sitting still and relaxing. Each subject was asked to sit quietly for 20-30 minutes, then meditate for 30 minutes, then just sit quietly for an additional 20-30 minutes.

Compared to periods of sitting quietly, Wallace and Benson noted the following physiological correlates of Transcendental Meditation:

1. Intensification of alpha waves
2. Increased skin resistance (decreased perspiration)
3. Decreased heart rate
4. Increased peripheral blood flow (vasodilation)
5. No change in arterial blood pressure

6. Decreased respiration rate
7. Decreased respiratory volume
8. Decreased oxygen consumption
9. Decreased carbon dioxide elimination
10. Decreased blood lactate levels

The significance of this cluster of somatic effects was best described by the experimenters themselves: "The pattern of changes suggests that meditation generates an integrated response, or reflex, that is mediated by the central nervous system. A well-known reflex of such a nature was described many years ago by the Harvard physiologist Walter B. Cannon; it is called the 'flight or flight' or 'defense alarm' reaction. The aroused sympathetic nervous system mobilizes a set of physiological responses marked by increases in blood pressure, heart rate, blood flow to the muscles and oxygen consumption. The hypometabolic state produced by meditation is of course opposite to this in almost all respects. It looks very much like a counterpart of the fight or flight reaction."

Based on this initial research into its physiological correlates, it appears that during meditation the body is in a state that is the antithesis of what we have described as human stress. It seems valuable, therefore, to offset our daily stress-related arousal with periods of meditation. It helps promote a healthy overall homeostatic balance. The next question is whether meditation training can influence stress reactivity or recovery during times when a person is not meditating.

To date, a handful of studies have investigated the ability of meditation training to produce a carryover effect for conditioning decreased stress reactivity. One of the most significant of these studies was performed by Daniel Goleman and Gary Schwartz (1976). They compared the reactivity of meditators (again they were practitioners of Transcendental Meditation) to nonmeditators while they watched a stressful film that described industrial shop accidents. They used heart rate and skin potential response (perspiration) as indicators of psychophysiological reactivity. One of their findings was surprising. Meditators reacted to the stressor with higher response amplitude than did nonmeditators. Other studies have confirmed that in response to relatively sudden stimuli, meditators initially show a greater somatic reaction.

Further analysis of Goleman and Schwartz's results, along with a careful look at data from similar studies, revealed an important facet of the meditator response pattern that was rarely discussed. The amplitude of response to sudden stimuli is greater in meditators than in nonmeditators, but the duration of response is significantly shorter for meditators. The two response patterns are illustrated in Figure 13.2. In this representation, level of arousal is plotted against time. The small arrow in the middle of the figure indicates the onset of the stressor. The normal, untrained individual's reaction to the stressor is indicated by the dashed line and the meditator's response is indicated by the solid line.

Notice that meditators recover from their arousal much faster than controls do. The high initial response amplitude and relatively rapid reaction on the part of meditators indicates something extremely important: Meditators are not oblivious to the external world. When not actually meditating, they are more sensitive and immediately reactive to changes in the environment than nonmeditators are. This is highly desirable as long as the cost is not increased disease susceptibility. Recovery rate now becomes important. A high response amplitude by itself does not represent a pathogenic response pattern. It is only specifically undesirable if a person already has a serious organ weakness that is close to the breaking point. The true indicator of pathogenesis is response duration. The longer an organ system stays aroused, the greater is the probability that it will contribute to a

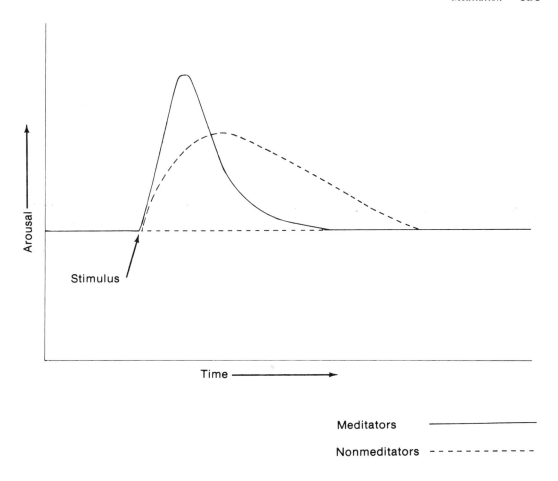

Figure 13.2. Stress reactivity patterns; meditators versus nonmeditators.

chronic imbalance resulting in disease. Look at Figure 13.2 again and notice that meditators recover quickly, whereas nonmeditators display the relatively pathogenic response pattern. It looks as though meditators get the best of both worlds. They are aware, alert, and sensitive to the environment, and when they are aroused, their reaction does not linger and hence induce a disease-fostering process. They react to the world and immediately relax.

If you remember our discussion of the impact of physical exercise on stress, you will note that meditation and aerobic exercise produce the same pattern of reactivity to stress. This should tell us something about the synchronous relationship of the mind and body. The same psychophysiological result can be achieved through both psychosomatic and somatopsychic pathways. We can think of all the stress control modalities as the spokes of a wheel, with perfect, adaptive mind-body integration at the center. Stress management devices can start at many different points, but they all meet at the center. Meditation is just one way to get there.

We have highlighted significant discoveries that are of particular concern to the management of psychophysiological stress. There are volumes of information on other facets of meditation. For example, many studies have been done to determine the effects of meditation on perception and perceptual performance. There is also a good deal of literature on the effectiveness of meditation training as a behavioral replacement for drug abuse. The conclusions that can be drawn from the rest of the meditation literature are that, although data are still inconclusive and highly contradictory, meditation has the apparent potential to alter positively numerous facets of human performance and may have some utility as a therapeutic tool for dealing with some maladaptive behavioral manifestations of excessive stress.

CONTRAINDICATIONS AND COMMON DIFFICULTIES

The general cautions given in Chapter 10 for the safe use of relaxation training also apply to meditation. If you have hypoglycemia (low blood sugar) or hypotension (chronically low blood pressure) or if you take regular medication for hypertension (chronically high blood pressure), diabetes, or epilepsy, you should contact your physician regularly while you are engaged in meditation training.

A good general guideline for the practice of meditation or any other related skill is that if any facet of a technique produces adversive or painful results, either physical or cognitive, you should stop using it and consult a knowledgeable expert for assistance. This could be the case if meditation training begins to unveil some repressed psychological trauma. Meditation awakens deep internal awareness, so it is not uncommon for long repressed thoughts to emerge. This is generally a positive effect, allowing one to air and hence deal with suppressed fears and anxieties, but many people react negatively. Psychological trauma or damage could result if a particularly strong negative reaction ensues. If this happens to you, either discontinue meditation practice or seek professional assistance with the problem that has been unearthed. If the problem is serious, do not try to deal with it alone. Get some expert guidance.

Although it is not specifically a contraindication to meditation training, we should restate that some people do not do well with this technique. Some people just cannot sit still. In general, meditation is not a good technique for Type A individuals. It is also not particularly effective for people who are accustomed to coping with stress by using active, behavioral devices like smoking or eating. In both of these instances, meditation is likely to lead to frustration or anxiety. Using other more behaviorally active techniques is recommended.

Because they have a limited attention span, children may have unique difficulties meditating. They also may experience unique rewards because of their relatively fresh, unhammered consciousness. If you wish to implement meditation with kids, see *Meditation for Children* by Rozman. It does a good job of explaining how to adapt meditation practice concepts to fresh minds.

People commonly encounter three difficulties during the initial phases of meditation training. These difficulties are not contraindications and should not be considered reasons to discontinue meditating. Each can be dealt with simply and effectively. In fact, it would be highly unusual if you did not experience them.

The wandering mind is an almost universal difficulty. Remember that the human mind is not designed to focus and maintain attention on repetitive or unchanging things. Your mind is going to wander. Simply remember to maintain a passive attitude, do not worry about it, and gently steer your attention back on track. Realize that it is a natural, unavoidable phenomenon, and do not let it trouble you further.

The second common meditation difficulty usually manifests itself a week or two after the start of a meditation program and persists for about a week at the most. Some people describe it by saying they feel as though they have been run over by a truck. It is not uncommon to experience aches, minor pains, and muscular discomfort a short time after starting meditation training. This seems disappointing when meditation is supposed to make you feel good.

At first, I thought that something about meditation was increasing muscular tension when I was investigating this in the Psychophysiological Research Laboratory at the University of Maryland. So I measured tension readings at various sites in the body of people who had no meditation training. After this group had been meditating for a couple weeks, the ones who complained of muscular discomfort returned to the lab for a second measurement while they were feeling rotten. I was surprised to discover that muscular tension was lower on the second reading. People who were experiencing tension problems as a result of meditation were actually more relaxed than they had been when they started.

Remember that besides helping you relax physically, meditation promotes enhanced somatic awareness. What seems to happen with people who have this difficulty is that their rate of increase in somatic awareness outpaces their ability to relax their body. They become aware of already existing muscular tension and related somatic difficulties. They had ignored their problems before, but meditation focuses their awareness on what is going on inside. The problem is usually solved in a few days, because the relaxation level of the body catches up with somatic awareness. Think of how your body reacts when you begin a physical exercise program. You are sore during the first few days, but if you stick with it, the discomfort soon fades. It is a good sign if meditation makes you feel physically strange after a week or so. It means you are learning to listen to your body.

The final problem is called the space cadet syndrome. Symptoms can appear anywhere from a few days to several months after one starts meditating. They can persist for just a few days, they can become chronic and remain with you for life, or they can be transient, coming and going without warning. Symptoms include glazed eyes, a spaced-out look, attempting to walk through closed doors, tripping over furniture, leaving home without putting on your clothes, difficulty in forming complex sentences, listening to brick walls, visually fixating on doorknobs, and responding to everything with a phrase like "Oh, wow." This syndrome is surprisingly common among novice meditators. It is due simply to an error in thinking. The afflicted person thinks meditation is supposed to numb your senses, place your consciousness permanently in the cosmic reaches, and keep you out of touch with your earthly existence. The altered state associated with meditation occurs only during meditation itself. It should not stay with you after your session is over. When you finish meditating, you should spend a moment returning your mind to the external world, and then arise feeling refreshed and alert, with an increased awareness of your external surroundings. Meditation is not withdrawal. It is a technique to enhance all aspects of life.

If you are meditating correctly, you can almost bet that one of these problems will affect you. Remember that they are common and often indicate that you are reacting naturally to a novel activity. Keep it up and the rewards will come.

WHAT TO EXPECT FROM MEDITATION

Meditation is a discipline of deep subtlety. Its effects and changes will come upon you quietly. Do not expect drastic, sudden shifts. Rather, expect the rough edges of your life to be smoothed over gradually from within.

First, expect to experience some of the characteristics of altered states of consciousness while you meditate. Some of these include a loss of time sense, perceptual alterations, changes in body image, and feelings of self-transcendence.

Meditation is fundamentally training in disciplined attention, so you will notice over time that your attention span increases. Tasks that you must attend to (like reading textbooks) will become more interesting; you will begin to see colors in areas you once thought were dark. Along with enhanced attentional ability will come an increased clarity of thought, sensation, and perception.

Most people report an increased ability to view life events in greater totality. They often say they can place events in proper perspective more easily. The result is that little things may stop bothering you as much as they did before, because your expanded awareness can better grasp how insignificant they are in relation to the totality of your life and happiness. Another manifestation of this effect may be a reduced desire to experience unnecessary stressors.

You will become aware that the arousal of your body to stress does not linger as it once did. You will still be aware and alert to external events, but you will begin to eliminate prolonged, maladaptive responses. You will clean the static from your mind and body and begin to experience a slowly growing inner calm that you will carry with you always.

SUMMARY

The ideas that led to the development of meditation were conceived more than 25 centuries ago. The techniques of meditation originally were designed to achieve an altered state of consciousness to facilitate spiritual awareness and integration. All meditative techniques involve the disciplined focusing of attention.

During this century, science discovered that meditative practice not only alters consciousness but also produces a profound alteration in somatic states. Meditation training helps create physiological states that can combat psychogenic stress. Because meditation training touches many facets of an individual's life, it can interrupt the psychosomatic chain of events at many levels. Regular practice of meditation may be the most valuable single technique we have for managing stress effectively.

REFERENCES

Allen, R. J. "Meditation," Autumn Wind, College Park, Md., 1979.

Allison, J. "Respiratory Changes During Transcendental Meditation," *Lancet*, v. 1(7651), 833-834, 1970.

Anand, B. K., et al. "Some Aspects of Electroencephalographic Studies in Yogis," *Electroencephalographology and Clinical Neurophysiology*, v. 13, 452-456, 1961.

———. "Studies on Shri Ramanand Yogi During His Stay in an Air-Tight Box," *The Indian Journal of Medical Research*, v. 49(1), 82-89, 1961.

Appelle, S., et al. "Simple Reaction Time as a Function of Alertness and Prior Mental Activity," *Perceptual and Motor Skills*, v. 38(3), 1263-1268, 1974.

Bagchi, B., and Wenger, M. "Electrophysiological Correlates of Some Yogi Exercises," *Electroencephalographology and Clinical Neurophysiology*, Supp. 7, 132-149, 1957.

Benson, H. "Decreased Alcohol Intake Associated With the Practice of Meditation: A Retrospective Investigation," *Annals of the New York Academy of Sciences*, v. 233, 174-177, 1974.

Benson, H., et al. "Continuous Measurement of CO_2 Elimination During a Wakeful Hypometabolic State, *Journal of Human Stress*, v. 1(1), 37-44, 1975.

———. "The Relaxation Response," *Psychiatry*, v. 37(1), 37-46, 1974.

Brosse, T. "A Psychophysiological Study," *Main Currents of Modern Thought*, v. 4, 77-84, 1946.

Childs, J. P. "The Use of Transcendental Meditation as Therapy for Juvenile Offenders," *Dissertation Abstracts International*, v. 34(8-A), 4732-4733, 1974.

Cowger, E. L. "The Effects of Meditation (Zazen) Upon Selected Dimensions of Personal Development," *Dissertation Abstracts International*, v. 34(8-A), 4734, 1974.

French, A. P., and Tupin, J. P. "Therapeutic Application of a Simple Relaxation Method," *American Journal of Psychotherapy*, v. 28(2), 282-287, 1974.

Goleman, D. J., and Schwartz, G. E. "Meditation as an Intervention in Stress Reactivity," *Journal of Consulting and Clinical Psychology*, v. 44(3), 456-466, 1976.

Kapleau, P. *The Three Pillars of Zen: Teaching, Practice, and Enlightenment*, Beacon Press, Boston, 1965.

Kasamatsu, A., and Hirai, T. "An Electroencephalographic Study of the Zen Meditation (Za-Zen), *Journal of the American Institute of Hypnosis*, v. 14(3), 107-114, 1973.

————. "Science of Za-Zen," *Psychologia: An International Journal of Psychology in the Orient*, v. b, 86-91, 1963.

Kuna, D. J. "Meditation and Work," *Vocational Guidance Quarterly*, v. 23(4), 342-346, 1975.

Linden, W. "Practicing of Meditation of School Children and Their Levels of Field Dependence-Independence, Test Anxiety and Reading Achievement," *Journal of Consulting and Clinical Psychology*, v. 41(1), 139-143, 1973.

Marcus, J. B. "Transcendental Meditation: A New Method of Reducing Drug Abuse," *Drug Forum*, v. 3(2), 113-136, 1974.

Maupin, E. W. "On Meditation," reprinted in Tart, C. T., *Altered States of Consciousness*, Doubleday, Garden City, N.Y., 1969.

Mishra, R. *Fundamentals of Yoga*, Julian Press, New York, 1959.

Naranjo, C., and Ornstein, R. E. *On the Psychology of Meditation*, Esalen Books, New York, 1971.

Orme-Johnson, D. W. "Autonomic Stability and Transcendental Meditation," *Psychosomatic Medicine*, v. 35(4), 341-349, 1973.

Penner, W. J., et al. "Does an In-depth Transcendental Meditation Course Effect Change in the Personalities of the Participants?" *Western Psychologist*, v. 4(4), 104-111, 1973.

Rahula, W. *What the Buddha Taught*, Grove Press, New York, 1959.

Rama, S., et al. *Science of Breath*, Himalayan Institute, Honesdale, Pa., 1979.

Ramsey, S. A. "Perceptual Style as a Predictor of Successful Meditation Training," Unpublished Master's Thesis, University of Maryland, College Park, Md., 1981.

Reps, P. *Zen Flesh, Zen Bones*, Doubleday, Garden City, N.Y.

Rozman, D. *Meditation for Children*, Celestial Arts, Millbrae, Calif., 1976.

Shafii, M. "Adaptive and Therapeutic Aspects of Meditation," *International Journal of Psychoanalytic Psychotherapy*, v. 2(3), 364-382, 1973.

Shafii, M., et al. "Meditation and Marijuana," *American Journal of Psychiatry*, v. 131(1), 60-63, 1974.

————. "Meditation and the Prevention of Alcohol Abuse," *American Journal of Psychiatry*, v. 132(9), 942-945, 1975.

Shah, I. *The Way of the Sufi*, Jonathan Cape, London, 1968.

Shapiro, D. H. "The Effects of Zen Meditation—Behavioral Self-Management Training Package in Treating Methadone Addiction: A Formative Study," *Dissertation Abstracts International*, v. 34(6-B), 2952-2953, 1973.

Smith, J. C. "Meditation as Psychotherapy: A Review of the Literature," *Psychological Bulletin*, v. 82(4), 558-564, 1975.

Stek, R. J., and Bass, B. A. "Personal Adjustment and Perceived Locus of Control Among Students Interested in Meditation," *Psychological Reports*, v. 32(3), 1019-1022, 1973.

Sugi, Y., and Akatsu, K. *Science of Za-Zen—Energy Metabolism*, Tokyo, 1964.

Suzuki, D. T. *What Is Zen?* Perennial Library, New York, 1971.

Swinyard, C. H., et al. "Neurological and Behavioral Aspects of Transcendental Meditation Relevant to Alcoholism: A Review," *Annals of the New York Academy of Sciences*, v. 233, 162-173, 1974.

Treichel, M., et al. "The Metabolic Effects of Transcendental Meditation," *Physiologist*, v. 16(3), 472, 1973.

Wallace, R. K. "Physiological Effects of Transcendental Meditation," *Science*, v. 167(3926), 1751-1754, 1970.

Wallace, R. K., and Benson, H. "The Physiology of Meditation," *Scientific American*, v. 226, 84-90, 1972.

Wallace, R. K., et al. "A Wakeful Hypometabolic Physiologic State," *American Journal of Physiology*, v. 221(3), 795-799, 1971.

Woolfolk, R. L. "Psychophysiological Correlates of Meditation," *Archives of General Psychiatry*, v. 32(10), 1326-1333, 1975.

Zuimonk, D. S., and Masunaga, R. *A Primer of Soto Zen*, East-West Center Press, Honolulu, 1971.

CHAPTER 14

Selective Awareness

. . . man is not something we know has to be surpassed; rather man is still something to be realized.

Robert Masters and Jean Houston

One of the most significant factors influencing the physical activity of our internal organs is the focus of our mental attention. The direction of our conscious thought via the neurological mechanisms of neocortical override can have a tremendous impact on all of our physiological processes. Psychogenic stress occurs when our minds focus attention on stimuli that foster worry, anxiety, fear, paranoia, or other forms of emotional upset. As we have learned, human beings have the power to choose where they direct their attention. This chapter will focus on several selective awareness techniques that can teach you how to gain control over the focus of your attention and then use this control to direct the internal activity of your body as an integrative psychophysiological means to combat stress.

HISTORICAL EMERGENCE
OF SELECTIVE AWARENESS TECHNIQUES

Perhaps the earliest known systematic form of selective awareness is **meditation**, which we have already discussed. In fact, most of the relaxation exercises discussed throughout this text involve elements of selective awareness. Most relaxation exercises include deliberate instructions for directing attention to specific sensations, which often enhances somatic awareness. This refers to the development of an increased awareness regarding the internal activities and sensations of the body. Selective awareness greatly enhances the effectiveness of all forms of systematic relaxation, even physical activities such as neuromuscular relaxation or aerobic exercise.

Hypnosis was one of the earliest systematic forms of selective awareness to emerge in the West. The principal figure credited with the early development and application of hypnosis was Anton Mesmer. Mesmer, an Austrian physician, practiced his technique during the late 18th and early 19th centuries. Mesmer's professional behavior deviated significantly from what was then considered appropriate clinical practice. Today we would call it quackery. Mesmer believed that organic disease was caused by an imbalance of universal magnetic fluids throughout the body. He thought that biological organisms had an innate balance of "animal magnetism." His therapeutic technique centered on restoring the balance of this magnetic flow in the body. During a treatment, Mesmer would place his patients inside a large tub (called a baquet) that resembled a horse trough. Inside the tub were several bottles filled with undefined chemicals; long iron rods protruded from each bottle. The tub was filled with water so that the bottles were totally submerged and only the ends of the iron rods remained above the surface of the water. Once the patient was situated in this tub, the lights would be dimmed and Mesmer would enter (wearing all manner of odd clothing). He would then remove the iron rods from the tub and touch them to various parts of the patient's body, informing the patient that this was to realign the flow of universal magnetic fluids.

Even though Mesmer's treatment was bizarre, it worked for many people who were suffering from the manifestations of hysteria (imagined physical problems). Mesmer's success had nothing to do with animal magnetism. The results he achieved have been attributed to his ability to convince his patients that the procedure was sound and would unquestionably cure them. It has been theorized that part of his effectiveness was due to the unusual setting he used for treatment and to his ability to induce, through this setting, a hypersuggestible state of consciousness within the afflicted individual. Mesmer purposely changed the focus of the patient's awareness in an effort to treat a perceived physical problem.

Mesmer, who was always regarded as a quack, purposely removed himself from the mainstream of medical science, but he had a steady flow of patients because his treatment was effective for many elements of hysteria.

A 19th century British physician named James Braid is credited with coining the term hypnosis. Braid was principally responsible for introducing hypnosis into accepted medical circles. Braid described the trance induced by hypnosis as "nervous sleep," from which the term neurohypnology was derived. This term was later shortened to simply hypnosis. Unlike Mesmer, Braid thought the origin of this trancelike state was within the subject rather than in an external source such as the therapist. Mesmer had believed that external factors, like the therapist and his magnetic rods, were the source of the therapeutic change. Through an understanding that the hypnosis phenomenon was one that took place within the mind of the subject through a shifting of attention, Braid was able to perform many public demonstrations of the techniques and gain the acceptance of his medical colleagues.

In 1842 a British physician named W. S. Ward performed a leg amputation on a patient who had been hypnotized. The patient reported that he felt nothing during the course of an operation capable of producing extreme physical pain. About 1849, a hospital in which operations were performed on hundreds of patients under hypnosis was opened in London. This selective awareness technique was found to be highly effective in altering or eliminating the subjective experience of physical pain under extreme conditions such as surgery. The discovery that ether could make a person insensitive to pain was made in this same decade, and ether quickly replaced hypnosis as a surgical anesthetic. Even though the chemicals were dangerous, the availability and reliability of chemical anesthetics severely hindered the further development of hypnosis as a therapeutic tool for helping patients handle pain and deal with physical disorders by changing their focus of attention.

Another systematic technique for using selective awareness to change consciousness or physiological states is called **autogenic training**. This system of exercises was developed in 1932 by the German psychiatrist Johannes Schultz. Schultz based this system on his early clinical experience with hypnosis. Autogenic training originated in part from the concept of autohypnosis, the induction of a hypnotic state without the external assistance of a therapist. From this, autogenic (auto: self; genic: genesis or origin) training derived its name. Autogenic training evolved as a series of techniques designed to induce states of deep mental and physiological relaxation. From his work with hypnosis and autohypnosis, Schultz noted that the two dominant sensations accompanying hypnotically induced relaxation were pleasurable feelings of overall warmth throughout the body and a pronounced feeling of heaviness in the limbs. Autogenic training was designed as a series of physical postures and mental focuses designed to build upon the two images of warmth and heaviness, thereby inducing deep relaxed states.

The late 1960s saw the expansion of specific techniques of visualization called **guided imagery**. Much of the pioneer work in developing guided imagery can be attributed to Robert Masters and Jean Houston. Masters and Houston began by studying the effects on consciousness and personality induced by psychoactive drugs, particularly LSD. In 1968, they published *Varieties of Psychedelic Experience*, which outlined the character of changes in consciousness a person experiences under the influence of psychedelic drugs. After their study of the qualitative changes in consciousness that accompanied hallucinogenic drug use, they designed a series of techniques called guided imagery. One early application of the guided imagery technique was as a behavioral replacement for the use of psychoactive substances. Subjects who had a long and maladaptive history of hallucinogenic drug abuse were taught the technique in an attempt to give them an alternative to using chemical substances for reaching an altered state. The theory was that guided imagery would be safer physiologically than the use of drugs and would give the individual a greater degree of control over the resulting state of consciousness. Guided imagery remains a dismal failure as a replacement for drugs. It does produce a profound altered state of consciousness, but the specific characteristics of that state do not mimic drug-induced states. Recently, however, a new therapeutic application has been discovered for directed imaginings. As we will discuss later in this chapter, guided imagery exercises are now being used effectively in the treatment of several forms of cancer.

From a historical perspective, selective awareness techniques emerged in disciplines such as meditation to facilitate mental discipline and to produce changes in the state of consciousness. The forms of selective awareness that emerged in the West have been applied largely to therapeutic situations. Although selective awareness techniques were originally used for treating hysterical disorders, they are now being applied to the treatment of somatic disease.

GOALS OF SELECTIVE AWARENESS TRAINING

There are two principal aims of selective awareness training as it applies to stress management. The first is to train your ability to concentrate and help you realize the potential you have for controlling the direction of your thoughts (as discussed in Chapter 8). The second aim is to provide you with tangible, positive mental stimuli that can compete with negative interpretations and sensations. Through hypnosis, autogenic training, and guided imagery, you can anchor in your consciousness positive thoughts and images that you can use as a focus of attention during times of stress.

Selective awareness training can help you reduce stress by training you to direct your mind, at will, to adaptive cognitive patterns. Theoretically, this will terminate the cognitive arousal, emotional responses, and resultant physiological changes that characterize psychogenic stress. Selective awareness techniques will help you achieve deep levels of psychophysiological relaxation as a buffer against stress, and they will condition your attentional skills so you can gain command over your mental responses to potential stressors.

THE ESSENCE OF SELECTIVE AWARENESS

Selective awareness is based on the idea that you can control your thoughts and the direction of your mental attention. We have discussed the basic elements of this idea in Chapter 8.

The first concept in the theory of selective awareness is that human beings are biologically designed to have a limited amount of awareness. We are capable of being aware of only a small amount of information that enters our sensory organs at any one time. This limited awareness facilitates our survival in a primitive physical world by making sure that when a threat is present our attention is not distracted from the immediate danger. Our limited awareness is one factor that helps us zero in on potential survival threats in order to have a reasonable chance of surviving physical combat. Do not consider this a disadvantage or a maladaptive limitation. Consider it a tool you can learn to use to your advantage.

The next theoretical component of selective awareness is that this limited amount of attention is usually directed toward the most dynamic or threatening element of the external environment. To ensure survival, our nervous systems were designed to focus attention on the most threatening aspect of the immediate environment so we could pay attention and respond appropriately to those things that might be life threatening. We also tend to pay automatic attention to dynamic stimuli, because a change in the environment, such as movement or noise, may be a warning signal that a survival threat is approaching.

The third component of selective awareness is that, although the limited scope of our attention is most often directed to the most dynamic or threatening stimulus present, we can choose what we think about. We can choose to focus on one source of stimulation rather than another. Rarely in life, however, do we exercise this power of choice. Selective awareness techniques can help train you to choose one thought or sensation over another. They will also provide focuses for your attention that will not trigger a physiological stress response. Rather, they will help induce a state of psychophysiological relaxation.

The final theoretical element in selective awareness is that the focus of our attention is a significant factor in determining the level of activity of our internal organs. What you think about helps determine the activity of your body. When your mind focuses on ideas or sensations that evoke fear, worry, anger, or apprehension, emotional arousal triggers the physiological stress response. If we can train the mind to redirect attention to events or thoughts that do not involve an emotional response, we can terminate physiological arousal within the body effectively. We can direct our attention to specific kinds of sensations or images that will produce a physiological response opposite to the stress response. During techniques such as autogenic training or visualization, the mind can be directed to relaxing images—such as images of heaviness and warmth—that will produce a trophotrophic physiological condition.

To summarize the theoretical bases of selective awareness: (1) we have a limited scope of attention, (2) the environment usually directs our attention to the most dynamic or threatening stimulus immediately present, (3) we can choose where to direct our attention and override our automatic biological programming, and (4) the direction of our attention has a direct influence on internal physiological functioning. We can choose to focus our minds away from sensations or thoughts that trigger a stress response, and direct them instead to thoughts or sensations or images that can induce a relaxation response.

THE ROLE OF SELECTIVE AWARENESS IN STRESS MANAGEMENT

Selective awareness techniques are forms of systematic relaxation. Through regular practice of any one selective awareness technique, you can begin to condition trophotrophically your psychophysiological response systems. Selective awareness training can also give you conscious control over the focus of your attention. Development of this type of control can help you divert your mind away from maladaptive sensations and thoughts that produce a stress reaction. Finally, selective awareness techniques can provide you with images and sensations that are associated with relaxation and can thereby give you competing mental stimuli that can help direct your attention away from disturbing thoughts toward more adaptive cognitive patterns that will help you relax and more effectively deal with the situation at hand. Developing these skills can help you combat stress through cognitive control.

HOW SELECTIVE AWARENESS WORKS

Although the diverse techniques of selective awareness have different origins, they all redirect awareness, usually toward sensations and images associated with deep relaxation. We will discuss three selective awareness techniques later in this chapter. The technique described below is a composite of several forms of selective awareness, including hypnosis and autogenic training. The best way to use this exercise is to have someone read the directions to you, or record them for yourself on tape. The instructions should be read slowly to allow you to experience each point fully.

Begin by sitting down. . . . Assume a relaxing yet reasonably erect posture so you'll feel comfortable and yet won't have a tendency to fall asleep.

Notice what you are aware of right now. . . . Scan your environment and notice all the things that are open to your senses at this moment. . . . What kinds of things are entering your awareness? . . . Now try to notice what you're ignoring. Most of these things must be mentioned to you. . . . Often we ignore sensations from our secondary senses, those other than vision . . . smells, for example . . . . When we mention the word smell, you can immediately notice the sensations of smell in the environment. . . . Clothing sensations. . . . What do your clothes feel like? What are the tactile sensations coming from your feet, from your legs, from your arms? . . . Sounds. . . . What things can you hear now that you were ignoring before? . . . Try to be as aware as you can of the subtle sensations in the environment, . . . the things you usually ignore, . . . the quiet spaces in the environment.

To help you relax from this point on, we'll use several selective awareness exercises. . . . To begin, scan the visual field immediately in front of you. . . . This could be a wall in front of you, it could be a painting, or it could be simply a part of your body—your hand, your lap, your legs. . . . Just passively scan the visual field in front of you and pick out one unique spot in that visual field . . . one thing you never noticed before . . . one definable spot in space that you can fix your eyes on and attend to for a period of time. . . . This could be a small spot on the wall or a definable area on the back of your hand. . . . Just pick out one thing you can see now that you've never noticed before.

When you've selected the spot you're going to focus your attention on, fix your eyes on that spot and don't take them away. . . . From this moment on, maintain your gaze on that one spot. . . . Don't let your eyes wander. . . . Fix your eyes on that one spot. . . . You'll soon feel the desire to look away, to glance from side to side, or to look momentarily away from the spot. This is a natural tendency. . . . Staring at any one thing for any period of time, no matter how interesting it is, becomes boring after awhile. . . . When you feel the desire to look away, to look to the side, to remove your gaze from that spot, resist that urge. . . . Use all your energy to keep your eyes fixed on that one spot. . . . Don't take them away. . . . Just keep your eyes on that one spot.

You'll notice that as you stare at anything for a long period of time, as you've been staring at that spot, certain visual changes begin to occur. There are many natural alterations that happen in the visual system when you stare at anything for a period of time. . . . You may be noticing some of them already. As you continue to stare, you may notice that the area surrounding the spot is slipping out of focus. . . . It may drift into a haze. . . . You may notice the spot itself begin to slip out of focus. . . . It may disappear altogether from your vision for just an instant. . . . It then takes conscious effort to bring it back, to readjust your eyes, and to focus on the spot again. . . . You may notice the spot slip in and out of focus and seem to move around a bit. . . . It may protrude from or recede into the background. . . . It may appear to change color. . . . These perfectly natural things happen when you stare at one spot for any length of time.

For a moment, just passively observe all the changes. . . . Notice how difficult it's becoming to keep the spot in focus. . . . You can't seem to focus on the area surrounding the spot at all. . . . Instead of passively being able to focus on the spot, you have to exert a conscious effort. . . . Your natural tendency is to let your eyes drift out of focus, to relax, and to let the entire visual image fade. . . . The longer you keep your eyes fixed on the spot, the more tired your eyes become. . . . You may have noticed this already, again another natural reaction to staring for any length of time. . . . Your eyes become fatigued. . . . The tiny muscles that you use to keep your eyes open are getting tired and sore. . . . You may feel a slight burning sensation. . . . Your eyes may be watering. . . . These are all natural reactions to staring. . . . Notice that the longer you stare at the spot, the more difficult it becomes to keep your eyes on that spot. . . . The more tired your eyes become, the more difficult it becomes to keep your eyes open. . . . Continue staring at the spot; continue to be aware of all the changes you see and all the sensations around your eyes.

Now imagine for a moment how nice it would be to close your eyes. . . . Think how good it would feel to let your eyes shut. . . .Keeping your eyes open and maintaining your gaze on that one spot, think how nice it would be to let your eyes close, to descend into that cool moist darkness inside your head, not to have to stare at the spot anymore, not to have to exert the effort to keep your eyes open. . . . Your eyes probably are becoming uncomfortable right now. . . . It's difficult to keep them open, perhaps even painful. . . . Your eyes may be watering or burning. . . . Think how nice it would be to close them, not to have to exert the effort to keep them open. . . . Soon you can.

You are going to count to 3. . . . When you hear the number 3, close your eyes. Keep them open until then. . . . Think how pleasant it will be to let your eyes close. . . . Notice how difficult it's becoming to keep your eyes focused and how difficult it is to keep them open. . . . You're feeling uncomfortable. . . . Think how nice it will be in only a few moments, when you can close your eyes, forget about the spot completely, and lie back and relax. . . . Ready? . . . *1* . . . *2* . . . *3* . . . Let your eyes drift shut. . . . Relax. . . .

Notice how different it feels, how much more pleasant it is to be inside that nice cool darkness, not to have to worry about staring at the spot anymore. . . . Notice all the sensations of having your eyes closed and how different it is from having them open. . . . Notice how much easier it is now to become aware of subtle sensations in the environment. . . . What can you hear right now? . . . What sounds are most obvious? . . . Try to listen beyond those. . . . Try to notice background sounds, those sounds that always seem to be there, that underlie all other sounds. . . . You may notice a humming sensation, a constant buzzing sound. . . . You may notice the rustling sound of the wind. . . . Try to be aware of all the sounds you have been ignoring. . . . With your eyes focused on that spot, it was difficult to be aware of anything else. Other sensations are now accessible to you. . . . Do you feel warm or cold? . . . Do your hands feel warmer than your feet? . . . What temperature sensations do you feel throughout your body? . . . What areas feel the warmest? . . . What areas feel the coolest? . . . Can you feel a shift over the surface of your body from the warm areas to the cool ones? . . . Notice any smells in the environment.

Notice that when you close your eyes, your other senses seem to blossom. . . . Try to notice all the things now accessible to your senses that you ignored before. . . . Most of all, notice how pleasant it is simply to sit quietly, your eyes closed, being relaxed.

Some of these new or awakened sensations (particularly sound) may distract you. . . . Television in another room or nearby may interrupt your relaxation. . . . Sudden loud sounds may distract or interrupt you. . . . The best way to deal with distractions is simply to accept that they'll always be there. If you hear a noise, simply note its occurrence and forget about it. Don't let it linger. Note the occurrence of the distraction and put it out of your mind. . . . Mental distractions can occur as well. You may be troubled by thoughts of work or things you have to do when you finish relaxing. Such mental distractions can be more disruptive than distractions from the environment. Remember that you don't have to pay attention to these mental distractions. Imagine that back in the dark spaces inside your head there's a little man who likes to antagonize you. Imagine he's the source of these mental distractions. He has a big mouth and he keeps talking. He won't be quiet. When mental distractions bother you, realize that it's just the little man with the big mouth. All you have to do to get rid of him is put him in a laundry bag, tighten up the drawstring, and toss him in a corner for awhile. He can talk as much as he wants later. For now, use your powers of selective awareness to get him to be quiet for a few moments.

Be aware that it's also easier now to notice what's happening inside you. . . . Be aware of small areas of pain or pressure within your body. If you pay close attention, you may notice your heart beating. You may hear it or feel it. Your body may seem to sway slightly with each pulsation. . . . Now focus your attention on your breathing. . . . Notice how each breath is unique. . . . Some are deep, some are shallow. . . . Some are long, some are quick and short. . . . Try not to analyze your breathing. Don't think about it. Just feel it. Notice all the sensations that accompany breathing. . . . When you inhale, your breath seems cool and crisp; when you exhale, it's warm and moist. . . . You may feel relaxed at this moment, but realize that it's possible to be even more relaxed.

Focus on one aspect of your breathing. Focus on exhaling. . . . As you exhale, the breath that comes out of your mouth and nostrils is warm and moist. Your muscles relax when you exhale. Let your body sink down a little bit each time you exhale. Count from 10 back to 1. With each number, take a deep breath and focus all your attention on exhaling. . . . Feel yourself becoming more and more relaxed. Feel yourself sinking deeper and deeper into your chair with each breath you take, as you count . . . *10*, inhale and exhale, feeling the warm air leaving and feeling your body relax . . . *9* . . . *8* . . . inhale deeply and slowly . . . *7* . . . with each breath feel warm and more relaxed . . . *6* . . . *5* . . . *4* . . . feel more and more relaxed . . . *3* . . . *2* . . . feel very relaxed and warm . . . *1*. Just sit quietly, feeling deeply relaxed.

Focus your attention on the spaces in your body that feel warm and relaxed. These quiet spaces are the ones we usually ignore. Focus your mind on those quiet spaces, those parts of your body that feel good, that feel comfortable, warm, free, and relaxed. Notice how good it feels to be relaxed, to be aware of all the sensations of being deeply relaxed. Focus your mind on quiet spaces in your body. They might be in your stomach, your chest, your arms, or your legs. Just focus your mind on wherever you feel quiet, peaceful, warm, and relaxed. . . . Imagine that this sensation of warmth and relaxation you feel in one part of your body is slowly spreading . . . slowly radiating warmth and relaxation. It reaches and spreads to every corner of your body, . . . radiating warmth slowly, growing, building, filling every portion of your body . . . every tiny space . . . until your entire body feels warm, peaceful, and relaxed. Feel yourself warm and relaxed.

No matter how disturbed your mind is, no matter how bothered you are by events of the day, there are always tranquil and peaceful spaces in your mind as well. Focus on one thought or image in your mind that's peaceful. It may be a sensation of relaxation in your body. . . . Imagine that the feeling of mental tranquility is growing and spreading throughout your mind, so that your entire body and mind feel warm and peaceful and relaxed. . . . Realize that you can recreate this sensation anytime you want to. The more often you practice, the better you'll be at recreating it. All you have to do is focus your attention on the part of your body or your mind that feels warm and relaxed. Then let the sensation spread. Let the feeling of warmth and relaxation spread and grow and radiate through your body.

To emerge from your relaxation, again focus your attention on your breathing. By paying attention to different phases of the respiratory cycle you can have varied effects on your level of arousal. So, instead of focusing on exhaling, focus on inhaling. Feel the sensations of expanding your chest and drawing in air. Focusing on inhaling can increase your level of arousal and help you wake up. Count from 1 to 10. With each number, take a deep full breath and exhale it completely. Feel more and more awake, more and more energized and refreshed with each breath. When you reach the number 10, take one last deep breath, blow it out completely, and open your eyes, feeling awake and refreshed. *1* . . . inhale and exhale completely, focusing your mind on inhaling, . . . *2*, breathe a little deeper this time . . . in and out . . . *3*, inhale . . . and exhale . . . *4*, feel more and more awake with each breath you take . . . *5*, in . . . and out . . . *6*, feel your chest expanding and your lungs filling with air; then exhale completely . . . *7*, in . . . and out . . . 8, think about what the room you're sitting in will look like when you open your eyes . . . *9*, as you inhale bring your mind back into the external world; think about what you have to do during the rest of the day; exhale . . . *10*, take one last breathe in . . . and exhale completely. Open your eyes, feeling relaxed, refreshed, awake, and ready to face the rest of the day.

VARIETIES OF SELECTIVE AWARENESS TRAINING

Of the three techniques we have discussed, the oldest (and most passive for the participant) is hypnosis. Hypnosis is simply an exercise in which a therapist places the subject in an altered state of consciousness, usually through relaxation or intensely focused visual concentration. While the subject is in this relaxed altered state, the therapist directs the person's focus of attention. Realize that during hypnosis subjects are never unconscious or unaware. If they were, the technique would be totally ineffective. Hypnosis relies on the subject's complete awareness. Its effectiveness lies in directing that awareness to specific stimuli. Hypnosis can be effective for focusing attention on troublesome psychological or physiological problems or for age regression situations, in which a person is asked to recall events they thought they had forgotten. Many facets of hypnosis, such as the ability to recall forgotten events and the hypersuggestibility we often associate with it, are simply manifestations that accompany the induction of any altered state of consciousness. The only distinction between hypnosis and altered states in general is that during hypnosis the subject receives specific directions for awareness. Hypnosis is simply an exercise in directing attention during an altered state of consciousness. This is naturally accompanied by perceptual changes, intensely focused attention, hypersuggestibility, and, often, deep relaxation.

Hypnosis is usually done with the aid of a therapist who verbally guides the subject into an altered state and then directs the focus of awareness during the session. Self-induced hypnosis, which is called autohypnosis, is an easy skill to learn. It involves learning to induce an altered state through focused visual concentration and then learning how to self-direct awareness during a deeply relaxed mental and physical condition.

Autogenic training, which evolved from hypnosis, involves a set of specific postures and cognitive exercises designed to help people self-induce states of deep relaxation and somatic control. Autogenic training constitutes one of the most rigidly specific systems of exercises in behavioral medicine. It involves highly specific postures and a specific sequence of mental images and activities that are used for a prescribed period of time. Johannes Schultz, who designed autogenic training, outlined the basic elements required for success as follows: (1) high motivation and cooperation of the subject, (2) a reasonable degree of subject self-control, (3) maintenance of specific body postures, (4) minimization of external stimuli and ability of subject to focus on endopsychic processes to the exclusion of external stimulation, (5) presence of monotonous input into many sensory receptors, and (6) ability of subject to maintain concentrated focusing of attention on somatic processes in order to effect internal focusing on consciousness. Given these conditions, there should be two results: the occurrence of an overpowering reflexlike psychic reorganization and the occurrence of disassociative and autonomous mental processes leading to an alteration of ego functioning and a dissolution of ego boundaries.

The mental images and suggestions prescribed by autogenic training focus attention on the physiological sensations associated with deep relaxation. Specifically, images of heaviness and warmth are used. In the first series of autogenic exercises, the person concentrates attention on the image "My arm feels heavy." Individuals may work on this particular image for months until they think they have mastered cognitively the induction of the sensation of heaviness within the limb. Before practicing specific images of heaviness or warmth, the practitioner must first learn to induce a deep, relaxed state of consciousness similar to that induced through hypnosis or meditation. Achieving such an altered state makes it easier for the practitioner to focus attention on the somatic sensations of autogenics and to internalize the suggestion deeply.

When a person repeats words or phrases such as "My left hand feels warm," a vasomotor response often occurs that causes a physiological warming of the surface of the hand. Phrases and images used in autogenic training not only help a person achieve states of deep relaxation cognitively but also seem to result in physiological changes. When used by itself, autogenic training requires considerable dedication and carefully directed practice over a long period of time. Some of its components can be used to enhance the effectiveness of other relaxation techniques. Biofeedback training often employs autogenic-type images and phrases to enhance conditioning of control over visceral responses. Even techniques like progressive neuromuscular relaxation (which we will discuss later) employ images similar to those used in autogenics to enhance the effort to relax.

Autogenic training places the subject in a more active and responsible role than does hypnosis training. During hypnosis, the subject is passive and often simply follows the direction of the therapist. During autogenic training, the subject is required to generate specific images and focuses for mental attention. This makes autogenic training a more difficult, yet ultimately more satisfying, technique for the individual who is using it to achieve and learn deep states of relaxation.

The most recent and most difficult (from the individual's standpoint) technique we have discussed is guided imagery. Guided imagery simply involves directed imaginings. The subject is placed in a relaxed state and vivid mental images that usually follow a specific pattern or sometimes a narrative line are suggested. Although assisted by a person who directs the course of events, subjects are required to use a high degree of imagination in creating for themselves most of the images they use as attentional focuses. This represents yet a further advance of hypnosis and autogenics, because it requires subjects not simply to direct attention to tangible sensations or memories pointed out by the therapist or to self-induce prescribed sensations such as heaviness or warmth, but rather it requires subjects to create their own comprehensive images as a focus for mental attention. Guided imagery is simply an exercise in sparsely directed, vivid mental imaginings. It most often takes on the character of imagining highly peaceful scenes that can serve as effective internal cognitive escapes.

APPLICATIONS OF SELECTIVE AWARENESS

Selective awareness techniques have been used for their therapeutic value since the 1840s. Hypnosis was probably the first selective awareness technique to find its way into therapeutic settings. Since its early use as an anesthetic, it has been applied in a wide variety of instances, most often for the treatment of psychological disorders. It also has been used frequently in the treatment of maladaptive behaviors related to personal health such as smoking or overeating.

Autogenic training has been used in a wide variety of therapeutic settings. Most recently it has been used in conjunction with biofeedback training to allow individuals to achieve a high level of conscious control over internal physiological processes. We will discuss this application in detail in Chapter 17.

One of the newest and most intriguing applications of selective awareness techniques has been the use of guided imagery training as part of cancer therapy. The application of imagery training as a potential treatment for cancer began with observations of the drawings made by children who were dying from cancer. In the 1970s, in an effort to understand a child's view of disease and death, Jean Achterberg decided to communicate with children using their drawings rather than words. She realized that a child's verbal skills are limited. She thought she could get the most meaningful information regarding their feelings if she asked them to draw pictures of what they thought was going on inside their bodies.

It was easy to evaluate the children's pictures in terms of which showed a positive outlook and which showed a negative or hopeless one. Factors that seemed to differentiate positive and negative illustrations included colors used and, in particular, the size of the child's depiction of the disease in relation to the representation of the child's own body. Positive pictures tended to be dominated by bright colors on the body of the child or by the portrayal of the child's somatic defenses as physically larger than the representation of the disease. Negative illustrations seemed to be dominated by dark colors and an indication that the disease was physically larger than the child. Positive images included such things as white knights stabbing tiny dark globs with their lances. One 11-year-old boy depicted himself as a large yellow bird flying high above the ground. "That's me," he said. "I'm up there flying high and nobody can catch me." Negative images were all characterized by the illustration of a hopeless condition. One 9-year-old girl with leukemia drew a picture of three children swinging. She herself was on the right swing. Bright yellow sunlight shone down on two of the children. The child on the right had a dark cloud over her head and dark purple rain streaming down on top of her. The three children looked exactly alike, except that the one on the right was wearing a black sweater. Another young girl drew seven flowers in a white field. Five of the flowers were pink and stood tall. Two of the flowers were dark blue. One of the blue flowers was cut off and lying on the ground. This child had had a very close friend in the hospital who had also died of cancer. She said her friend was the blue flower lying on the ground and she was the blue flower that was still standing. She died two weeks after Christmas and was buried beside her friend. Another negative illustration depicted the disease as a large black military tank about to run over a small child who is directly in its path. In another drawing, the disease was represented as a large porcupine with stick figures of children impaled on its large quills. One child drew himself lying on the ground with his body being pecked apart by large black birds that represented cancer.

The most interesting finding from this study was that the children who drew positive images lived much longer than those who drew negative ones. At the time the illustrations were done, the children in the positive illustration group had on the average the same prognosis as the children in the negative illustration group, yet the children who had drawn positive images lived longer, and the disease progressed more slowly in them than in the children who had drawn negative images. The progress of a disease was clearly associated with how a person visualized the disease process. Therapists began to wonder whether people could be trained to have positive images of their physical disease and hence enhance the ability of their body to combat the disease.

Working under this theory, Bolen tested the effects of a meditation program on 152 cancer patients. This program employed relaxation and visualization of peaceful scenes. He reported that 150 out of the 152 patients responded to treatment in direct correlation with subjective assessments of their degree of participation in the meditation program.

Two oncologists, Simonton and Simonton (1975, 1978), employed imagery training as adjunct therapy in the treatment of cancer. The program they used was similar to that described by Masters and Houston. Although little research exists on the efficacy of their visualization treatment, their clinical observations indicate that when individuals learn to relax and are trained to produce positive visual images regarding their physical disease state, their response to traditional cancer therapy is greatly enhanced.

To date, it cannot be established that imagery programs can effect a change in the progress of cancer. Clearly, however, relaxation and imagery therapy have helped patients reduce the stress associated with the disease. Using such techniques may minimize the psychogenic impairment of the body's natural immunity, thereby maximizing the ability of patients to defend themselves against cancer by using natural mechanisms.

SUMMARY

Selective awareness techniques help train individuals to gain conscious control over what facets of thought or sensation they pay attention to from moment to moment. During psychogenic stress, the most common type of stress experience, the focus of attention automatically migrates to threatening or emotionally arousing aspects of events. Through selective awareness techniques, we can learn how to control our attention so we can direct it consciously to elements that are positive and adaptive rather than to elements that are threatening and capable of triggering the physiological stress response. Selective awareness techniques also provide us with focuses for attention that facilitate the induction of deep states of mental and physical relaxation. Selective awareness techniques can therefore help us control stress by giving us control over the focus of our mental awareness and by providing an increased awareness of the images and sensations that can help promote states of deep relaxation and trophotrophic physiological responses.

REFERENCES

Achterberg, J., and Lawlis, G. *Imagery of Cancer*, Champaign, Ill., Institute for Personality and Ability Testing, 1978.

Achterberg, J., et al. *Stress Psychological Factors and Cancer*, New Medicine Press, Ft. Worth, 1976.

————. "Psychological Factors and Blood Chemistries as Disease Outcome Predictors for Cancer Patients," *Multivariate Experimental Clinical Research*, v. 3(4), 109-122, 1977.

Amkraut, A., and Solomon, G. "From the Symbolic Stimulus to the Pathophysiologic Response: Immune Mechanisms," *International Journal of Psychiatry in Medicine*, v. 5(4), 541-563, 1974.

Barber, T. X. "Responding to 'Hypnotic' Suggestions," *American Journal of Clinical Hypnosis*, v. 18(1), 6-22, 1975.

Barber, T. X., and DeMoor, W. "A Theory of Hypnotic Induction Procedures," *The American Journal of Clinical Hypnosis*, v. 15(2), 112-135, 1972.

Barber T., and Spanos, N. "Toward a Convergence in Hypnosis Research," *American Psychologist*, v. 29(7) , 500-511, 1974.

Bolen, J. S. "Meditation and Psychotherapy in the Treatment of Cancer," *Psychic*, v. 4(6) , 19-22, July 1973.

Bry, A. *Directing the Movies of Your Mind*, Harper and Row, New York, 1972.

Davison, G., and Neale, J. *Abnormal Psychology*, John Wiley and Sons, New York, 1974.

Giusto, E., and Bond, N. "Imagery and the Autonomic Nervous System: Some Methodological Issues," *Perceptual and Motor Skills*, v. 48, 427-438, 1979.

Holt, R. "Imagery: The Return of the Ostracized," *American Psychologist*, v. 19, 254-264, 1964.

Horowitz, M. *Image Formation and Cognition*, Appleton-Century-Crofts, East Norwalk, Conn., 1970.

Klisch, M. "The Simonton Method of Visualization: Nursing Implications and a Patient's Perspective," *Cancer Nursing*, v. 33, 295-300, 1980.

Kolata, G. "Texas Counselors Use Psychology in Cancer Therapy," *Smithsonian*, v. 11(5) , 49-54, 1980.

Leuner, H. "Guided Affective Imagery: An Account of Its Development," *Journal of Mental Imagery*, v. 1, 73-92, 1977.

Luthe, W. *Autogenic Therapy*, Grune and Stratton, New York,
  Vol. 1, Schultz, J., and Luthe, W. *Autogenic Methods*, 1969.
  Vol. 2, Luthe, W., and Schultz, J. *Medical Applications*, 1969.
  Vol. 3, Luthe, W., and Schultz, J. *Applications in Psychotherapy*, 1969.
  Vol. 4, Luthe, W. *Research and Theory*, 1970a.
  Vol. 5, Luthe, W. *Dynamics of Autogenic Neutralization*, 1970b.
  Vol. 6, Luthe, W. *Treatment for Autogenic Neutralization*, 1973.

————. *Autogenic Training: Correlativeness Psychosomaticae*, International Edition, Grune and Stratton, New York, 1965.

————. "Method, Research and Application of Autogenic Training," *American Journal of Clinical Hypnosis*, v. 5(1), 17-23, 1962.

Masters, R., and Houston, J. *Mind Games: The Guide to Inner Space*, Delta, New York, 1972.

————. *Varieties of Psychedelic Experience*, Delta, New York, 1966.

Miller, N. "Learning of Visceral and Glandular Responses," *Science*, v. 163, 434-445, 1969.

Paivio, A. *Imagery and Verbal Processess*, Holt, Rinehart and Winston, New York, 1971.

Pelletier, K. R. *Mind as Healer, Mind as Slayer*, Delta Books, New York, 1977.

Price, A. "Heart Rate Variability and Respiratory Concomitants of Visual and Non-visual Imagery, and Cognitive Style," *Journal of Research in Personality*, v. 9, 341-355, 1975.

Richardson, A. *Mental Imagery*, Springer Publishing, New York, 1969.

Samuels, M., and Samuels, N. *Seeing With the Mind's Eye*, Random House, New York, 1975.

Scarf, M. "Images That Heal: A Doubtful Idea Whose Time Has Come," *Psychology Today*, v. 14, 33-46, 1980.

Schultz, J. *Das autogene Training*, G. Thieme Verlag, Leipzig, 1932.

Schultz, J., and Luthe, W. *Autogenic Training: A Psychophysiologic Approach in Psychotherapy*, Grune and Stratton, New York, 1959.

Segal, S. *Imagery: Current Cognitive Approaches*, Academic Press, New York, 1971.

————. *The Adaptive Functions of Imagery*, Academic Press, New York, 1971.

Sheehan, P. *The Function and Nature of Imagery*, Academic Press, New York, 1972.

Simonton, 0. , and Matthews-Simonton, S. *Getting Well Again*, St. Martin's Press, New York, 1978.
Simonton, 0. C., and Simonton, S., "Belief Systems and Management of the Emotional Aspects of Malignancy," *Journal of Transpersonal Psychology*, v. 7(1) , 29-48, 1975.
Singer, J., and Pope, K. *The Power of Human Imagination*, Plenum Press, New York, 1978.
Worthington, E. "The Effects of Imagery Content, Choice of Imagery Content, and Self-Verbalization on the Self-Control of Pain," *Cognitive Therapy and Research*, v. 2(3), 225-240, 1978.

CHAPTER 15

Yoga and Breath

Sun's glow in face
Fill the lungs lift your hands in praise
as you feel the spine curve back in warmth
In springtime
Exhale   Exhale lower in surrender
Surrender all tension   Surrender the past
Surrender the cold the pain   Spring is here

Anne Adams

Yoga represents perhaps the oldest assemblage of exercises designed to enhance human health. The activities collectively labeled yoga touch and integrate all facets of human health—the body, the mind, and the spirit. Because it is truly holistic, yoga is of great value for stress reduction and for the overall enhancement of your quality of life.

We have discussed psychosomatic forms of relaxation training (i.e., meditation and selective awareness). With this chapter, we begin a presentation of somatopsychic techniques or stress control skills that operate first on the body. As we will present it, yoga represents a scheme for achieving tranquility by working principally with posture and breathing. Realize, however, that yoga is truly an integrative discipline that affects the mind-body system directly at many levels. As you will discover, even psychosomatic techniques like meditation are integral parts of yoga. In this text, we will emphasize its somatopsychic facets.

Mastery of breathing is fundamental and essential in yoga training. In fact, simply learning to control your pattern of breathing can be of direct, immediate value for reducing stress-related autonomic arousal.

What follows is a grossly oversimplified explanation of a highly involved discipline. Use the material presented here as an introduction to some of the basic concepts and techniques of yoga. If you decide to pursue yoga on a regular basis, seek additional, comprehensive instruction. The manuscripts by Swami Rama are highly recommended for accuracy, thoroughness, clarity of presentation, and practical application.

HISTORICAL EMERGENCE OF YOGA

In the sixth century B.C., Kapila founded the Sankhya school of philosophy. The basic postulate of Sankhya was that there are two ultimate realities: cosmic consciousness (purusha) and elemental matter (prakriti). According to Kapila, life and the elemental universe evolved out of a union between prakriti and purusha, "matter permeated by consciousness" (Swami Rama 1979). Most genuine scholars of yoga think the Sankhya teachings of Kapila are the most direct historical root of yoga.

The actual method of yoga comes from Patanjali, who lived approximately 400 years after Kapila. Patanjali compiled the *Yoga Sutras*, a work of four chapters (padas), totaling 196 aphorisms (sutras). This work describes the states, methods, effects, and goals of Raja yoga.

Raja yoga, or the royal path, is often called astranga yoga, meaning the eightfold path, because there are eight elements (angas) to it. According to Swami Rama, the angas include yama, niyama, asana, pranayama, pratyahara, dhrana, dhyana, and samadhi. The first two, yama and niyama, involve attitudes and the moral foundations of yoga. Asana refers to the physical postures, the element we commonly associate with yoga. Pranayama refers to control of the first energy, the breath. Pranayama involves understanding and learning mastery of the process of breathing. Pratyahara involves withdrawal from the sensations of the external physical environment. This was the facet of yoga investigated by Anand in his study of meditating yogis, which we discussed in Chapter 13. Dhrana is the ability to focus mental attention on a single thought or stimulus. Dhyana is meditation, or simply prolonging dhrana. According to Swami Rama, prolonged dhyana may lead to samadhi, or a transcendent state of complete self-realization, the aim of yoga.

GOALS OF YOGA TRAINING

Classically, yoga is one of several Eastern disciplines designed to help human beings realize their true nature by transcending limitations. Swami Rama (1979) best explains the aim of yoga. "The main teaching of yoga is that man's true nature is divine, but that he is unaware of his true nature and therefore falsely identifies with his body and his intellect—both of which are within prakriti, or matter, and hence subject to decay and death. All of man's misery is therefore, a consequence of this false identification. Yoga leads one to realization of the Self, and with such realization comes liberation from all human imperfections."

The two angas of Raja yoga that we will discuss have immediate influence on physiology and stress reactivity. Our goal for this limited presentation of yoga is to use it to develop styles of breath control that are useful in stress management and to introduce techniques that will promote balanced, integral physical well-being.

THE ESSENCE OF YOGA

Raja yoga works to attain self-realization, or samadhi, by operating on the body, the mind, and the spirit. It is much more than simply the attainment of seemingly painful, pretzel-like, contorted postures. Yoga involves elements of philosophy, attitude, concentration, discipline, meditation, and transcendence as well as breathing and bodily postures.

Raja yoga is but one of several dominant variations of yoga. In this chapter, we will discuss only two of its facets, **asana** and **pranayama**. These two angas represent the essence of Hatha yoga, a branch of Raja yoga that has gained popularity in the West. As I have mentioned, yoga involves much more than posture and breath. I encourage you to explore it beyond the limited scope of this presentation.

THE ROLE OF YOGA IN STRESS MANAGEMENT

The first element in our somatopsychic presentation of yoga is breath control. Mastery of the recommended diaphragmatic breath aids in trophotrophic response tuning. Additionally, the rapid arousal reduction techniques derived from this style of breathing are of great benefit for calming yourself in suddenly tense situations. We will discuss one such technique later in this chapter.

Practice of the asanas presented in this chapter will help develop and integrate your body. Yoga will not necessarily enhance skeletal muscle strength, as is the aim of other physical conditioning approaches. Yoga practice facilitates somatic balance, coordination, and adaptive physical integration. Subjectively, you will feel a keener motor integration and a sense of increased somatic clarity. With practice, you will begin to feel the static clear out of your body. You will have the sense of living inside a cleaner and fresher body.

Yoga promotes a high degree of comprehensive somatic awareness. You will gradually learn to listen to your body and be keenly aware of its subtle tensions, changes, and needs. This facet has considerable utility for allowing early recognition of a stress-related problem and the capacity to correct the pathogenic imbalance before it produces pain or discomfort or gets out of control.

As part of a comprehensive stress management program, yoga should be practiced every day. It takes about half an hour to perform the initial exercise, run through the asanas, and close. If you practice each day, you will soon notice results.

THE TECHNIQUES OF YOGA

The first essential component in the practice of yoga is mastery of the diaphragmatic breath.

Right now, in your normal fashion, take a deep breath. Do it again. What part of your body expands as you inhale deeply? Your chest? Your stomach? Breathe deeply again and pay attention.

Most Americans (about 75 percent) are thoracic or chest breathers. If you fall into this category, you will notice your chest expand as you inhale deeply. Thoracic breathing may be a learned phenomenon. Infants are diaphragmatic breathers, but in this culture, they often switch to thoracic breathing as they grow older. One possible reason that we learn to breathe this way is because our culture considers it attractive to have a small, slender waistline and a large chest. We often suck in our stomachs and puff up our chests in an unconscious effort to look more attractive. Even our clothing styles reflect this preference by being tight around the waist, which restricts mobility and discourages diaphragmatic breathing.

One way to draw air into the lungs is through the lateral expansion of the ribs during thoracic inhalation. You can also inhale effectively by dropping your diaphragm. All you need to do is push out your stomach. This may seem strange, because when you breathe thoracically, you pull your stomach in during inhalation. To breathe diaphragmatically, all you need to do is push your stomach out to inhale, and pull it in to exhale.

Try breathing with your diaphragm now. It helps to place your hands lightly across your stomach, one on top of the other. Use your hands simply as an indicator of what is going on. Imagine that you have a pouch in your stomach. Imagine that each time you inhale, you are going to fill that pouch under your hands with air, drawing it all the way into your stomach. (You will not get any air in your stomach, but it is a useful image.) Now, inhale by pushing your stomach out and exhale by pulling it in. Let your stomach move out . . . and in, . . . as you breathe in . . . and out. If you normally breathe this way, fine. If not, practice this diaphragmatic style until you feel comfortable with it. You need to master this style of breathing before proceeding with yoga practice. In fact, simply learning to control your breathing may be the single most important facet to yoga and the overall enhancement of your personal health.

The asanas, or positions, represent the one characteristic most commonly associated with yoga. The asanas of Raja yoga are thought to have significant influence on cognitive and somatic functioning, as well as nebulously defined therapeutic effects. In this chapter, we will show you most of the asanas of Raja yoga and present simple guidelines on how to use them.

Some of the asanas are easy to achieve; others appear to be strange and difficult. The first important guideline is never to strain yourself. Never push yourself beyond what feels reasonably comfortable for your body. The initial aim of yoga is not to have you achieve all the asanas. You must ease into them, always balanced, always relaxed, always able to breathe freely. Do not push or strain. Do not overexert yourself. Gradually acquire the skill to master all the postures. If you are doing them correctly, it will take many years. Use the asanas to help you slowly, gently, deeply evolve your physical self into adaptive, integrated functioning.

We will discuss two types of asanas: those used as meditation postures and those used to promote physical well-being.

The meditative postures are used to stabilize the body by aligning the torso, neck, and trunk. They are designed to provide an erect, very stable posture that allows meditation to be practiced with a minimum of somatic distraction. These asanas are also said to facilitate a clear pathway for breathing and the transmission of nervous messages and the flow of other energy systems within the body.

There are four meditative postures: sukhasana, or easy posture; swastikasana, or auspicious posture; siddhasana, or accomplished posture; and padmasana, the lotus posture. The four meditation asanas are presented here in order of increasing difficulty. Use whichever one feels comfortable to you. Over time, develop the others so you will be able to meditate comfortably in the more stable (yet difficult) positions. The last posture, padmasana, is mastered by few individuals and takes many years to develop properly. Do not rush. Do what feels comfortable and let yourself progress slowly. The meditative postures are shown in Figures 15.1 through 15.4.

The remainder of the asanas are designed to enhance physical well-being. They can be performed in the order given during a single setting. Stay in each posture for at least several breaths. When you have mastered an asana, you will be able to maintain it effortlessly for hours. Practice the asanas in either the morning or the evening, several hours after your last significant meal. (This is important, because these postures alter gastrointestinal alignment and motility.) It is nice to precede the asanas with aerobic exercise or a long, warm bath so your muscles are relaxed and supple.

There are five phases to performing each asana. Move into and through each one gently, slowly, carefully, without unnecessary effort or strain. Always stay relaxed.

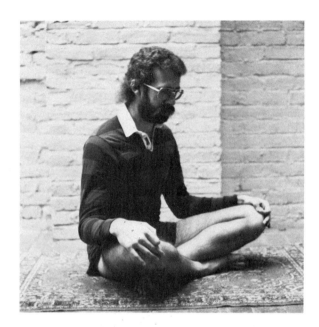

Figure 15.1. Sukhasana: The easy posture.

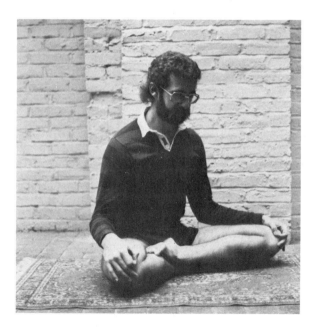

Figure 15.2. Swastikasana: The auspicious posture.

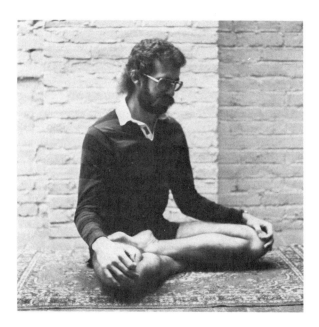

Figure 15.3. Siddhasana: The accomplished posture.

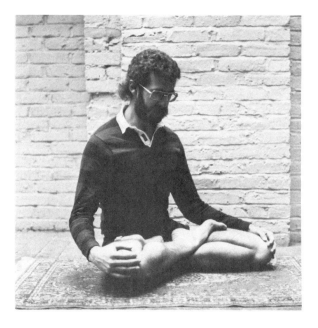

Figure 15.4. Padmasana: The lotus posture.

1. *Posture.* Slowly, without straining, move your body into each pose. One at a time, duplicate the positions shown in the photographs that follow. (Note: It is essential that you obtain step-by-step instructions on how to assume the more difficult asanas from a comprehensive yoga text.) Always stay balanced and stable while moving into the posture. *Never* push your body beyond reasonable limits of comfort. If you cannot attain a position, do not worry. Make a relaxed, balanced attempt. It will develop with time.
2. *Balance.* When you have attained a position, take a moment to balance your body. You should use no muscular effort whatsoever to hold the pose. Balance yourself so you could maintain it for hours if you wished.
3. *Breath.* When you have comfortably balanced yourself in the posture, breathe easily from your diaphragm. (Many of the asanas require a lot of flexibility. You can extend your range of motion by breathing properly. As you exhale, stretch and reach further; as you inhale, hold your position. Do this with every breath. Muscle tissue should be stretched or lengthened while it is relaxed. When you exhale, your entire body can relax, so stretch or move during that phase of breathing. Then hold while you inhale. In several breaths, you will stretch beyond what you thought you could. You will begin to see your greater physical performance potential.)
4. *Relaxation.* Balance, breathe, and let yourself relax in the position for the span of five to ten diaphragmatic breaths. Do not use any effort. Just relax in the pose.
5. *Focus.* While you relax in the asana, focus your awareness on all your somatic sensations. Notice how it feels to breathe. Observe the quiet sensation of balance, stability, and integration. Listen to your body.

Gracefully crawl out of the posture and move on to the next asana.

You should open and conclude each yoga practice session with an exercise called **salute to the sun.** There are many variations of this standard exercise, which involves moving gracefully through a number of postures. Each posture should be accomplished as an asana, involving attainment of the position, balance, breathing, relaxation, and focus prior to moving to the next step. Figure 15.5 illustrates the sequence of postures in one variation of the salute to the sun. For each picture with an asterisk (*), hold that pose as an asana for three or four diaphragmatic breaths. Move from one asana to the next within the span of just one complete breath.

The remainder of the physical well-being asanas are shown in Figures 15.6 through 15.21. Practice them according to the guidelines just discussed. Remember, the aim is not to show the world how good you are. Instead, balance yourself, breathe freely, relax, and listen to your body. Do not push or strain. You will not be able to assume all the asanas right away. Give yourself plenty of time and your body will gradually grow strong.

VARIETIES OF YOGA TRAINING

Raja yoga has six other facets that deal with philosophical and spiritual foundations and that involve exercises in concentration and meditation designed to lead to transcendent states of consciousness and being. There are many other forms of yoga besides Raja yoga. According to Swami Rama, there is Karma yoga, the yoga of action; Bhakti yoga, the yoga of devotion; Jnana yoga, the yoga of knowledge; and Kundalini yoga, the yoga of awakening latent power (a powerful discipline that is potentially dangerous unless practiced with master guidance and total devotion). As we have noted, Hatha yoga, which

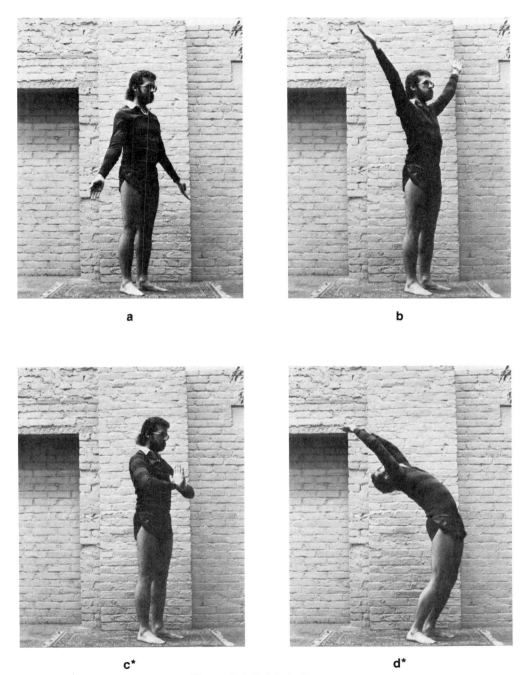

Figure 15.5. Salute to the sun.

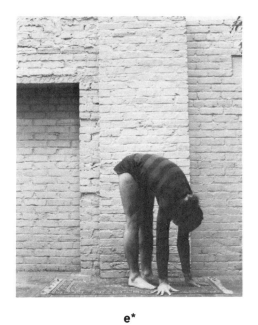

e*

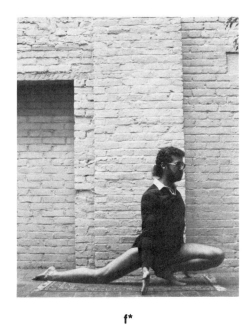

f*

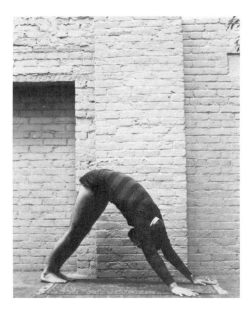

g*

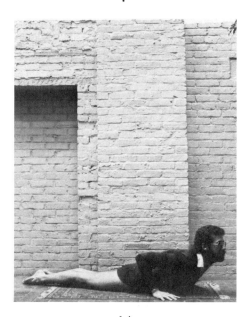

h*

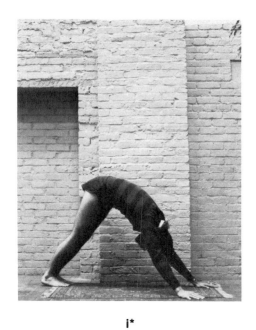

i*

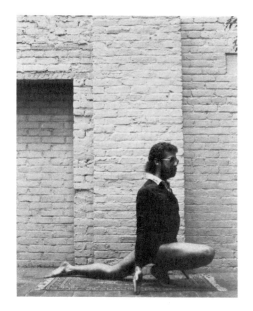

j*

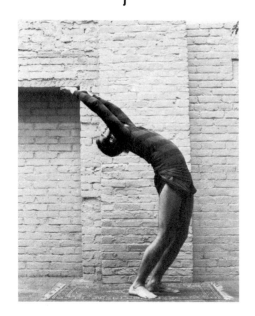

k*

l*

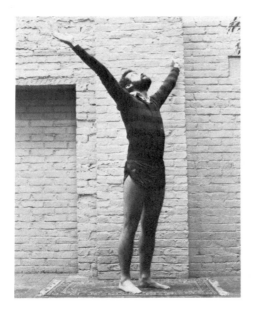

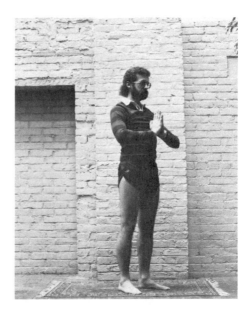

m   n*

we have looked at briefly, seems to agree with the Western mind set because it presents the tangible techniques and exercises without delving heavily into philosophy or spiritual development. Despite its limitations, it is beneficial, and instruction in Hatha yoga is easily accessible in this country (although instructor qualifications vary widely).

Many of the techniques used to reduce psychophysiological arousal have their roots in yoga. Specifically, the diaphragmatic breathing component of pranayama is central to several techniques for rapidly relieving maladaptive arousal. One of these techniques, called **calming down**, was developed by George Everly (1979). It was derived from a series of exercises, designed to elicit a **quieting response**, that were originally outlined by Charles Stroebel (1978).

In designing this technique, Everly recognized that Americans have trouble with techniques like meditation because we think they take too much time. We prefer to do everything in a hurry. What Americans need, he thought, is a "quick fix." His maneuver was designed to require only a minute or so and yet effectively reduce arousal. We will refer to the technique simply as calming down.

The calming down technique is effective for reducing autonomic arousal quickly, but it does not condition long-term trophotrophic tuning. Use it anytime you are presented with a sudden stressor and feel a need to calm down fast. Examples of such times might include right before taking an examination, before giving a speech or performance, when you want to reduce the physiological effects of sudden embarrassment, or when you need to reset your autonomic systems in the middle of a trying day.

There are two components to calming down: diaphragmatic breathing and autogenic phrases. To begin, breathe with your diaphragm. Push your stomach *out* and *inhale*, and pull it *in* to *exhale*. Place your hands over your stomach and use them as an indicator if you find it helpful. Just breathe in and out this way until it feels comfortable and natural.

Next, each time you *inhale*, say silently to yourself, "I feel calm." Do not just say it, however; make this phrase a statement about how you feel right now. No matter how uptight or tense you feel, somewhere in your body a calm spot exists. Focus your mind on that spot. With each breath, as you repeat "I feel calm," feel a sensation of calm spreading throughout your body from that small spot you have been focusing on. Feel the calm spread farther and farther with every breath.

Now, as you *exhale*, say to yourself silently, "I feel warm," with every breathe. Each time you exhale, feel your warm breath as it leaves your mouth or nostrils. Feel the sensation of warmth radiate throughout your body each time you exhale and repeat "I feel warm." Feel the warmth melting away all your tension, helping you relax. Repeat these phrases with each breath. "I feel calm," . . . "I feel warm," . . . as you breathe in . . . and out, . . . feeling ever calmer and warmer with each breath.

Practice this simple exercise a couple times each day, under reasonably stress-free circumstances, until you feel proficient. Then try to use it several times a day. It is a quick and temporary measure, without much conditioning capability. The more often you use it, however, the more effective it will be for you. After only a couple days of practice, this technique will calm you down within five to ten breaths (from 30 seconds to a minute). It works. Try it.

The breathing components of yoga can be used to enhance performance in nearly any human endeavor, from musical virtuosity to athletic excellence. Learn to master your breath, and you can move, act, and perform within your breath. You may be amazed at the sudden ease and grace with which you can undertake the challenges of life.

THEORETICAL MECHANISM OF EFFECTIVENESS

Research on the effects, mechanisms, and applications of yoga is almost nonexistent. Although it is a highly effective discipline from a subjective standpoint, its physiological mechanisms have never been studied in appropriate scientific settings. This void, it is hoped, will be filled in the near future.

The only area of yoga that has been researched involves the physiological changes associated with breathing. There is evidence in the available literature to indicate that diaphragmatic breathing stimulates activity of the parasympathetic nervous system. Diaphragmatic breathing changes the pattern of intrathoracic pressure in a manner somewhat different from thoracic breathing. It has been suggested that the pattern of intrathoracic pressure change elicited by diaphragmatic breathing causes sodium leakage of the vagus nerve and hence vagal discharge. The vagus nerve is the main branch of the parasympathetic system. It innervates most of the autonomic organs. If diaphragmatic breathing stimulates vagal activity, it would result in a rapid reduction in overall visceral arousal. This theory seems plausible because, unlike the sympathetics tracts, the parasympathetic tracts nearly all emanate from one location in the cranial region of the spine (refer back to Figure 5.7). It would be possible, therefore, for a change in pressure within the body cavity to stimulate parasympathetic discharges without significantly affecting sympathetic activity. This mechanism is purely theoretical, since no research has yet established its validity. This theory might represent the reason you feel a little sleepy after breathing from your diaphragm for a few minutes. Breathe thoracically for awhile, and then take 10 to 20 diaphragmatic breaths. Notice that a drowsy sensation comes over

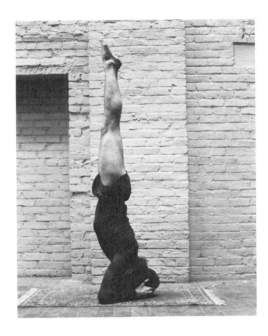

Figure 15.6. Shirshasana (headstand).

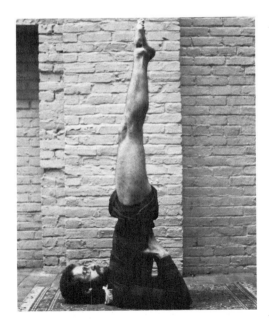

Figure 15.7. Sarvangasana (shoulderstand).

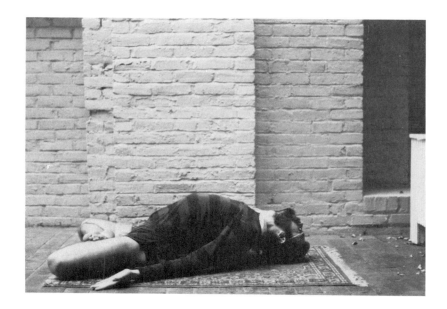

Figure 15.8. Matsyasana (fish).

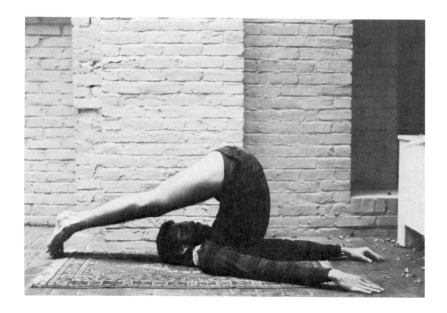

Figure 15.9. Halasana (plow).

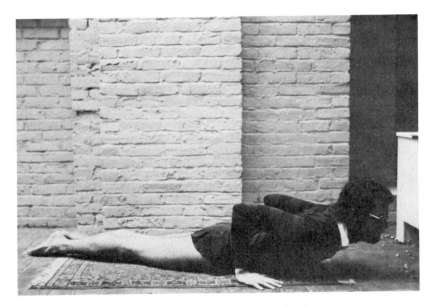

Figure 15.10. Bhujangasana (cobra).

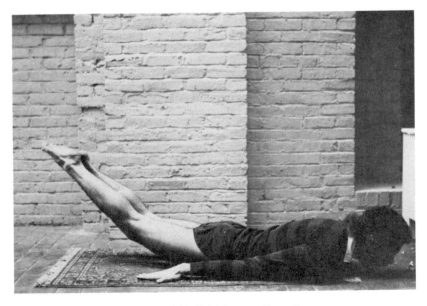

Figure 15.11. Salabhasana (locust).

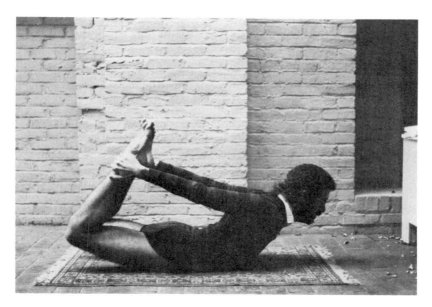

Figure 15.12. Dhanurasana (bow).

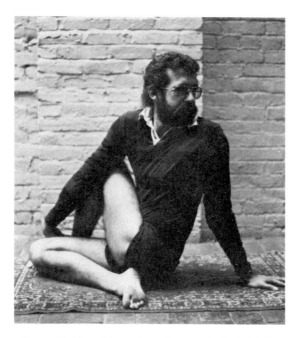

Figure 15.13. Ardha-matsyendrasana (spinal twist).

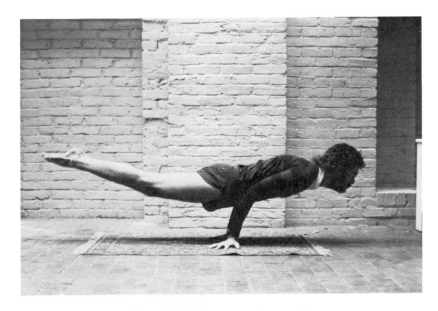

Figure 15.14. Mayurasana (peacock).

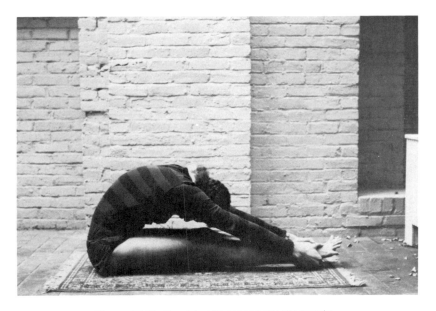

Figure 15.15. Paschimottanasana (back stretch).

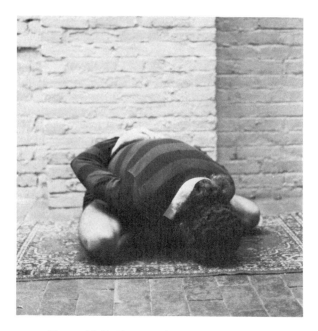

Figure 15.16. Yoga mudra (symbol of yoga).

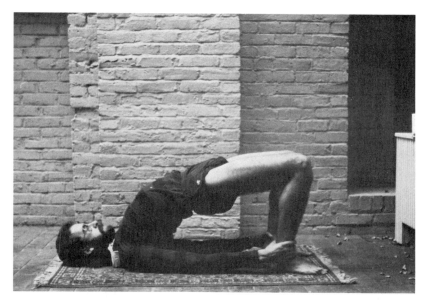

Figure 15.17. Chakrasana (wheel).

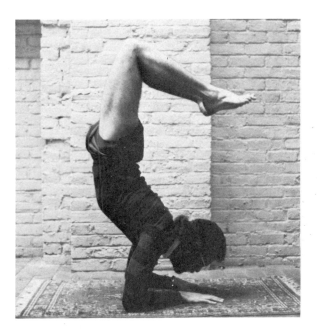

Figure 15.18. Vrischikasana (scorpion).

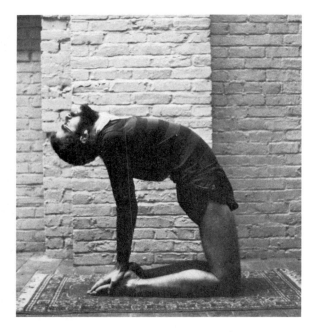

Figure 15.19. Ustrasana (camel).

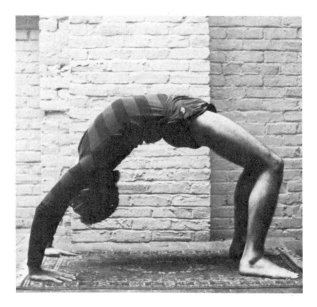

Figure 15.20. Setu-bandhasana (bridge).

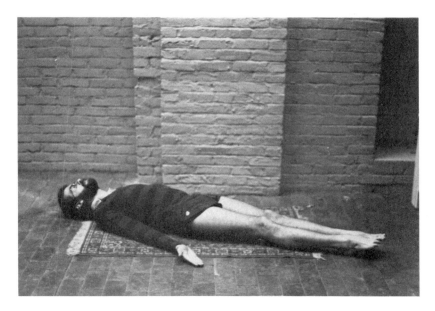

Figure 15.21. Savasana (corpse).

you. More research is needed to determine the reason for this phenomenon, but there are indications that vagal stimulation is a probable mechanism.

There are numerous claims for the benefits of yoga. Many of them cite lining up the visceral organs or the chakras as the mechanism of effect. As yet, there is no scientific literature on the mechanisms by which specific asanas produce physiological or therapeutic effects. They clearly alter the system, but science does not know how or why.

CONTRAINDICATIONS AND COMMON DIFFICULTIES

One problem that plagues Westerners who practice yoga is our need to be competitive. We try too hard. We associate physical activity with competition, strain, and exertion. We believe you have to do it till it hurts or it will not do any good at all. This is absolutely *not* the way to practice yoga. You must never push, strain, or compete when attempting to assume or maintain the asanas. Effort and strain can damage muscle and connective tissue. When you stretch to assume a posture, do so only to the limits of reasonable comfort. Do not strain yourself. Always stay balanced and maintain breath control. The aim is not to be able to attain and hold the posture (as in gymnastics), but ultimately to be able to maintain it in a comfortable, relaxed, balanced, and breathing condition. Westerners need to liberate themselves from their maladaptive, competitive nature to learn that yoga can be used effectively by anyone, regardless of physical condition.

WHAT TO EXPECT FROM YOGA AND BREATH CONTROL

You will notice many tangible benefits as you continue to practice yoga. You will first notice an enhanced somatic awareness. You will be clearly in touch with your body, sensitive to its states, changes, and needs. You will notice an evolving grace that allows you to perform your everyday physical activities with greater ease, less effort, and smoother motor coordination. You may begin to feel more comfortable in your physical body. It may seem to "fit" better. You will seem more at ease within your physical self. This somatic integration will begin to clear the maladaptive tensions, static, and imbalances from your body, resulting not only in enhanced physical performance but in increased mental clarity and tranquility as well. You will feel wonderful.

Many of these same expectations apply to breath control as well. If you coordinate physical action properly with breathing, your performance will increase and your frustration and the effort you have to put forth will decrease.

By practicing the calming down technique regularly, you can become highly proficient at quickly reducing unexpected, or sudden, arousal. As you condition yourself to the diaphragmatic breath and autogenic phrases, you will be able to calm yourself after only a few breaths.

SUMMARY

Yoga is one of the most effective tools ever devised to enhance human health. It operates on the body, the mind, and the spirit. We have limited our discussion of yoga to pranayama (breath control) and asana (postures), just two of the eight facets of Raja yoga. The practice of yoga, in its correct and comprehensive sense, is so effective that it can be used as a single modality for managing stress. Readers interested in pursuing yoga should seek qualified instruction that presents the discipline in totality.

Yoga forms the basis of several Westernized forms of quick relaxation. The calming down technique combines diaphragmatic breathing with autogenic phrases to reduce arousal in sudden, tense situations.

REFERENCES

Aurobindo, Sri. *Essays on the Gita*, Sri Aurobindo Library, New York, 1950.

Ballantyne, J. (trans.) *Sankhya Aphorisms of Kapila*, Chowkhamba Sanskrit Series, Varanasi, 1963.

Bolton, B., et al. "Vasoconstriction Following Deep Inspiration," *Journal of Physiology*, v. 86, 83-94, 1936.

Chaudhuri, H. "Yoga Psychology," in Tart, C. T., *Transpersonal Psychologies*, Harper and Row, New York, 1975.

Datey, K., et al. "Shavasan: A Yogic Exercise in the Management of Hypertension," *Angiology*, v. 20, 325-333, 1969.

Engle, B. T., and Chism, R. A. "Effects of Increases and Decreases in Breathing Rate on Heart Rate and Finger Pulse Volume," *Psychophysiology*, v. 4, 83-89, 1967.

Everly, G. S. "A Technique for the Immediate Reduction of Psychophysiological Stress Reactivity: A Pilot Study," *Health Education*, v. 10(3), 44, 1979.

Harris, V. A., et al. "Paced Respiration as a Technique for the Modification of Autonomic Response to Stress," *Psychophysiology*, v. 13(5), 396-405, 1976.

Helbick, T. M. "The Effects of Thoracic and Diaphragmatic Breathing on Cardiovascular Functioning," Unpublished Doctoral Dissertation, University of Maryland, College Park, 1980.

Holmes, D. S., et al. "Control of Respiration as a Means of Controlling Responses to Threat," *Journal of Personality and Social Psychology*, v. 36(2), 198-204, 1978.

Krishna, G. *The Kundalini: The Evolutionary Energy in Man*, Shambala, Berkeley, 1971.

———. *The Secret of Yoga*, Harper and Row, New York, 1972.

Kuvalayananda., *Pranayama*, Popular Prakashan, Bombay, 1966.

Mishra, R. *Fundamentals of Yoga*, Julian Press, New York, 1959.

Radhakrishnan, S. (trans.) *The Bhagavadgita*, Harper and Row, New York, 1952.

———. (trans.) *Principal Upanishads*, Harper and Row, New York, 1953.

Schneider, E. C. "A Study of Respiratory and Circulatory Responses to a Voluntary Gradual Forcing of Respiration," *American Journal of Physiology*, v. 91, 390-398, 1930.

Schulte, H. J., and Abhyander, W. "Yoga Breathing and Psychologic Status," *Arizona Medicine*, v. 36(9), 29-34, 1979.

Segesman, M. (trans.). *Wings of Power*, Hill of Content, Australia, 1973.

Sharpey-Schafer, E. P. "Effect of Respiratory Acts on the Circulation," in Hamilton, W. F., and Dow, P., *Handbook of Physiology*, s. 2, v. 3, American Physiological Society, Washington, D.C., 1875-1886, 1965.

Shean, G. D., and Stange, P. W. "The Effects of Varied Respiratory Rate and Volume Upon Finger Pulse Volume." *Psychophysiology*, v. 8(3), 401-423, 1971.

Sivananda, S. *Raja Yoga*, Yoga Vendanta Forest University, Rishikesh, 1950.

Stern, R. M., and Anschel, C. "Deep Inspirations as Stimuli for Responses of the Autonomic Nervous System," *Psychophysiology*, v. 5, 132-141, 1968.

Stroebel, C. F. *Quieting Response Training*, Biomonitoring Applications, New York, 1978.

Stroufe, L. A. "Effects of Depth and Rate of Breathing on Heart Rate and Heart/Rate Variability," *Psychophysiology*, v. 8, 648-655, 1971.

Swami Karmananda. "Relaxation Through Yoga," in White, J., and Fadiman, J., *Relax*, Dell, New York, 1976.

Swami Rama. *Lectures on Yoga*, Himalayan International Institute of Yoga Science and Philosophy, Honesdale, Pa., 1979.

Swami Rama et al. *Science of Breath*, Himalayan International Institute of Yoga Science and Philosophy, Honesdale, Pa., 1979.

Woodroffe, J. *The Serpent Power*, Ganesh, Madras, 1964.

CHAPTER 16

Progressive
Neuromuscular Relaxation

TENSION does not come from outside you, it is something that you produce. Excessive TENSION is a non-verbal message from your body asking you to become more receptive, permissive, to let go and relax.

Bernard Gunther

Progressive relaxation is a somatopsychic technique designed to reduce tension levels in the skeletal muscles. It provides an option that is particularly useful for those who find passive activities like meditation to be exercises in frustration. It is useful for reducing muscle tension and for treating stress-related muscular disorders. Neuromuscular relaxation is ideally suited to Type A individuals and others who are accustomed to coping in active, yet maladaptive, ways.

Anyone who hopes to learn to manage stress should experience progressive relaxation, because it facilitates a recognition of the sensations that accompany deep physical relaxation. The resulting general increase in overall somatic awareness may later prove to be highly valuable in recognizing the early physical precursors of stress-related disease, permitting the problem to be dealt with before it gets out of hand.

HISTORICAL EMERGENCE OF PROGRESSIVE RELAXATION

In 1929, Edmund Jacobson published a book entitled *Progressive Relaxation* that described the practice and application of a technique for neuromuscular tension reduction. Jacobson was a physician who recognized that muscular tension was associated with many somatic diseases. (Ironically, Selye was at this same time noticing the constellation of symptoms in somatic disease called the "syndrome of just being sick.") Jacobson also noted that the presence of excess tension seemed to exacerbate the disease condition. He reasoned that a mechanism capable of reducing muscular tension could have broad therapeutic utility. Jacobson may have been the first Western medical practitioner to

222

recognize the medical value of relaxation and design a systematic relaxation technique to be used as a therapeutic modality in the treatment of somatic disease.

In designing his relaxation technique, Jacobson found that people were unaware of the sensations of muscular relaxation. To most people, relaxation simply meant the absence of tension. He decided to teach people to relax by first inducing tension, on the theory that you cannot recognize and produce relaxation until you first experience tension. The resultant technique was a progressive series of tension/relaxation intervals performed bilaterally (on both sides of the body at the same time), one major muscle group at a time. As it turned out, this tension/relaxation approach was effective for physiological reasons beyond the promotion of the sensory and cognitive awareness of relaxation sensations.

Jacobson tried his new technique on patients manifesting diverse medical problems. As a result of the progressive relaxation technique, he reported either marked or very marked improvement for the following disorders treated: nervous hypertension (31 cases), acute insomnia (6), anxiety neurosis (2), cardiac neurosis (1), chronic insomnia (12), compulsive neurosis (1), convulsive tic (3), cyclothymic exaltation (2), cyclothymic depression (7), esophageal spasm (3), Graves' disease (3), hypochondria (2), mucous colitis (2), spastic paresis (1), stuttering or stammering (3), unclassified psychosis (1), and cardiac asthma (1). Of 81 cases studied, he reported either no improvement or slight improvement in only 17 instances.

It has been popular to criticize Jacobson's early findings because he used no controls. All the patients treated were undergoing other medical treatments as well. We must interpret Jacobson's initial data from the perspective of the time during which they were generated. His empirical observations on treatment efficacy suggested the possibility that relaxation can be of therapeutic value.

GOALS OF PROGRESSIVE RELAXATION TRAINING

The initial purpose of progressive relaxation is to reduce unnecessary, maladaptive neuromuscular arousal. It can also decrease overall stress reactivity and contribute to trophotrophic conditioning by eliminating much of the principal, exacerbating, end-organ feedback in the psychosomatic model. Another goal of neuromuscular relaxation is to teach the practitioner to recognize the sensations of deep physical relaxation and thus increase general somatic awareness.

The overall purpose of progressive neuromuscular relaxation is for the practitioner to manifest a dynamic condition called **optimal tonus** in all facets of human movement and skeletal muscle activity. Gunther (1968) describes optimal tonus as "a dynamic concept in which the organism automatically adjusts to the amount of tension necessary to perform each particular act. The best example is a cat, sitting at ease, completely alive, eyes open or closed, breathing easily; ready in an interested instant to spring into action. Complete involvement, absorption in any activity or inactivity. Never pushing or straining unnecessarily. No excessive effort, allowing the organism to operate with a minimum of energy expenditure. Muscles are firm-soft and resilient, allowing coordination, sensitivity, integration."

THE ESSENCE OF PROGRESSIVE RELAXATION

As we have noted, Jacobson designed a technique that involves a progressive series of tension/release intervals. The practitioner first contracts isometrically specific major muscle groups on both sides of the body at the same time. After holding a near maximal contraction for 5 to 10 seconds, the practitioner releases the tension and then relaxes the previously tensed muscles for about 45 seconds and notes the difference in sensation between the tension phase and the release phase. The technique operates on one muscle group at a time, progressing to each major muscle site throughout the body. Neuromuscular relaxation progressively builds complete muscular relaxation through a series of individual tension/release intervals. Soon, by comparing the somatic sensations of tension and relaxation, the practitioner becomes aware of the unique sensations of relaxation as an autonomous state. This awareness of the feelings of deep, somatic relaxation is one of the most valuable components of progressive relaxation.

THE ROLE OF PROGRESSIVE
RELAXATION IN STRESS MANAGEMENT

Progressive relaxation should be practiced daily, as part of a comprehensive stress management program, to facilitate trophotrophic tuning and optimal tonus. It is particularly well suited for active people who have difficulty settling into the more passive relaxation techniques. Everyone can benefit from some exposure to progressive relaxation, because it teaches recognition of the somatic sensations that accompany deep relaxation and it promotes enhanced somatic awareness.

As we will discuss shortly, this technique can be done in small pieces anytime during the day. As you notice tension building somewhere in your body, you can relieve it by simply performing one or two of the tension/release intervals on that site. You can thus prevent tension from building as the day goes on, minimizing the possibility that your overall psychosomatic arousal will accelerate and leave you close to your tolerance limit by the day's end. Performing a few simple intervals of progressive relaxation periodically will help to keep you at a healthy, safe level of psychophysiological arousal.

THE TECHNIQUE OF PROGRESSIVE RELAXATION

Neuromuscular relaxation is practiced as a series of progressive tension/release intervals. The character and steps of each interval are essentially the same. Each interval contains the following five elements:

1. *Awareness.* Notice how each body part, or muscle group, feels right now. Open your awareness to all somatic messages and sensations coming from a specific area. Pay particular attention to any tension sensations.
2. *Tension.* Isometrically contract the muscle group to a near maximal state. Pull very hard. If you feel cramping, however, back off a little. Hold the tight, isometric contraction for 5 to 10 seconds. While it is tense, note the sensations of muscular tension in the area.
3. *Relaxation.* Release all the tension from the muscles you have been contracting. Just let it go. Do not exert any muscular effort whatsoever, not even the effort to maintain position. Just relax. Let all the tension float away.
4. *Listening to the body.* Notice how different the muscles feel in their relaxed state compared to the previous tension. What does it feel like to be relaxed? What are the unique sensations of relaxation? Learn to recognize and feel the sensations of deep relaxation.
5. *Focus.* Direct all your awareness to this feeling of relaxation. Become totally aware of your internal sensations. Immerse your mind in the feelings of being very, very relaxed.

This five-step procedure is repeated on each muscle group in a progression throughout the body.

Neuromuscular relaxation should be practiced lying down, not sitting. In order to release tension as completely as possible, your body must be in a position that requires no muscular effort to maintain. Performing individual intervals periodically during the day does not require a reclined posture. If you are going to practice the complete series of exercises to condition muscular hypoarousal and optimal tonus, do it with your eyes closed lying in the savasana posture shown in Figure 15.21.

The following activities, outlined by Allen and Hyde (1980), can be used for the individual tension phases of the technique. Maintain contraction for 5 to 10 seconds for each muscular site. Then relax for about 45 seconds before moving on to the next body part.

1. *Feet and lower legs*

    Point your feet and toes.

    Pull back on your feet. Try to touch your knees with your toes (most people cannot do this, but try anyway) and fan your toes out as wide as possible.

2. *Thighs*

    Straighten your legs and, using the muscles in the front of your thighs, lock your knees tightly. Make them unbendable.

3. *Buttocks*

    Tighten these large muscles as much as possible. If you are sitting, imagine that you will sit up a little higher and straighter in your chair as you contract. Imagine severe constipation.

4. *Abdomen*

    Tense your stomach muscles as though you were preparing for the blow of someone about to throw a basketball into your stomach.

5. *Chest and shoulders*

    Place the palms of your hands together, with your arms outstretched. Press your palms together as hard as you can.

6. *Back and shoulders*

    Tighten the muscles of your lower back as though someone were about to give you a stiff slap on the back.

    Pull back on your shoulders, trying to touch them together behind you.

7. *Upper arms, forearms, and hands*

    Bend your elbows until your hands are close to your shoulders, and form a fist with each hand. Clench your fists and pull as hard as you can with your arms. Imagine that, with a reverse grip, you are holding onto reins and pulling hard against a runaway team of horses.

    Pull your wrists backward and spread your fingers out as wide as possible. Try to touch your elbows with the backs of your hands.

8. *Neck and face*

Press your chin into your chest.

Clench your teeth.

Close your face tightly, as though a drawstring were pulling it shut. Squeeze your eyes, ears, mouth, and nostrils tightly closed, as if you were preparing to have hot coffee thrown in your face.

With your eyes still closed, stretch your face open. Open your mouth wide, pull your ears back, open your nostrils, and raise your eyebrows.

When you have finished this sequence of 14 intervals, keep your eyes closed and relax for a few moments. Notice how relaxation feels. Scan your body for any lingering muscular tension and simply release any that you find. Familiarize yourself with this sensation of deep, thorough muscular relaxation. Before opening your eyes, spend a few moments lifting your awareness from internal sensations and bringing it back to the outside world. When you feel comfortable, refreshed, and reoriented, open your eyes.

For a more complete description of the practice of neuromuscular relaxation, refer to Jacobson's latest volume on the subject, *You Must Relax*. The effort involved in trying to remember the sequence of intervals and specific activities is not conducive to effective relaxation. Many people find it helpful to listen to taped directions. You can purchase a tape or an audio cassette such as "Progressive Neuromuscular Relaxation," by Allen, or, better yet, you can make your own tape. This way, you will consider your ability to relax something you control completely independent of someone else's directions.

VARIETIES OF PROGRESSIVE RELAXATION

The progressive relaxation scheme just presented moved from the feet upward. Some variations begin with the hands, and others begin with the face. It does not seem to matter, as long as the progression of interval sites makes either logical or intuitive sense to the practitioner. If you wish to pursue the technique further, look over *You Must Relax*. The book tells you how to do it, straight from the pen of its originator.

Many people think that performing tension/release intervals as needed throughout the day represents the most useful aspect of the technique. You can use it whenever you notice unnecessary tension building, or you can use the exercises to fill down times—those moments when you have no choice but to be inactive for awhile. Next time you have to stop your car at a long red light, do some neuromuscular exercises with your arms or hands against the steering wheel. Next time you have to stand and wait in a long line at the grocery store, do some of the leg intervals. Not only will it help you relax, but it will minimize fatigue and help prevent the development of varicose veins.

It is highly desirable that you combine appropriate breathing with the tension/release intervals of neuromuscular relaxation. Inhale as you tense your muscles, and exhale as you release the tension. By properly matching your breath with the phases of relaxation, you can immeasurably enhance the psychophysiological effectiveness of the technique.

THEORETICAL MECHANISMS OF EFFECTIVENESS

By design, neuromuscular relaxation is primarily effective at the physical effects stage of the psychosomatic model.

There are three principal mechanisms by which neuromuscular relaxation reduces stress-related psychophysiological arousal. The first of these is through a reduction in tension levels of the skeletal muscles. This is accomplished through the isometric contraction phase of the exercise, followed by the tension release. This type of activity alters the biasing of the muscle spindle fibers. The spindles are the control mechanisms inside the muscle that set the level of contractility for the muscle fibers. The isometric contraction/ release of neuromuscular relaxation resets the bias of the spindle at a lower level, thereby reducing the basal contractility of the muscle fibers and resulting in overall decreased tension.

Lowering muscular tension is the primary aim of neuromuscular relaxation. As discussed earlier, muscular tension is the principal source of exacerbating feedback within the psychosomatic model. As muscular tension is reduced, this feedback is shut off and a generalized reduction in psychosomatic arousal may soon follow. A somatopsychic technique thus may have a generalized effect in reducing overall psychophysiological arousal and stress reactivity.

A centralized element of the effectiveness of progressive relaxation is enhanced somatic awareness. Regular practice of this technique promotes greater somatosensory awareness, particularly of subtle muscular states. This is valuable for two reasons. First, it teaches the sensations of deep physical relaxation that can be used as sensory cues to enhance the effectiveness of any relaxation activity. Second, somatic awareness allows the detection of muscle tension problems in their early stages, permitting a person to deal with a problem easily, before it builds to a point that is painful and difficult to manage. Somatic awareness is the first step in the personal prevention of stress-related disease.

The final mechanism of effectiveness, which elicits a generalized somatic reduction in arousal, seems paradoxical at first. The tension phase of each interval produces a sharp *rise* in blood pressure. Ironically, this can help you relax. A sudden increase in arterial pressure is sensed by the baroreceptors (pressure sensors) of your carotid arteries, which are located in the neck and supply blood to the brain. The purpose of the baroreceptors is to monitor and help regulate arterial pressure and thus protect the delicate vascular structures of the brain from high-pressure damage. When you contract your muscles isometrically during progressive relaxation, blood pressure rises quickly. The baroreceptors sense this increase and send a message to the hypothalamus to lower blood pressure immediately. The hypothalamus then triggers activity to the vagus nerves, the main tracts of the parasympathetic nervous system. The vagal discharge lowers blood pressure through cardiodeceleration and vasodilation. Since the vagus nerves also innervate most of the other visceral organs of the body, there will be an overall reduction of somatic arousal. Neuromuscular relaxation increases blood pressure temporarily and the result is a decrease in visceral arousal. This is an immediate homeostatic reaction of the body. Think of it in terms of this example. Suppose your house was too hot and you wanted to cool it off (lower its arousal). You would not think that turning on a blow dryer (like raising blood pressure) could help cool the house. If, however, you turn on that dryer and aim it at the thermostat (baroreceptor), the thermostat will think the house is hot and turn on the air conditioning. This is just what happens in the body. By temporarily raising blood pressure, neuromuscular relaxation triggers the regulatory mechanism that lowers arousal all over the body.

This last mechanism suggests that the timing and duration of tension phases of the technique may be important. Ideally, you would want to release tension so that it coincides with vagal discharge. Unfortunately, no research yet exists to indicate the appropriate timing for producing this synergistic result.

Putting this all together, there are three mechanisms through which progressive relaxation can help you manage stress and lower arousal:

1.   Decreased skeletal muscle tension
2.   Increased somatosensory awareness
3.   Temporary sudden increase in arterial blood pressure

APPLICATIONS OF PROGRESSIVE RELAXATION

Clearly, progressive relaxation is useful in preventing and treating stress-related muscle tension problems such as muscle tension headaches, chronic low back pain, and tendonitis. It is also a highly effective technique for the treatment of insomnia. The most interesting facet of its application, however, is not so much what it does but who it works for.

There are three basic types of people who can derive significant benefit from progressive neuromuscular relaxation. The first of these is the Type A individual. Type As characteristically have trouble with passive forms of relaxation because they feel guilty or anxious when they have to sit still and do nothing. Type As usually do not care what they are doing as long as they are doing something. To this type of person, progressive relaxation seems like a legitimate way to spend time because it involves continual activity.

Many Americans have learned to cope with stress by using behavioral crutches—activities that provide minor attentional diversion from stress. Some of these include nervous habits like nail chewing, pencil tapping, or beard stroking. Others are maladaptive habits like cigarette smoking or overeating—habits that can actually harm human health. Both smoking and overeating have tranquilizing effects on the nervous system, so it is easy for people to fall into the habit of using them to cope with stress. It is estimated that at least 40 percent of all cigarette smokers are stress smokers. Stress is a common stimulus for them to light up, and their cigarette consumption significantly increases during times of stress. People who have learned to handle stress with such maladaptive habits have great difficulty in trying to replace their habit with quiet, passive relaxation.

I tried once to help a group of stress smokers quit by teaching them meditation. I gave them the mantra "I don't need a cigarette." They were told to sit quietly, focus on breathing, and meditate with this mantra whenever they felt stressed and needed a cigarette. You can imagine what happened when a smoker in a nicotine fit sat down to meditate on breathing. My little program dramatically increased cigarette consumption in all participants. Many began complaining of severe chest pains, shortness of breath, and increased nicotine cravings. They said their mind readily changed the mantra from "I don't need a cigarette" to "I wish I had a cigarette."

A physically active form of relaxation is needed to combat the itching desire to revert to the old coping habit. Progressive relaxation reduces stress and provides an attentional diversion for smokers, eaters, chewers, tappers, and strokers.

Studies of the carryover capability of neuromuscular relaxation have shown that only about one in four persons manifests a significant trophotrophic conditioning effect as a result of progressive relaxation training. Most people get something out of the experience, but only about 25 percent seem to be able to use it to condition low psychosomatic reactivity. For those in that quarter of the population, however, the technique produces a dramatic reduction in maladaptive reactivity. What makes some individuals react so positively to neuromuscular relaxation? From subjective observation of the characteristics of experimental subjects, it seems that this technique works best for people who are athletic or who regularly participate in physical activities.

There are two theories to explain why this might be the case. The first is that physically active people may have an inherently higher somatic awareness or identification with their bodies. This could mean that they associate stress with muscular tension states, so any technique that eases muscular tension minimizes their subjective experience of stress. It also is possible that most physically active people are more physically fit than their sedentary counterparts. This could mean that their bodies possess a greater capacity to alter spindle biasing or to produce quick changes in arterial blood pressure due to isometric exercise. In other words, the body of the physically fit individual may be better able to elicit the mechanisms of physiological effectiveness for the technique, just as the mind of the Zen roshi has a greater concentration capacity than does the mind of the average person, permitting the roshi to meditate effectively and think clearly. We do not yet understand why progressive relaxation works well for people who are physically active, but research into this phenomenon is being conducted.

To summarize, progressive neuromuscular relaxation is particularly effective for:

1. Individuals suffering from stress-related muscle tension problems
2. Individuals suffering from insomnia
3. Type A individuals
4. Individuals accustomed to active, maladaptive coping habits
5. Physically active individuals

CONTRAINDICATIONS AND COMMON DIFFICULTIES

Because one mechanism of this technique involves sharp increases in blood pressure, progressive relaxation training is contraindicated for people with hypertension or a history of myocardial infarction. The danger is that neuromuscular relaxation techniques will suddenly raise blood pressure too high in an already elevated, weak, or vulnerable cardiovascular system. If you are hypertensive or have had one or more heart attacks, consult your physician first and, if you choose to use neuromuscular relaxation at all, use only gentle contractions.

For some people, neuromuscular relaxation results in immediate physical pain, most often headaches. This happens to about 1 person in 40 or 50. If you develop a severe, persistent headache shortly after completing a sequence of neuromuscular intervals, stop using this technique and try another. No one yet knows why this phenomenon occurs, but it represents a good reason for not using the technique.

WHAT TO EXPECT FROM PROGRESSIVE RELAXATION

With regular practice of this technique, you will become increasingly aware of the internal state of your body, particularly muscular sensations. You will be more aware of such things as muscular tension, postural imbalances, unnecessary contractions, and minor twitches and tremors. In other words, when you first start noticing training effects, you may feel lousy. You will be aware of tension sources and muscular problems that have always existed in your body and that unconsciously increased your stress reactivity, but that you always ignored. Do not confuse this reaction with the contraindicated pain of severe headaches. Although increased somatic awareness may feel strange for awhile, it is a good sign. The first step in dealing with old muscular problems is to become aware of them. Continued practice of neuromuscular relaxation will help you learn to cleanse your body of this maladaptive tension.

Also look for indications of the development of optimal tonus. You will gradually notice the disappearance of some old habits associated with tension. You may, for example, no longer wrinkle your forehead, clench your fists, grip the steering wheel too tightly, grind your teeth, or sit on the edge of your chair. In time, you will notice a growing grace in your movement. You may begin to flow rather than stumble, fumble, and jerk through physical activity. You will perform muscular tasks with greater ease, simplicity, and efficiency. You may also become ever more aware of how your muscles feel as they move and of the beauty of the dynamic integration and coordination that produces the miracle of human movement.

Finally, if progressive relaxation is facilitating trophotrophic conditioning, you will soon become aware that you respond to stress in a more relaxed manner, both cognitively and physically.

SUMMARY

Progressive neuromuscular relaxation was one of the first therapeutic relaxation techniques to emerge from Western medical sciences. It was born of the realization that excess muscular tension is a significant exacerbating factor in somatic disease and that the reduction of that tension could have broad therapeutic utility. This somatopsychic technique is an active one, so it is effective for individuals who become frustrated with passive techniques. Progressive relaxation decreases arousal at the skeletal muscles but, through several mechanisms, can produce a generalized reduction in psychosomatic arousal and contribute to trophotrophic conditioning. A primary aim of neuromuscular relaxation training is the development of a dynamic, optimal tonus condition for all facets of human movement and muscular activity.

REFERENCES

Allen, R. J., "Progressive Neuromuscular Relaxation," Autumn Wind, College Park, Md. 1979.
———. "The Relative Effectiveness of Progressive Relaxation, GSR Biofeedback, and Meditation for Reducing Psychophysiological Stress," University of Oregon Microforms, Eugene, 1979.
Allen, R. J., and Hyde, D. H. *Investigations in Stress Control*, Burgess, Minneapolis, Minn., 1980.
Gellhorn, E. "The Influence of Baroreceptor Reflexes on the Reactivity of the Autonomic Nervous System," *Experientia*, v. 13, 259-260, 1957.
———. "The Influence of Curare on Hypothalamic Excitability and the Electroencephalogram," *Electroencephalographology and Clinical Neurophysiology*, v. 10, 697-703, 1958.
———. "The Physiological Basis of Neuromuscular Relaxation," *Archives of Internal Medicine*, v. 102, 392-399, 1958.
———. *Principles of Autonomic-Somatic Integrations*, University of Minnesota Press, Minneapolis, 1967.
Gunther, B. *Sense Relaxation*, Macmillan, New York, 1968.
Jacobson, E. *Modern Treatment of Tense Patients*, Charles C Thomas, Springfield, Ill., 1970.
———. *Progressive Relaxation*, University of Chicago Press, Chicago, 1929.
———. "The Technique of Progressive Relaxation," *Journal of Nervous and Mental Disease*, v. 60, 568-578, 1924.
———. *You Must Relax*, McGraw-Hill, New York, 1978.
Langbein, W. "Comparison of Two Approaches for Teaching Neuromuscular Relaxation," Unpublished Master's Thesis, George Williams College, Chicago, 1969.
Mathews, A. M., and Gelder, M. G. "Psychophysiological Investigations of Brief Relaxation Training," *Journal of Psychosomatic Research*, v. 13, 1-12, 1969.
Rathbone, J. L. *Relaxation*, Columbia University Press, New York, 1943.

Reinking R. H. "Effects of Various Forms of Relaxation Training on Physiology and Self Report Measures of Relaxation," *Journal of Consulting and Clinical Psychology*, v. 43, 595-604, 1975.

Steinhaus, A. H., and Norris, J. E. *Teaching Neuromuscular Relaxation*, George Williams College, Chicago, 1964.

Voight, R. A. "The Effect of Cardiorespiratory Fitness Level on the Physiological Arousal Response After Neuromuscular Relaxation Training," Unpublished Doctoral Dissertation, University of Maryland, College Park, 1982.

———. "Physiological Processes Involved in Lowering Hypothalamic Excitability: A Physiological Basis for Neuromuscular Relaxation," Unpublished Monograph, University of Maryland, College Park, 1980.

CHAPTER 17

Biofeedback

. . . a powerful and effective tool for the future of the mind. Its potential may be unlimited, or it may be merely a step toward a new reality. Beyond this we cannot predict. What new resources man will find within the depths of his mind cannot be foretold. One can guess that new forces of mental energy will be unleashed, for we are all familiar with the repressive constraints exerted upon our minds during the entire age of materialism and technology. Now technology has come full circle and is allowing us to begin the exploration of the recesses of our inner space.

Barbara B. Brown

The relatively recent applications of biofeedback training have begun to expand our concepts of the limitations of the human mind with reference to the degree of control that it can exert over the internal organs of the body. Through the use of biofeedback, it is now possible for the average person to perform feats of visceral control once thought to require decades of rigorous disciplines and practice in techniques like yoga. Biofeedback training helps us realize innate human potential; our conscious minds can regulate the activities of the so-called autonomic organs. This training can be applied to the treatment of disease and the prevention of stress-related disorders by placing the individual in control over the internal workings of the body and the physiological processes that can precipitate disease.

Biofeedback is simply receiving immediate information on the dynamic state of a given physiological parameter. As we will soon discover, this feedback is an essential component in learning to control internal organ activity. Since most of the visceral organs have identifiable lines of innervation, it is theoretically possible that the brain could override their autonomic activity and control their functioning via conscious thought. The only missing element is the ability to sense the constantly changing state of an organ. We cannot readily perceive changes in visceral phenomena like heart rate, arterial blood pressure, or fine muscular tension, so we are not yet in a position to see the immediate results of our efforts to alter consciously such physiological activity. Biofeedback fills this gap by telling us what the organs of the body are doing. We then have the information necessary to learn to regulate the physiological behavior of these organs. Once we can consciously learn to regulate the activity of our internal organs, we can learn to regulate our predisposition to disease and even control the body's responses to disease once it has begun. Biofeedback is beginning to teach us how to gain a measure of control over our physical health by placing us in personal control of our internal physiology.

HISTORICAL EMERGENCE OF BIOFEEDBACK

Biofeedback, as an essential component in the visceral learning process, seems to have been stumbled upon by many different investigators from many different settings at the same moment in history. Identifying one individual or one line of research as the beginning would be impossible. The following discussion is merely representative of the persons and directions of initial research that helped the biofeedback phenomenon emerge and evolve into a powerful therapeutic tool.

One of the first investigations into the ability of animals to gain control over visceral processes was conducted by Neal Miller and Leo DiCara in the mid 1960s. Initially, they were interested in exploring whether classical conditioning and instrumental conditioning were two separate phenomena or merely two manifestations of the same phenomenon. During the course of their investigations, they reported success in setting up conditions under which rats could learn to regulate their heart rate, blood pressure, rate of urine formation, vasomotor activity, and intestinal contractions.

Under one set of experimental conditions, Miller and DiCara monitored the heart rates of rats injected with curare, a highly toxic botanical extract that effectively blocks all skeletal muscle activity. (The use of curare meant that if rats trained under these conditions could show a significant change in heart rate, the change could be attributed not to muscular manipulations but to cognitive control. Since their skeletal muscles were paralyzed, the animals were attached to a respirator to sustain life.) An electrode was implanted in the medial forebrain bundle of each rat's brain. The medial forebrain bundle is loosely (but accurately) labeled the pleasure center of the brain. When this area is electrically stimulated, the subject (human or any other animal) feels an ineffable sensation of intense pleasure, providing an excellent vehicle for communicating the experimenter's wishes to an animal subject.

During a 90-minute training session, rats were reinforced (via medial forebrain bundle stimulation) for either increases or decreases in heart rate. The level of heart rate change required to elicit the reward stimulus was raised continually throughout the session. After the 90-minute session, rats in the group that were rewarded for increases were showing heart rates of about 500+ beats per minute, whereas rats rewarded for heart rate decreases were averaging about 320 beats per minute. (The rats began the experimental sessions with resting heart rates of between 400 and 430 beats per minute.)

DiCara (1970) described some of the findings in this way:

We worked with curarized rats, which we trained to increase or to decrease their heart rate in order to obtain pleasurable brain stimulation. First we rewarded small changes in the desired direction that occurred during "time in" periods, that is, during the presentation of light and tone signals that indicated when the reward was available. Then we set the criterion (the level required to obtain a reward) at progressively higher levels and thus "shaped" the rats to learn increases or decreases in heart rate of about 20 percent in the course of a 90-minute training period. . . . By the end of the training they were changing their heart rate in the rewarded direction almost immediately after the time-in period began. . . . Our animals learned to respond with the proper visceral behavior to one stimulus (such as a light) and not to respond to another (such as a tone). . . . To test for retention we gave rats a single training session and then returned them to their home cages for three months. When they were again curarized and tested, without being reinforced, rats in both the increase group and the decrease group showed good retention by exhibiting reliable changes in the direction for which they had been rewarded three months earlier.

In reference to the possible implications of these findings, DiCara (1970) stated:

The evidence for instrumental learning of visceral responses suggests that psychosomatic symptoms may be learned. . . . If visceral responses can be modified by instrumental learning, it may be possible in effect to "train" people with certain disorders to get well. Such therapeutic learning should be worth trying on any symptom that is under neural control, that can be continuously monitored and for which a certain direction of change is clearly advisable from a medical point of view. . . . It is far too early to promise any cures. There is no doubt, however, that the exciting possibility of applying these powerful new techniques to therapeutic education should be investigated vigorously at the clinical as well as the experimental level.

Miller and DiCara's work came under severe criticism during the 1970s because no one was able to replicate their findings. Recent research, however, has clearly demonstrated that animals can learn to control what were once thought to be autonomic functions when given appropriate feedback via reinforcement for success. The early work of investigators like Miller and DiCara opened up the tremendously exciting possibility that the conscious mind could control the internal workings of the body.

Encouraged by success with the visceral learning phenomenon in animals, many investigators either accidentally or intentionally began exploring the possibility that humans could override and control involuntary physiological behavior. Numerous investigators made significant, almost simultaneous, contributions. Two outstanding examples are Joe Kamiya and Elmer Green.

Kamiya was interested in the ability of subjects to detect when they were and were not producing specific brainwave patterns. He arranged a monitor stimulus so that a light would go on when the subject produced alpha waves from the occipital region of the brain. He found that by giving subjects feedback related to the presence or absence of their own alpha wave activity at a given moment, subjects could alter the amount of time they spent producing this pattern of brainwave activity. The feedback information allowed Kamiya's subjects to begin to regulate their own patterns of brainwave activity.

Green demonstrated that when given appropriate physiological feedback, subjects could learn to regulate skeletal muscle tension and peripheral blood flow. The discovery of these human abilities led to revolutionary new treatments for muscle tension and vascular migraine headaches. These headache treatments are now considered to be among the most effective approaches known to contemporary medicine.

During Green's attempts to train subjects to gain conscious control over physiological processes, he discovered that the most important external component to provide to the subject was feedback on the dynamic state of the parameter under study. No matter what strategy was tried, subjects found it difficult to regulate internal activity consciously unless they had immediate information available to inform them as to when their efforts were moving the activity of the parameter in the desired direction and when their efforts were changing the parameter in an undesired direction. In other words, information feedback is essential to control.

During roughly this same time period, Green was validating physiologically some of the unusual feats of visceral control that were being demonstrated by the Indian yogi Swami Rama. He learned that the practice of yoga can result in the acquisition of specific voluntary control over certain visceral functions after years of dedicated training, whereas the same degree of visceral control could be achieved in only a matter of weeks using biofeedback assistance. According to the yogis, the element of visceral control that requires much time and dedication to master is the ability to mentally shut out external stimuli and quiet the mind so the yogi can "listen to the body." Once that ability has been achieved, visceral control is relatively easy. With biofeedback assistance, subjects can begin working toward visceral control without spending decades in meditation practice just becoming sensitized to internal changes.

GOALS OF BIOFEEDBACK TRAINING

The aim of biofeedback training is to provide immediate physiological information feedback that can be used in acquiring conscious control over visceral parameters. This control can be applied in three basic directions. First, it can be used in the treatment of disease states. An afflicted individual can voluntarily alter the activity of the problematic system and thereby either aid the body in resisting further damage or effect a cure for acute conditions. Second, control can be used by healthy individuals to reduce disease probability or reverse a pathogenic physiological trend at its earliest stages. This application is of particular interest, because it allows people to deal with disease while the organ structures are still healthy and responsive to learning and conditioning and before actual systemic damage or suffering has occurred. Finally, gaining conscious control over physical functions can help us achieve new potentials for positive states of performance, well-being, and health beyond the mere elimination of physical disease. Biofeedback, then, can be used to treat physical disease, help prevent the appearance of psychosomatic problems, and open up new possibilities for human potential.

THE ESSENCE OF BIOFEEDBACK TRAINING

Biofeedback has always been an integral part of our everyday lives. Biofeedback simply refers to receiving information feedback on some aspect of physical functioning. We usually use this information to help us control facets of our physical selves. A bathroom scale is one example of a biofeedback instrument. We use it to determine whether our activities are making us fatter or skinnier. A mirror is also a biofeedback device. Imagine how difficult it would be to arrange your hair in the morning if you could not see how it looked. If you have ever had dirt on your face and been unable to find a mirror to check it out, you know how helpless you can feel in controlling (or fixing) your appearance in the absence of biofeedback. Biofeedback is essential to any meaningful level of control over the state of our physical selves.

We now relate biofeedback to the use of electronic instrumentation. To gain control over internal processes, we must first be able to monitor them. Most internal physiological processes are not directly accessible to our senses. Instrumentation is required to sense internal organ activity and then create a presentation that reflects the activity of the organ in a manner accessible to the subject's senses. Typically, biofeedback instruments convert physiological signals into changes such as variation in the pitch of an auditory tone or variations in the display of flashing lights. Biofeedback instruments convert physiological events that are not available to our senses into stimuli that we can readily perceive, thereby allowing us access to control over aspects of our physiological funtioning previously thought to be beyond the reach of cognitive control.

Theoretically, since nervous pathways of control extend from our brains to our internal organs (via the sympathetic and parasympathetic nervous systems), we can control internal organ activity if we have some means of monitoring internal changes immediately. Biofeedback represents that component.

THE ROLE OF BIOFEEDBACK TRAINING IN STRESS MANAGEMENT

Biofeedback training can play three basic roles in an overall program of stress management. First, as previously discussed, biofeedback can be used in treating psychosomatic disorders. When used for conditions such as vascular migraine headaches, Raynaud's syndrome, muscle tension headaches and other related muscle tension disorders, hypertension, and tachycardia, biofeedback training can give individuals some measure of voluntary control over the problematic organ system, allowing them to effect a cure or mediate the course of the disorder.

Biofeedback also can be used effectively in preventing stress-related disorders, as mentioned previously. Current research is seeking to identify "weak organs" within given individuals. It may be possible at some point in the near future to administer a psychophysiological stress assessment to healthy persons and predict, based on the person's pattern of stress reactivity, which of his or her organ systems is most likely to fail in the future due to stress. Theoretically, then, it would be possible to curb disease predisposition with biofeedback training that focused on controlling the potentially pathogenic system. The thinking is that if weak organs can be identified in advance of the actual manifestation of disease, the person can learn to control the activity of the system while it is still healthy and responsive to learning and conditioning and thus avoid the appearance of the disease altogether. This approach to preventive medicine is still in its early development phases, yet biofeedback is already an essential tool for learning the type of autonomic control useful in preventing psychosomatic disease.

Finally, biofeedback can be valuable in augmenting the effectiveness of systematic relaxation techniques. Biofeedback involves monitoring the body for immediate assessment of the physiological impact of activities potentially capable of effecting internal arousal. It can therefore be used to determine which forms of systematic relaxation are the most physiologically effective for a given individual. It is often ineffective and inaccurate to rely on subjective sensations to tell us when we are aroused or relaxed physiologically. Biofeedback provides accurate information about whether a relaxation strategy is lowering visceral arousal effectively. Biofeedback also can be used to help refine and enhance relaxation skills and achieve levels of low arousal and internal control not accessible in the absence of physiological information feedback. In fact, some people find biofeedback highly useful as simply a validation tool to establish that systematic relaxation does indeed produce measurable physiological effects within their bodies.

THEORETICAL MECHANISM OF EFFECTIVENESS

The implication of the theoretical approach to brain organization (discussed in Chapter 5) was that conscious thought can control physiological processes. This phenomenon works against our health and physical well-being during the psychogenic stress response. It seems plausible, using this same theoretical brain-to-body connection, that conscious thought can regulate internal processes. The lines of innervation exist between the brain and the body. All that is needed is some means of information feedback that allows the brain to monitor the results of its control efforts.

We have stated that it is impossible to be in control of any aspect of the physical body without continual information feedback regarding the ever-changing state of the physical parameter. To illustrate this point, let us take a simple example and outline the essential steps involved in controlling a physical outcome.

Suppose Sidney has just read an article on ideal body weights. According to this report, a man of his age and height should weigh 165 pounds. Let us further suppose that Sidney is so impressed by this article that he is going to try to bring his body around to this ideal weight by altering some minor facets of his life-style. What can we recommend that Sidney try? Obviously, the first information we need is how much Sidney currently weighs. In other words, the first step in controlling any physical condition is to observe its current status. Suppose that we get a scale and learn that Sidney weighs about 184 pounds. Now we can hypothesize that Sidney could lose weight if he altered his diet. We recommend that he eat only organically grown alfalfa sprouts fried in peanut oil for four months. Will this diet help Sidney lose weight? More importantly, will this alteration place him in control of his body weight? We do not know the answer to the first question, but the answer to the second is no. To determine whether this behavior change is helping Sidney get closer to his desired body weight, we must again check his weight. By continually acting and then observing the results of our actions, we can realize some measure of control over the physical condition we are trying to influence.

Controlling any physical condition (whether it be body weight, hair color, blood pressure, or muscular tension) involves observing the current state of the physical parameter, proposing an action that is likely to change the parameter in the desired direction, and then taking that hypothesized action. This action may or may not change the state of the physical parameter, so a second observation is necessary, followed by an evaluation of the effect of the original action and a further hypothesis and action, and so on. In other words, the process of controlling anything involves both action and observation of the results. We might consider control to be a continuous feedback loop composed of these elements. The more times we go around the loop, the more we refine our control over the physical event and the closer and closer we get to our desired outcomes or states. Figure 17.1 illustrates this control loop.

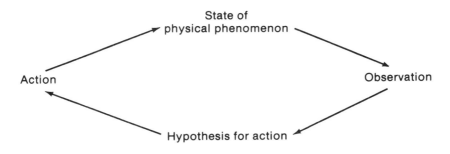

Figure 17.1. Control loop.

This same feedback loop applies to learning to control the internal workings of the body, but we are here faced with a serious difficulty. The problem is that we cannot observe changes in visceral phenomena readily. We are not equipped to be able to perceive changes within the body to the degree necessary to achieve effective control.

When you were in grade school, were you taught that there are voluntary and involuntary functions of the human body? Were you ever told that things such as heart rate or blood pressure were outside the reaches of voluntary control? Were you ever given the impression that these phenomena could not be controlled consciously by the human mind? The reason we have grown up with this belief is that it is impossible for us to observe internal activity directly. In other words, a gap exists in our feedback loop between the state of the phenomenon and our observation of it.

Biofeedback instruments bridge this gap. We can refer to a biofeedback instrument as a perceptual transducer: something that converts a phenomenon we cannot directly perceive into a form we can. A compass is one common example of a **perceptual transducer**. We cannot directly perceive magnetic fields, but when a magnetized needle lines itself up with magnetic lines of force, we can see the deflection. A compass converts something we cannot perceive directly into a visible form. A biofeedback instrument works the same way. For example, although we cannot sense changes in arterial blood pressure directly, with the aid of a stethoscope and sphygmomanometer, we can use audible arterial sounds and the visually observable deflection of a gauge to perceive internal pressure. Biofeedback instruments first sense physiological events and then transduce them into a form that is readily accessible to our sense organs so the activity of the measured parameter can be displayed and ultimately controlled. Figure 17.2 indicates how a biofeedback instrument, or perceptual transducer, fits into our feedback loop to facilitate control over a physical phenomenon.

With electronic biomonitoring devices, which allow us to perceive direct and immediate changes in the activity of the internal organs, we can realize our potential to achieve conscious control over what were once considered the "involuntary" organs of the body. In fact, many researchers in the area of biofeedback now believe that any aspect of the human body that is innervated by the nervous system can be brought under conscious control if its activity can be monitored and the information returned to the subject. The only factor now limiting our ability to control internal physiology with the conscious mind is the capability of biomonitoring technology.

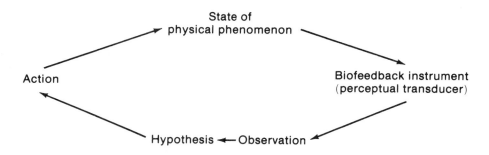

Figure 17.2. Biofeedback-assisted control loop.

Theoretically, this is how biofeedback operates. How a person actually uses physiological feedback to effect control over an internal process is still a mystery. This unresolved question is of current interest to basic researchers in the field.

According to Barry Gruber (1981), there are four possible mechanisms of action for using biofeedback information to facilitate visceral control. We can label them the direct afferent, indirect afferent, direct efferent, and indirect efferent mechanisms.

The direct afferent theory of internal regulation supposes that the subject learns to regulate the activity of the internal organs by attending to the feedback signal itself. Subjects who use this approach to a visceral learning task cannot explain what they do to effect control over the parameter. They indicate that they just pay close attention to the feedback display and "will it to change." Surprisingly, some of the most accomplished visceral learners use this approach.

Subjects who use the indirect afferent approach make associations between changes in activity of the parameter of interest and related physical sensations from other systems of the body. A person using this strategy may discover, for example, that increases in peripheral blood flow are associated with feelings of warmth. To learn to regulate peripheral blood flow, this individual may direct efforts toward imagining sensations of warmth in the hands and feet.

The direct efferent method may be the most infrequently used method (if it is even possible to use at all). This strategy involves deliberate efforts directed at changing the activity of the target organ itself. For example, in learning to regulate fine skeletal muscle tension, a subject might manipulate the muscles or limbs to alter the tension level of the muscles. Using this strategy with visceral parameters is difficult to conceptualize.

The indirect efferent strategy is commonly used to effect changes in the activity of internal organs. Using this method, subjects identify manipulations of bodily systems other than the one being monitored that measurably alter the monitored parameter. For example, breath morphology changes can alter blood pressure. So, if someone is trying to lower blood pressure via biofeedback assistance, the person may try different styles of breathing, thus using the respiratory system (easily accessible to voluntary control) to effect desired changes in blood pressure.

Regardless of the strategy employed by an individual using biofeedback information, it is clear that by providing information feedback on the dynamic state of internal physiological happenings, conscious control of the autonomic organs can be achieved.

HOW BIOFEEDBACK IS ACCOMPLISHED

To begin biofeedback training, sensors are attached to the body of the subject to pick up the physiological activity. These are most often electrical sensors, since many physiological processes (myocardial activity, muscular tension, brainwave activity, etc.) generate electric current, and the character of the electrical signal coming from the body itself is indicative of the physiological activity of the organ. Some other types of sensors are called transducers, because they convert a physiological happening that is not inherently electrical into electricity so the biofeedback instrument can process the signal. Examples of transducer sensors include electrically active sensors, which pass a minute current across the skin surface to facilitate electrodermal measurement (assessments of perspiration); thermistors and thermocouples, which are sensitive to changes in temperature and are used to make assessments of superficial peripheral blood flow; and photoplethysmographs, which pass infrared light through the skin to a photoelectric cell, permitting measurement of pulse pressure curves by converting beat-to-beat changes in coloration density into electrical waveforms. To start this biofeedback process, the instrument must first sense or "perceive" the physiological event.

The electrical signal from the sensors passes along a cable to the instrument itself. Here, the electrical signal is processed and converted to a form that the subject can perceive and understand. The physiological event is then displayed for the subject in an auditory fashion, a visual fashion, or both. The display changes in a perceptible way as the activity of the monitored organ site changes. For example, if muscle tension of the frontalis is being measured, the instrument may display to the subject an auditory tone that varies in pitch as the tension level of the measured muscle site changes. As another example, a subject may watch a column of lights that increases or decreases its span of illumination as blood flow to a peripheral site increases or decreases.

Figure 17.3 pictures a subject receiving biofeedback training to assist in the control of a forearm supinator muscle. Note the sensors on her arm and the cable carrying the muscle tension signal to the instrument. In this instance, the instrument is providing both auditory and visual displays. The headphones in the picture present an oscillating tone that shuts off when her muscle tension goes below a preset level. The meter displays absolute tension readings for her by moving its needle to the right as tension increases and to the left as tension decreases. By attending to the displays, the subject pictured here can begin to learn how to regulate her skeletal muscle activity to a fine degree.

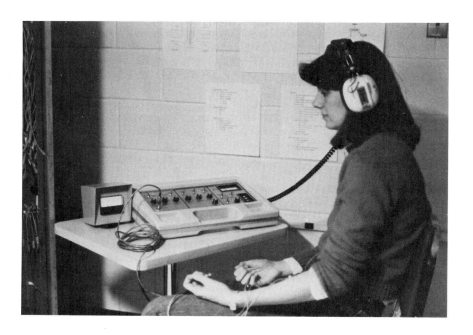

Figure 17.3. Electromyographic biofeedback arrangement.

Once the subject is being monitored by the instrument, the real training begins. The instrument, remember, does nothing to the subject; it merely reflects the activity of the subject's body. If changes in internal activity are to occur, they must be accomplished by the subject. With biofeedback, the subject is an active participant in the control process (a sharp contrast to traditional medical methods, which tend to separate the subject's actions and volition from the therapeutic process).

The training process itself may involve any (or a combination) of the control strategies discussed earlier in this chapter. Essentially, the subject can explore different schemes and observe their effect on the parameter of interest. After experimenting with different techniques or strategies, the subject can focus on those that move the parameter in the desired direction and learn to avoid those that produce the opposite result.

No one knows exactly what one should do to control a given parameter in either direction. Clinicians and therapists can make initial suggestions, but individuals must discover which approach is most effective for them.

Biofeedback training sessions usually last from 20 to 30 minutes. The precise number of sessions required to learn a particular autonomic control task varies according to the parameter and the subject. Typically, muscular tension is the parameter that can most readily be brought under significant voluntary control. Usually, four to six training sessions are required before a subject achieves the level of control required to produce deep relaxation at will. Parameters such as peripheral blood flow are more intangible physiological dimensions in the mind of the subject and require significantly more training time for measurable control to be achieved.

Actual training with an instrument does not go on indefinitely. (If it does, subjects can acquire a sense of instrument dependence.) Once a subject has acquired control of the parameter, there is no further need for training with the external instrument. By its nature, biofeedback trains you to be aware of your own internal sensations and indicators of visceral change. A biofeedback instrument is analogous to training wheels on a bicycle. The instrument helps you get started, but your ability to control your internal body is a skill that lies within yourself.

VARIETIES OF BIOFEEDBACK TRAINING

There are diverse varieties of biofeedback training. Essentially, any innervated physiological event that can be monitored and fed back to the subject can be considered a form of biofeedback training. The most commonly employed varieties of feedback training include electroencephalography, electromyography, cardiovascular parameters, and electrodermal activity.

Electroencephalographic Biofeedback. Electroencephalographic (EEG) biofeedback refers to monitoring brainwave activity. EEG monitoring was one of the earliest forms of biofeedback training and investigation conducted with human subjects. In this type of training, sensors are placed on the subject's scalp and the underlying electrical activity of the brain is monitored. The subject is given information on the nature of the dominant waveforms appearing on the EEG record from moment to moment. Usually the goal of EEG biofeedback training is to teach subjects to control the pattern of brainwave activity from specific regions of the brain. Several different brainwave patterns have been associated with subjective states of consciousness. The task for the subject is to learn to access these states of consciousness by learning to regulate the underlying brainwave activity.

Electromyographic Biofeedback. Electromyographic (EMG) refers to the electrical activity of the muscles. As muscle fibers contract, the signal that initiates contraction gives off a small amount of electric current that can be measured on the surface of the body. Muscular tension is related directly to the amount of measured electrical activity on the skin surface immediately above the underlying muscle mass. This type of feedback training is used to help individuals gain control over the precise activities of individual muscles, coordinate patterns of muscular interrelations during specific actions, and facilitate control over the general level of muscular arousal in the body.

Cardiovascular Biofeedback. Cardiovascular biofeedback can provide information on the activities of the heart, the vascular system, or arterial blood pressure. Each of these three feedback modalities has been used in clinical settings to treat cardiovascular pathologies. Cardiovascular disease is so widespread in this country that cardiovascular biofeedback is the focus of serious attention in the medical community.

Electrodermal Biofeedback. Electrodermal biofeedback involves measuring the ability of the skin surface to conduct electricity. This ability is greatly influenced by perspiration and is therefore an excellent indicator of sweat gland activity. There are many variations in measurement technique for assessing electrodermal response. This parameter used to be labeled G.S.R., galvanic skin response. More specific terms describe the specific measurement methodologies of the individual approaches, such as S.C., skin conductance; S.R., skin resistance; S.C.R., skin conductance response; S.P.R., skin potential response, and so forth. Regardless of the style in which it is measured, electrodermal biofeedback is a means of assessing superficial perspiration, one of the most labile of all the psychophysiological response systems.

Several other feedback modalities exist, but these four have the most widespread current applications. Biofeedback involving gastrointestinal activity is currently being developed, but all measures of this parameter involve invasive techniques. The trauma created is not conducive to relaxation and learning. The future should bring the development of methods for monitoring many functions currently out of the grasp of our technical and conscious control.

APPLICATIONS OF BIOFEEDBACK TRAINING

Most current applications of biofeedback involve the treatment of psychosomatic disease.

Electromyographic Feedback Applications

Muscle tension biofeedback has been applied to a wide variety of stress-related muscle tension dysfunctions, including muscle tension headaches, low back pain, tendonitis, and a range of spasmodic problems. In general, learning to relax the affected muscle site with biofeedback augmentation brings great relief from the physical disorder. EMG biofeedback also has tremendous and virtually unlimited applications in physical therapy and muscular rehabilitation. When a patient has temporarily lost the use of a given muscle, a feedback instrument can accelerate restoration by letting the patient know when the muscle is active and when it is at rest long before the person can generate enough force with it to produce movement. This type of feedback also has been used with great success in helping children with cerebral palsy coordinate their motor activity.

EMG biofeedback often is used to indicate states of general relaxation or arousal. It is used when general relaxation is deemed valuable for a patient. It also is useful as an indicator of success with systematic relaxation skills. By monitoring muscular tension, an individual can learn to refine the ability to relax physically when using techniques such as meditation or neuromuscular relaxation.

An exciting application of EMG feedback training is in the area of enhancement of athletic performance. For a given action, biofeedback can be used to train maximum contractility in the prime movers and maximum relaxation in the antagonistic muscles. This means that it is possible to train increased kinesiological efficiency for athletic performance tasks. Theoretically, athletes could be taught to jump higher and throw farther if their antagonistic muscles are given relaxation feedback. The possibilities for this type of feedback training have yet to be explored.

EMG training is so tangible and effective that it represents one of the most widely used techniques and perhaps the one with the greatest immediate application potential.

Cardiovascular Feedback Applications

One of the earliest therapeutic applications of biofeedback training was in the treatment of vascular migraine headaches. Essentially, pain is created during a migraine by a vascular imbalance, as discussed in Chapter 6. With biofeedback, the surface temperature of the forehead and hands is monitored and fed back to the subject. The surface temperature of these areas is directly related to the underlying blood flow. The subject is then instructed to "warm" the hands in relation to the head. If a subject is successful in accomplishing this, the result will be a net movement of blood from the cranium to the periphery. There will be a resultant decrease in cranial fluid pressure and a reduction in the level of pain experienced. Currently, this type of thermal (referring to surface temperature changes, related to underlying blood flow) biofeedback is the single most effective medical treatment for migraine headaches.

A relatively recent application of thermal biofeedback is for the treatment of Raynaud's syndrome. This vascular disorder, which is probably caused by an overactive sympathetic nervous system is characterized by extreme vasoconstriction in the periphery, particularly the hands and feet. By learning to raise superficial hand temperature, Raynaud's patients can use biofeedback to help them treat this serious disorder. Before the development of the thermal biofeedback approach, this disease was considered untreatable. The only solutions were sympathectomy (surgical removal of the sympathetic nerves) or progressive amputation (to remove fingers, toes, feet, and hands that had died from suffocation due to lack of blood flow).

Cardiac arrhythmia (variation from normal rhythm of the heartbeat) and hypertension also seem treatable using biofeedback technology. Treatment of these conditions with biofeedback is still in the developmental phase, however, due to the still-primitive nature of measurement and display of the parameter. Soon, however, blood pressure biofeedback will be accessible to most hypertensive people and should become an effective treatment for the self-management of one of the most common life-threatening diseases in this country.

Electrodermal Feedback Applications

This type of biofeedback is rarely used in treating somatic disease. Perspiration, as we have noted, is an excellent indicator of transient emotional arousal because it is so labile. Since it is unaffected by medullary catecholamines, perspiration changes rapidly with sudden shifts in cognitive activity. For this reason, its prime therapeutic application is in psychotherapy. An electrodermal monitor can indicate when a patient is focusing cognitive activity on emotionally arousing stimuli. With this type of instant information, a therapist can direct the course of sessions with a subject more effectively, and a patient can explore areas of personal emotional difficulty more efficiently. The same type of information feedback can be used as an objective measure of psychotherapeutic progress. Odd as it may seem, sweat is our clearest window to the mind.

Electroencephalographic Feedback Applications

EEG biofeedback has been widely applied and widely misunderstood. Initially, it was used to help people reach transcendent states of consciousness. The classic "alpha training" allowed people easier access to meditative-like states of consciousness. Green's work with theta brainwave training gave some early hints that it might be possible to train people to reach a brainwave state that was the domain of visual imagery, imagination, and creative thought. The results of this work are numerous but are often difficult to interpret. Just as people can feel relaxed and pleasant in "alpha states," they also can feel upset and nauseated, depending on other variables in their minds and the immediate environment.

This type of biofeedback has been tried for everything from accessing extrasensory perception to getting people to stop smoking. Much of the EEG application literature brings fascinating possibilities to mind and it may someday prove to be a valuable tool for achieving transcendent consciousness, but most of its applications are inappropriate and peripheral, because we do not know what the significance of brainwaves is. Some associations exist between brainwave patterns and subjective states of consciousness, but the real meaning of these waveforms is not clearly understood.

As we have discussed, applications of this phenomenon are not limited to treating disease. Biofeedback has great potential for disease prevention and for helping humans realize their optimal potential. This discussion should merely give you an idea of the range of possibilities.

COMMON DIFFICULTIES

The first and almost universal difficulty with biofeedback is that people try too hard. Visceral learning is a paradoxical phenomenon. Subjects find that they are most effective at controlling internal activity when they relax and "just let things flow." When we try hard to perform a given task, we increase mental arousal effectively, which triggers a somatic arousal response that washes away any success we may have had up to that point. In this way, biofeedback can often be a frustrating experience. In biofeedback training you must exert your will without *trying* in order to be successful. The best way to handle this difficulty is to adopt a mind set similar to the passive attitude discussed in Chapter 13. In biofeedback training, this is called **passive volition.** You must learn to exert your will over your body's internal activity without trying too hard. The more you are able to sit back, enjoy the experience, and concentrate in a relaxed fashion, the faster you will learn. Above all, you must not try to compete with yourself, others, or nebulous performance standards.

If you would like to try biofeedback training and particularly if you seek biofeedback treatment for a clinical disorder, go *only* to a qualified professional. Anyone can buy some biomonitoring instruments and hang out a shingle, but you need the kind of service that a certified professional can give. The Biofeedback Research Society of America has established competency guidelines and certifies people who know what they are doing. Biofeedback can be a positive, life-altering experience or a frustrating waste of time and money. If you choose to pursue it, do it right.

WHAT TO EXPECT FROM BIOFEEDBACK TRAINING

Biofeedback can help validate for you that the stress control measures we have discussed in this text really work. It can therefore give you an increased measure of confidence that you can be a controlling factor in your own health. For this reason, Type As relate well to biofeedback. It provides an objective, quantitative assessment with external monitors, flashing lights, and even numbers to tell you just how relaxed you are!

By the nature of biofeedback practice, you will develop a keen and accurate somatic awareness capability. Many of the relaxation techniques covered in this text have emphasized the development of somatic awareness. Biofeedback sharpens that awareness and provides you with objective information to refine the accuracy of your internal perceptions.

Finally, biofeedback will help you develop a greater sense of control over your existence. Many clinicians cite this as the greatest benefit derived from biofeedback training. When individuals learn to control the internal workings of that "black box" they live in, it often gives them a profound sense that they are the real master of their life. It has been noted that success breakthroughs often occur when subjects stop referring to the instrument as the agent that must be changed and realize that they are working with their own body. When a subject stops asking questions like "Why can't I make the needle on this machine move?" and starts asking questions like "What am I doing to change my body?" measurable success soon follows. Biofeedback training helps many people see that regardless of what the outside world does, it is possible to master the internal self.

SUMMARY

Biofeedback training represents a new facet of human learning that allows human organisms to realize a new level of their innate potential: the ability to control the internal workings of the body with the conscious mind. This phenomenon has direct applications for the treatment of psychosomatic disease, the prevention of stress-related disease, the enhancement and validation of the physiological effectiveness of systematic relaxation techniques, and the expansion of human potential to gain tangible control over personal health, performance, and well-being. Although the biological evolution of the human organism may currently be at a standstill, techniques such as biofeedback training give us tools by which we can evolve by continually developing the vast untapped potential of our minds.

REFERENCES

Basmajian, J. "Control of Individual Motor Units," *Science*, v. 141, 440-441, 1963.

Basmajian, J. V., and Newton, W. "Feedback Training of Parts of Buccinator Muscle in Man," *Psychophysiology*, v. 11, 92, 1974.

Blanchard, E., et al. "Awareness of Heart Activity and Self-Control of Heart Rate," *Psychophysiology*, v. 9, 63-68, 1972.

Brener, J., and Hothersall, D. "Heart Rate Control Under Conditions of Augmented Sensory Feedback," *Psychophysiology*, v. 3, 23-28, 1966.

Brown, B. *New Mind, New Body*, Harper and Row, New York, 1974.

————. *Stress and the Art of Biofeedback*, Harper and Row, New York, 1977.

Budzynski, T., et al. "EMB Biofeedback and Tension Headache: A Controlled Outcome Study," *Psychosomatic Medicine*, v. 35, 484-496, 1973.

Calder, N. *The Mind of Man*, Viking Press, New York, 1970.

DiCara, L. V. "Learning in the Autonomic Nervous System," *Scientific American*, v. 222 (1), 30-39, 1970.

Engel, B., et al. "Operant Conditioning of Retrosphincteric Responses in the Treatment of Fecal Incontinence," *New England Journal of Medicine*, v. 290, 646-649, 1974.

Gaarder, K., and Montgomery, P. *Clinical Biofeedback: A Procedural Manual*, Williams and Wilkins, Baltimore, 1977.

Green, E., et al. "Feedback Technique for Deep Relaxation," *Psychophysiology*, v. 6, 371, 1969.

————. "Voluntary Control of Internal States: Psychological and Physiological," *Journal of Transpersonal Psychology*, v. 11, 1-26, 1970.

Gruber, B. "Development of an Animal Model to Study Mechanisms Mediating Biofeedback Learning," Unpublished Doctoral Dissertation, University of Maryland, College Park, 1981.

Jonas, G. *Visceral Learning*, Viking Press, New York, 1972.

Kamiya, J. "Operant Control of the EEG Alpha Rhythm and Some of Its Reported Effects on Consciousness," in Tart, C., *Altered States of Consciousness*, John Wiley and Sons, New York, 1969.

Katkin, E., and Murray, E. "Instrumental Conditioning of Autonomically Mediated Behavior: Theoretical and Methodological Issues," *Psychological Bulletin*, v. 70, 52-68, 1968.

Miller, N. "Learning of Visceral and Glandular Responses," *Science*, v. 163, 434-445, 1969.

Patel, G. "Yoga and Biofeedback in the Management of Hypertension," *Lancet*, v. ii, 1053, 1973.

Sargent, J., et al. "The Use of Autogenic Feedback Training in a Pilot Study of Migraine and Tension Headaches,' *Headache*, v. 12, 120-124, 1972.

Schwartz, G. "Voluntary Control of Human Cardiovascular Integration and Differentiation Through Feedback and Reward, *Science*, v. 175, 90-93, 1972.

Shapiro, D., et al. "Effects of Feedback and Reinforcement on Control of Human Systolic Blood Pressure," *Science*, v. 163, 588, 1969.

Shearn, D. "Operant Conditioning of Heart Rate," *Science*, v. 137, 530-531, 1962.

Stern, R., and Ray, W. *Biofeedback and the Control of Internal Bodily Activity*, Learning Systems Co., Homewood, Ill., 1975.

Taub, E. "Self Regulation of Human Tissue Temperature," in Schwartz, G. E., and Beatty, J., *Biofeedback Theory and Research*, Academic Press, New York, 1977.

PART IV

What Next?

Once you learn to manage stress effectively, you will be well on your way to becoming a nearly disease-free organism. If you have followed and practiced the ideas and activities presented in this text, you are learning to become the master of your biological destiny. So, what else is there? Does "healthy" mean simply ridding yourself of disease, or is there something more to human health than just not being sick? Could there be such things as positive states of health beyond mere diseaseless conditions?

Most people just try to get by in life. If nothing hurts, that is good enough. What a low-life attitude. If you are just "not sick," then what are you? Nothing? Nothing yet! There exist states of human potential far beyond mere diseaseless states. Further, there may be contagious, transpersonal states of positive human health. Further still, our evolving attitudes, realizations, and manifestations of this high-order health may reshape our sociobiological destiny and the future quality of human life.

CHAPTER 18

Human Potential and Transpersonal Health

What one believes to be true, either is true or becomes true in one's mind,
within limits to be determined experimentally and experientially. These limits
are beliefs to be transcended.

John Lilly

We have used a physical disease orientation in this text to understand and control stress. Throughout the book, we have emphasized that the problems associated with the experience of human stress lie with the manifestation of physical disease. We have also indicated that the principal reason for learning stress control techniques is to reduce the probability of physical disease occurring later on in life. Such thinking represents a radical change. Traditionally, medicine waits until a disease manifests itself before taking action. If you can learn how to control stress effectively, you will be taking a significant step in the direction of preventing disease before it blossoms in your body, before you must suffer, and before physical damage occurs. Preventing disease from happening rather than treating it after its occurrence is a valuable way to approach health, but is this all there is to human health? Are persons deemed healthy simply by virtue of the fact that they are not sick? Are persons in a state of optimal health simply because their behavior, life-style, and attitudes place them at a low probability for becoming physically ill? Physical disease and its prevention through stress management has been the main focus of this book. The concept of human health, however, extends far beyond the simple elimination of physical illness.

The stress management techniques we have discussed were designed and presented in the interest of lowering your probability of encountering somatic illness. If you practice them, they will be effective toward this end. If you have been using any of the techniques, you may already have noted that there are positive benefits or side effects that accompany them. They do much more for you than simply change the physiological stress reactivity of your body. Their value extends beyond your capability to reduce the probability of encountering disease. With a technique like meditation, for example, you may have noticed an increase in your clarity of thought, an increased ability to concentrate, and an increased sense of overall tranquility in life. In fact, if you have been practicing these techniques regularly, you may already have noticed that they help you attain an ineffable feeling of balance, integration, and well-being. In other words, there is far more to the practice of these stress management techniques than simply fostering an ability to reduce your probability of encountering psychosomatic illness. The practice of these techniques will take you along a path of development toward the attainment of a state of optimal health and well-being.

Being healthy involves far more than being free of physical disease problems. It involves far more than simply living a long life. Human health cannot be described in quantitative terms such as the length of time a person is expected to live or the incidence of physical disease. Rather, human health relates to the quality of an individual life. It relates not simply to the absence of suffering and death but to maximizing well-being and the individual potentials of each human organism.

WHAT IS OPTIMAL HEALTH?

No one yet understands what the term optimal health means. It is easy to define health in terms of disease. Your physician will tell you that you are healthy if he cannot detect a disease problem in your systems. There are no tangible effects and no descriptors of positive health. No one has yet been able to define or understand the characteristics of positive health or well-being, although many people have experienced it. Optimal health is often experienced as a state of balance within the organism. All facets of human existence seem to be functioning in harmony with each other. Many philosophers have suggested that a human being is composed of body, mind, and spirit. In this book, we have used the body as our basic measurement for determining when stress is becoming a problem or whether stress management techniques are working. We have considered the mind to be an intervening variable capable of triggering or mediating the disease process and capable of controlling the physical body in a positive way. We have not touched on the construct of spirit so far. This term could have many possible interpretations.

In terms of human health, the spiritual dimension seems to relate to one's drive for life and existence. It could be discussed in terms of one's will to live or the belief that one is the co-creator of one's life and its quality. In one sense, human health can be viewed as a synergistic balance among mind, body, and spirit. We can conceive of a healthy human condition as one in which all three elements work together to enhance the functioning of each. The spirit provides the drive for life, the will to live, and an attitude that one's own actions can help shape the quality of individual life. The mind develops interpretive styles that are capable of meeting one's continually evolving needs for cognitive adaptation. The body serves as our vehicle, an exquisitely designed machine capable of carrying our consciousness through all of life's experience as long as we keep it well maintained. These elements are perpetually intertwined. By enhancing the functioning of one component, we can derive positive benefits in the other two. Conceptually, learning to intergrate mind, body, and spirit so they work together is a basic facet of optimal human health.

As you recall from the earlier chapters of this book, our stress problems are rooted in the fact that our biological systems were designed to function in a primitive environment much different from the social settings in which we now find ourselves. By integrating forces of the mind, body, and spirit, we can achieve new levels of adaptation so we can cope in a positive way with the challenges presented by our contemporary environment.

Stress problems arise because the design of our body is somewhat out of place with our current environmental setting and mental operations. Through the activities of this textbook, we have learned how to use the mind and body relationship to help promote physical health and well-being. Part of the overall integration that characterizes human health is helping us to evolve in an integrated fashion that transcends the simple design of our biological machinery. We can take charge of our own destiny if we understand how mind, body, and spirit operate together. An imbalance of this interaction can damage us severely; a proper integration can help us attain new levels of positive evolution in human potential. The healthy human organism is one that can reach optimal potentials of somatic control, physical performance, and creative thought, thereby stimulating continued positive growth.

GROWTH OF THE HUMAN POPULATION

The idea of optimizing human health applies not just to the individual but to the human population as a whole. It is highly possible that as attitudes for promoting states of positive well-being begin to develop and manifest themselves within more and more individuals, there will be a resultant enhancement of the overall quality of life within the human population.

The direction of the overall human condition in relation to the health construct has been explored by Jonas Salk in his treatise *The Survival of the Wisest*. Salk expresses the view that we can use what we know of living systems to direct our efforts toward defining and optimizing human health. From a biological perspective, Salk's model for an understanding of health is not difficult to understand and apply.

Salk begins by presupposing that health is related to life. His paradigm is built around the growth characteristics of a living system. The growth of any living population of organisms starts out slowly and gradually accelerates as more and more individuals within the population become available to contribute to the overall reproductive effort. After a given period of time, the growth in the number of individuals within the population shows an exponential increase. This is illustrated in Figure 18.1.

The population size cannot continue to rise forever in this exponential fashion. Ultimately, limits of available necessary resources will be reached, or pollution from the waste products of the population will begin to slow down the rate of growth. As the rate of population growth begins to slow, the growth curve will change direction and soon peak or level off, resulting in a situation termed logistic growth, which is illustrated in Figure 18.2.

Almost without exception, growing natural populations display this type of growth pattern. Yeast cells in a closed container will reproduce and grow until they have polluted their environment with alcohol waste to about 14 percent concentration. When this level is reached, the environment the yeast population has created for itself is now toxic. Growth of the population will slow and then most of the cells will die. A few cells will be left to begin reproducing when the environment has been cleared of toxins. The growth cycle will then repeat. Consider the example of rabbits inhabiting a small grassy island. Theoretically, the rabbit population will grow and eat grass until the grass population declines significantly. A decline in the growth rate of the rabbit population will soon follow. Most of the rabbits will then starve. When most of the rabbits are dead, the grass population will increase, followed by a renewed increase in rabbits. The cycle repeats. The growth patterns in these two examples are a function of different conditions, but the

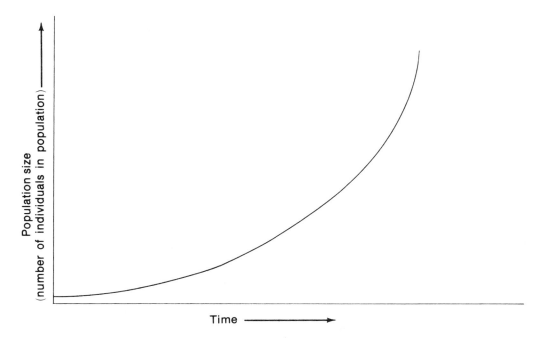

Figure 18.1. Exponential growth.

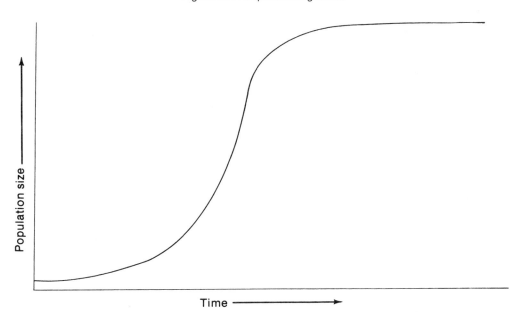

Figure 18.2. Logistic growth.

resulting growth curves are the same, as they are for any living system. This population growth cycle is illustrated in Figure 18.3.

There are three critical points labeled on this curve. Point A is the point of inflection, the point at which the rate of growth begins to decline (illustrated by the curve changing direction), characterized in a natural system by the beginning of resource depletion or the accumulation of toxic waste. This is the phase of the growth cycle identified as the "optimal growth period" by population biologists. Point B represents the point at which resources are functionally depleted or the polluted environment becomes lethal for most members of the population. This level represents the "carrying capacity," or the maximum number of individuals of that population that the system or environment can support or tolerate. At Point C, the population has reached its lowest value. If resources are restored or the environment is cleared, the cycle of growth will continue with renewed reproduction by survivors. This pattern of dynamic balance represents the cycle of growth in a natural system.

The human population conforms to the same rules of supply and demand, pollution and death, that the rest of nature adheres to. The growth of the human population, however, is still in the exponential growth phase. The growth curve for the human population is illustrated in Figure 18.4.

Salk has observed that the growth of the human population is rapidly approaching (and perhaps already may have reached) the "point of inflection," the point at which the rate of population growth will begin to decline and soon level off. This perhaps has been stimulated by the onset of the depletion of resources such as food and energy and by the beginning accumulation of toxic wastes such as hydrocarbons, industrial pollutants, and spent nuclear fuels. If we follow our current behavior as a growing mass of hedonistic, autistic human individuals, we will soon meet our biological destiny as a population: we will decline in numbers through starvation, poisoning, and death.

Hope for the future of human existence is simply a matter of developing and applying a sound knowledge and understanding of life and health. In *The Survival of the Wisest*, Salk

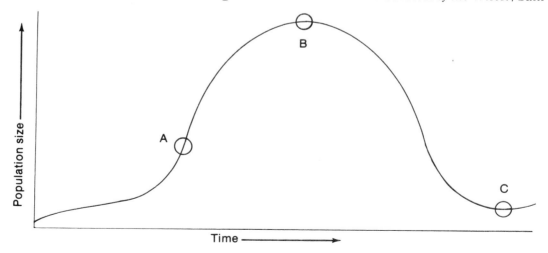

Figure 18.3. Population growth cycle.

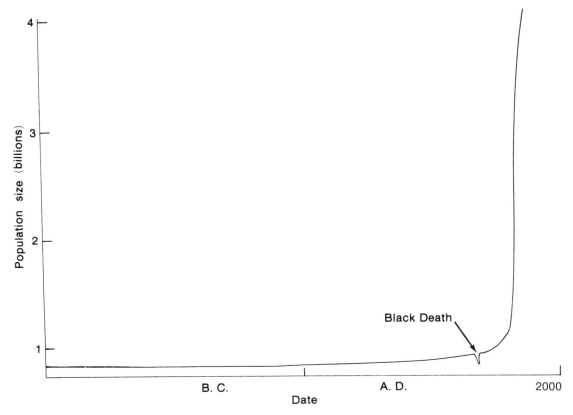

Figure 18.4. Human population growth.

has provided the insight required to save human existence from its biologically predictable catastrophic decline. If the basic logistic growth curve is divided at the point of inflection into two halves, two distinctly different biological situations are delineated. The two halves of the curve represent not only different biological sets but potentially different social and cultural conditions with different goals, values, and potentials. In relation to human population growth, Salk has discussed this dichotomy as two epochs of human existence, one that we are reaching the end of and another that is just beginning. He has labeled them **epoch A** and **epoch B**, as illustrated in Figure 18.5.

Consider the predominant human condition throughout most of epoch A. This phase of the existence of our species has been characterized by the need to survive. Efforts to facilitate individual survival in a difficult environment have dictated the nature of the human condition. With survival the dominant issue, competition for available resources has been the principal style of living. Some have won and some have lost. Even in the health sciences, the chief concern has been to survive, to simply eliminate disease and suffering. The only health concerns have been to delay the onset of death and minimize suffering. In epoch A, health has been viewed as a disease-free condition, nothing more.

As the growth rate for our population begins its decline, we may find ourselves in epoch B. According to Salk, as epoch B unfolds, basic survival will no longer be a critical

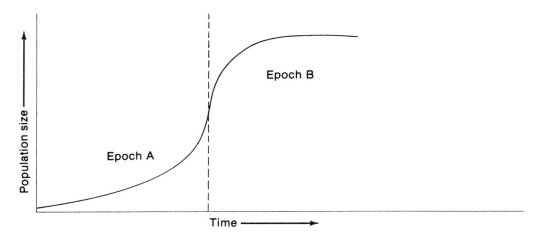

Figure 18.5. Epoch A and B dichotomy.

issue. As we have witnessed over the past century, medical science and technology have made marked progress toward the elimination of most life-threatening diseases of the human organism. In epoch B, with individual survival no longer a daily dominant worry, cooperation will replace competition.

In epoch B, health will take on an expanded meaning. Health will be viewed as a positive state beyond simply a disease-free condition. Consider human well-being as a numerical continuum. The negative values indicate disease. In epoch A, health has been viewed simply as the zero point on the scale. Now, however, as ever-increasing numbers of human beings reach that zero point, we can reach higher, to positive values of the scale, to an as yet undefined level of existence—optimal health. This concept is illustrated in Figure 18.6.

Salk (1978) has stated:

> I regard health not as an abstraction but as something specific and concrete, not in terms of the absence of a negative condition (i.e., disease), but as a positive state (i.e., health). By this I mean a state in which the potential of the individual is developing in a balanced way, that he may cope with the vicissitudes of life and function fully in the service of life in evolution.

THE CAPACITY TO CHOOSE

A dominant theme throughout this book has been that human beings have the capacity to choose to take command of their psychosomatic well-being and reach high levels of human potential. The human population also has the capacity to choose. The choice is one between catastrophic destruction of the species or a high level of positive self-directed evolution. According to Salk's model, if we follow our biological destiny, the human population is headed for a catastrophic collapse. When we reach the carrying capacity of our environment, we may pollute our environment to toxic levels beyond survival limits, we may destroy ourselves through nuclear war, or we may deplete the world's supply of consumable resources like food and energy. We are unique, however, because we do not have to follow a biological destiny; we can exercise our power of choice and ensure a high level of quality of life for the population, or we can choose to sit back

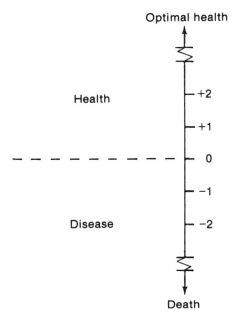

Figure 18.6. Human health continuum.

passively and destroy ourselves. The first factor involved in implementing this decision is simply realizing that we do have a choice and that we can self-direct our evolution and our future, just as we can now self-direct our individual health.

There are a number of possible mechanisms by which we can begin to take charge of the future quality of life of the human population. One of these is simply through the enhancement of individual human life. A number of thinkers have suggested the enticing idea that, like infectious disease, human health may be a contagious condition. Many forms of illness can spread from one individual to another. How nice it would be if the attitudes that foster a high level of personal health were contagious as well.

The ideas and techniques presented in this book have been part of an effort to provide you with the attitudes, ideas, and skills necessary to begin to take charge of your own quality of life. The techniques discussed and the ideas presented can do much more for you than simply reduce your chances of getting sick. They can start you off on a pattern of self-exploration, self-realization, and an optimizing of your individual human capabilities. The human organism is perhaps nature's finest creation. You may be capable of far more than you can yet imagine.

REFERENCES

Antonovsky, A. *Health, Stress, and Coping*, Jossey-Bass, San Francisco, 1979.

Ardell, D. B. *High Level Wellness*, Rodale Press, Emmaus, Pa., 1977.

Cousins, N. "The Anatomy of an Illness," *Health Education*, v. 1(9), 8-13, 1978.

————. *The Celebration of Life: A Dialogue on Immortality and Infinity*, Harper and Row, New York, 1974.

Dubos, R. *Beast or Angel? Choices That Make Us Human*, Charles Scribner's Sons, New York, 1974.

————. *Man, Medicine, and Environment*, Frederick Praeger, New York, 1968.

Fuchs, V. R. *Who Shall Live? Health Economics and Social Choice*, Basic Books, New York, 1974.

Girdano, D. A. "Preventive Treatment: An Intermediate Step," *Health Education*, July/Aug. 1977.

Hoyman, H. S. "Human Ecology and Health Education II," *Journal of School Health*, v. 41, 538-546, Dec. 1971.

————. "Rethinking an Ecologic-System Model of Man's Health, Disease, Aging, Death," *Journal of School Health*, v. 45, 509-518, 1975.

Illich, I. "Medicine Is a Major Threat to Health," *Psychology Today*, v. 1, 66, May 1966.

Lily, J. *The Center of the Cyclone*, Bantam Books, New York, 1972.

Salk, J. *Man Unfolding*, Harper and Row, New York, 1972.

————. *The Survival of the Wisest*, Harper and Row, New York, 1973.

————. "What Do We Mean by Health," *Health Education*, v. 9(1), 14-16, 1978.

Tiger, L. *Optimism*, Simon and Schuster, New York, 1979.

Epilogue

In this text, we have presented lots of ideas related to the nature and control of human stress. The overall aim of the book has been to provide you with the understanding and techniques you need to manage stress effectively in your life. All the ideas discussed can be distilled into a concise listing of the components of a comprehensive personal stress control program. So if you truly wish to control the stress in your life, just follow this recipe.

1. Understand —the nature of the physical stress phenomenon and why it exists in human beings.
   —the nature of the mind-body interaction.
   —what constitutes a stressor.
   —the facets of the stress-prone personality.
   —the basic somatic pathways and effects of the stress response.
   —the basic mechanisms by which states of mind can contribute to somatic disease.

2. Identify —the dominant stressors in your life.
   —facets of your own personality that relate to your experience of stress.
   —your own physical symptoms of excessive stress.

3. Do —reengineer your daily behavior to minimize your encounters with unnecessary stressors and to achieve your life goals in the most stress-efficient manner possible.
   —appraise every potential stress situation in a manner that is positive, adaptive, and growth promoting.
   —engage in vigorous aerobic physical activity at least three times a week.
   —open up your senses by drowning your perceptual ignorance in floods of sensory experience and becoming aware of life's perpetual, effervescent diversity.

—learn to listen to your body.

—select a form of systematic relaxation that fits your personal style and practice it daily.

—grin, because you will feel good and it will make everyone wonder what you have been up to.

This stuff really works. If you decide to use it, you *will* become a healthier human being. The choice is yours.

Index

Benson, Herbert, 109, 140, 167, 179–180
Beta cell depletion, 75–76
Bhakti yoga, 206
Bhujangasana, 214
Bimodal consciousness, theory of, 143–155
Biofeedback, 103, 140, 195, 196, 232–245
    applications, 242–244
    cardiovascular, 242–243
    defined, 232, 235
    EEG, 241–244
    Electrodermal, 242–244
    EMG, 240, 242–243
    history, 233–235
    mechanisms, 236–241
    modalities, 241–244
Biofeedback Research Society of America, 244–245
Birth weight, 109
Blood pressure, 227–229, 233. *See also* Hypertension, Physiological effects of stress, Disease
Bodhidarma, 166
Body temperature, effects of stress on, 78
Body weight, effects of stress on, 74–76, 106–108
Bogen, J. E., 148
Bohr, Niels, 155
Bolen, J. S., 197
Boyle, Robert, 54
Bradbury, Ray, 158
Braid, James, 188
Brainstem, 57–58, 59, 63
Brain structures
    amygdala, 58–59, 60
    brainstem, 57–58, 59
    cerebellum, 57–58, 60
    cingulate gyrus, 58–59, 60
    corpus callosum, 58–59, 60, 147–149
    cortex, 58–59, 60
    fornix, 58–59, 60
    hippocampus, 58–59, 60
    hypothalamus, 57–58, 60
    limbic system, 59, 60
    medulla oblongata, 57–58, 59
    mesencephalon, 57–58, 59
    pons, 57–58
    thalamus, 57–59, 60
Brainwaves. *See* Electroencephalography (EEG)
Brautigan, Richard, 115

Breath control, 140, 177, 200, 202–203, 206, 210–211, 220, 226
Breathing, 172–173, 193–194, 202–203, 206, 226
Brosse, Theresa, 178
Brown, Barbara, 232
Buddha, 165, 166
Buddhism, 124, 151, 166
Buerger's disease, 102–103

Calcitonin, 77
Calming down, 210–211, 220
Cancer, 42, 86–94, 196–197
    defined, 86
    imagery therapy, 196–197
    influence of stress on, 93–94
    malignant cells, 86–89, 108
    stages, 89–91
Cannon, Walter B., 4, 9, 20, 45, 180
Carcinogens, 90
Cardiac failure, 78, 101. *See also* Physiological effects of stress, Disease
Cardiovascular disease, 94–103, 109, 130, 134
Cardiovascular effects of stress. *See* Physiological effects of stress
Carrying capacity, 252
Carryover effect, 140, 170, 180, 228
Catecholamines, 33, 68–72, 78, 79, 81–82, 96–97, 110, 132, 133
Cerebral cortex, 58–59, 60, 63, 81–82, 147–150
Cerebral organization, 56–63
    integral model, 56, 59–62
    pathways during stress, 63
    reductionist model, 56–59
Cerebral palsy, 242
Cerebration, rate of, 78
Challenge, 14–15, 47
Chakrasana, 217
Children, 109–110, 182, 196–197
Choice, 123–127, 190–191, 254–255, 258
Cholesterol, 33, 99–100, 108
Chuang-Tzu, 167
Clark, Frank A., 28
Classical conditioning, 233–234
Confucius, 165
Cognitive reappraisal, 123–127
Competitiveness, 49
Contact inhibition, 88–89

Student Survey

Roger J. Allen, *HUMAN STRESS: ITS NATURE AND CONTROL*

Students, send us your ideas!

The author and the publisher want to know how well this book served you and what can be done to improve it for those who will use it in the future. By completing and returning this questionnaire, you can help us develop better textbooks. We value your opinion and want to hear your comments. Thank you.

Your name (optional) _____ School _____

Your mailing address _____

City _____ State _____ ZIP _____

Instructor's name (optional) _____ Course title _____

1. How does this book compare with other texts you have used? (Check one)
   ☐ Superior   ☐ Better than most   ☐ Comparable   ☐ Not as good as most

2. Circle those chapters you especially liked:
   Chapters: 1 2 3 4 5 6 7 8 9 10 11 12 13 14 15 16 17 18
   Comments:

3. Circle those chapters you think could be improved:
   Chapters: 1 2 3 4 5 6 7 8 9 10 11 12 13 14 15 16 17 18
   Comments:

4. Please rate the following (check one for each):

	Excellent	Good	Average	Poor
Logical organization	( )	( )	( )	( )
Readability of text material	( )	( )	( )	( )
General layout and design	( )	( )	( )	( )
Match with instructor's course organization	( )	( )	( )	( )
Illustrations that clarify the text	( )	( )	( )	( )
Up-to-date treatment of subject	( )	( )	( )	( )
Explanation of difficult concepts	( )	( )	( )	( )
Selection of topics in the text	( )	( )	( )	( )

OVER, PLEASE

5. List any chapters that your instructor did not assign. _____

_____

6. What additional topics did your instructor discuss that were not covered in the

text? _____

_____

7. Did you buy this book new or used?   ☐ New   ☐ Used

Do you plan to keep the book or sell it?   ☐ Keep it   ☐ Sell it

Do you think your instructor should continue to
assign this book?   ☐ Yes   ☐ No

8. After taking the course, are you interested in taking more courses in this field?

☐ Yes   ☐ No

Are you a major in health education?   ☐ Yes   ☐ No

9. GENERAL COMMENTS:

May we quote you in our advertising?   ☐ Yes   ☐ No

To mail, remove this page and mail to: Mary L. Paulson
Burgess Publishing Company
7108 Ohms Lane
Minneapolis, MN 55435

THANK YOU!